The Principles and Practice of Nurse Education

Fourth Edition

Francis M Quinn
University of Greenwich, London, UK

First published in 2000 by:
Stanley Thornes (Publishers) Ltd

Reprinted in 2001 by:
Nelson Thornes Ltd
Delta Place
27 Bath Road
CHELTENHAM
GL53 7TH
United Kingdom

02 03 04 / 10 9 8 7 6 5 4 3

A catalogue record for this book is available from the British Library

ISBN 0-7487-3895-9

Typeset by Acorn Bookwork, Salisbury, Wiltshire
Printed and bound in Italy by G. Canale & C.S.p.A., Borgaro T. se, Turin

CONTENTS

PREFACE TO THE FOURTH EDITION

It seems to me very appropriate that the fourth edition of *The Principles and Practice of Nurse Education* should be published in the millennium year, this being the 20th year since it first appeared in print. Over that period the book has achieved worldwide sales, attracting interest not only from nurses, midwives and health visitors, but also from other health professionals including physiotherapists, osteopaths and medical educators.

In order to take into account the changes that have occurred in nurse education since the third edition was published, I have added new chapters on Continuing Professional Development, and Teaching Patients, Clients and their Families. I have also undertaken extensive revision and updating for this new edition, but have retained the blend of theoretical principles and practical applications that has proved so successful over the past two decades.

Once again I am pleased to acknowledge the debt I owe to colleagues and students for providing me with ideas and experiences that have informed my writing. I must also express my thanks to Tony Wayte, List Development Manager at Stanley Thornes Publishers, for his unstinting support and encouragement throughout the process of writing this fourth edition.

Finally, I must acknowledge the help and support of my family in the preparation of this book. Firstly, to my wife Carole, a paediatric liaison Health Visitor, and secondly to my daughter Tara, a qualified psychologist, both of whom provided me with important clinical and community background material, as well as keeping my nose to the grindstone; thirdly, to my son Hamnet, a geography graduate, whose regular provision of soccer results and cricket scores, plus the occasional beer, helped to remind me that there is more to life than writing books!

Francis M. Quinn
Fleet
Hampshire, UK

INTRODUCTION: NURSE EDUCATION IN THE UNIVERSITY AND THE WORKPLACE

1

The focus of this book is education within nursing, midwifery and health visiting, and this introductory chapter identifies some key developments relevant to these professions. The aim of the introduction is to provide signposts for the reader, by indicating where each issue is further explored within the chapters of this book.

Variety is one of the hallmarks of nurse education, consisting as it does of a variety of disciplines, engaging in a variety of activities, carried out by a variety of staff, in a variety of settings. The disciplines involved are nursing, midwifery and health visiting, but within these main groups there are numerous sub-groupings such as community midwives, intensive care nurses, liaison health visitors and so forth.

The activities of nurse education range from the formal, academic type of teaching through to the impromptu teaching that occurs spontaneously in the day-to-day work. The former includes a range of academic awards including NVQ awards, diploma of higher education, bachelor's degrees, postgraduate diplomas, master's degrees, and research degrees at master's and doctoral levels.

This teaching is delivered by nursing personnel such as university lecturers, lecturer/practitioners, mentors, clinical and community practitioners, students themselves, and also by a range of non-nursing personnel including medical practitioners and members of the professions allied to medicine.

The settings in which nurse education takes place include university departments of nursing, hospitals in both public and private sectors, clinics, GP surgeries, prisons, nursing homes, and patients'/clients' own homes.

THE INSTRUMENTAL IDEOLOGY OF NURSING CURRICULA

Nurse education comes under the overall umbrella of post-compulsory education and training, i.e. education that takes place after completion of compulsory schooling at age 16. The principles of nurse education are based upon the theory and practice of adult learning, and as such differ significantly from the education of children in school. One of the main differences between curricula in nursing and the national curriculum for children is that nurse education curricula are instrumental, i.e. their purpose is the production of a nursing workforce that is equipped to deal with the demands of the role, and vocational relevance is therefore a key principle.

This is not to say that nursing curricula omit the wider aspects of education such as the needs, aspirations and personal growth of the individual, but these considerations are secondary to the main purpose.

Nurse education takes place within two major contexts, the National

Curriculum ideologies are discussed in Chapter 6

Health Service and the University Sector within the UK, and each of these is subject to continuing development and change. There are also important developments in professional nursing that have a major impact on the design and delivery of nurse education. The following sections will highlight some of these current developments, and reference will be made to the appropriate chapters of this book in which further discussion of the issues can be found.

DEVELOPMENTS IN THE NURSING PROFESSION

Perhaps the most significant developments affecting the nursing profession are the proposals for restructuring the regulation of nurses, midwives and health visitors, which include replacing the UKCC and the National Boards with a new Nursing and Midwifery Council. However, a number of other important developments relating to the United Kingdom Central Council for Nursing, Midwifery and Health Visiting (UKCC) are included here also.

Review of Nurses, Midwives and Health Visitors Act 1997

In summer 1997, JM Consulting was commissioned to review the system of professional regulation of nurses, midwives and health visitors. Its report highlighted a number of weaknesses in the current Act; for example, its unhelpful complexity, the fact that it does not take account of devolution, and the difficulties of having five separate bodies setting and monitoring standards. The Government has accepted a number of its recommendations (DoH, 1999a) including:

- A single, UK-wide regulating body to replace the UKCC and the four National Boards. This will be the 'Nursing and Midwifery Council'.
- The new body will have offices in all four countries in the UK, with equal representation of elected nurses, midwives and health visitors from each country.
- The current fifteen parts of the register will be reduced to three parts: registered nurse (RN), registered midwife (RM) and registered health visitor (RHV).
- Marks will be used on the register to indicate specialism, higher qualifications, and enrolled nurse status.
- The new Council will have additional legal powers for dealing with poor performance, misconduct, and issues relating to fitness to practice.
- The Government will commission a review to explore the issue of regulation for health care assistants.

It is interesting to note that JM Consulting recommended only two parts to the register, omitting health visitors. However, the Government disagreed with this recommendation, and it was overturned. The new Council will be funded by registration fees, and implementation will be overseen by a steering group with an independent chair.

UKCC Commission for Education Report: 'Fitness for Practice'

In 1998 the UKCC established a Commission to examine the future direction of pre-registration nursing and midwifery education, and its terms of reference were as follows (UKCC, 1999a):

'To prepare a way forward for pre-registration nursing and midwifery education that enables fitness for practice based on health care need. The Commission will have particular regard to:

- *the contemporary and anticipated needs of health care;*
- *an outcomes based competency approach to fitness for practice;*
- *sound assessment of practice and its integration with theory;*
- *the nature of and standards for the teaching of nursing and midwifery;*
- *positioning in relation to possible inter-professional approaches where appropriate.'*

The Commission membership included ten Council members and five non-Council members, and reported in September 1999 (UKCC, 1999b). Referring to the evidence obtained, the Commission commented that 'There are significant strengths within current programmes but it was also recognized that there are problems which are clearly impacting upon fitness for practice at the point of registration'. The report identifies a number of key issues that constantly emerged:

- the variable quality of careers advice;
- under-utilization of the wide entry gate;
- lack of opportunities for branch selection during nursing programmes;
- overlap between entry qualifications and parts of pre-registration nursing programmes;
- the perceived imbalance of the common foundation programme (CFP);
- the perceived imbalance between theory and practice;
- the variable nature of practice placements;
- variable support for student learning in practice placements;
- management of the student experience;
- the more complex nature of decision making which is now required in practice;
- the need to move towards inter-professional learning and working;
- the requirements for evaluation of outcomes;
- the requirement for joint working between health services providers and higher education institutions;
- reciprocity of support for lecturers and practice staff;
- the changing nature of educational purchasing arrangements.

The Commission made a wide range of recommendations based upon the evidence gathered, and these include:

- changes to the common foundation programme, i.e. reducing it to one year, integrating it with branch programmes, and the introduction, early in the programme, of clinical skills and practice placements;
- the stating of standards for registration as a nurse should be in the form of outcome competencies;
- a portfolio of practice experience should be used to demonstrate students' fitness for practice, evidence of rational decision making and clinical judgement, and should be assessed using rigorous tools for practice assessment.

Other recommendations relate to the use of learning contracts for clinical placements that give outcomes and competencies to be achieved; curricula should utilize experiential and problem-based learning to facilitate development of interpersonal and practice skills; health care providers and institutions of higher education should work closely together on a range of aspects such as curriculum development, student support, placements, and mentor preparation and support.

One report that informed the work of the Commission is *Healthcare Futures 2010*, prepared by the Welsh Institute for Health and Social Care. This report identifies a number of paradoxes that may intensify over the next decade (UKCC, 1999c):

- a growing emphasis on prevention, yet a great demand for cure and palliation;
- public reliance upon professionalism within the workforce, yet greater lay assertiveness;
- a greater demand for technical competence and scientific rationality among nurses and midwives, yet a continuing need for traditional nursing qualities and the time to express them.

Department of Health: 'Making a Difference: Strengthening the Nursing, Midwifery and Health Visiting Contribution to Health and Healthcare'

This comprehensive new strategy was launched by the Government in July 1999, and recognizes that 'nurses, midwives and health visitors are crucial to the Government's plans to modernise the NHS and to improve the public's health' (DoH, 1999b). The strategy identifies the need for action to be focused on the following:

- recruiting more nurses;
- strengthening education and training;
- developing a new more flexible career structure;
- improving working lives;
- enhancing the quality of care;
- strengthening leadership;
- modernizing professional self-regulation;
- supporting new roles and new ways of working.

The section on strengthening education and training includes a plan to facilitate career pathways from health care assistant to registered nurse by strengthening the links between vocational training and pre-registration nurse education, and by offering more part-time training. 'Stepping on' opportunities will enable health care support workers to fast-track nurse training; 'stepping off' opportunities will allow them to interrupt nurse training to work as a support worker, and return to education later. This section also addresses issues of student placements and supervision, and the strategy aims to boost teacher support for students on placements, and to increase the pace of joint appointments. There is a commitment to enhance the status of those who provide practice-based teaching.

The strategy addresses a new career structure that replaces clinical grading, consisting of four levels of practitioner. The progression is as follows:

1. Health Care Assistant;
2. Registered Practitioner;
3. Senior Registered Practitioner;
4. Consultant Practitioner.

Each level subsumes the competencies of the levels below, with each level requiring more complex competencies than the ones below. The qualifications for each level also reflect the demands of that level, and range from National Vocational Qualifications through to master's and doctoral degrees.The structure is linked to new pay proposals.

UKCC: 'A Higher Level of Practice'

The UKCC completed a consultation process within the profession in autumn 1998, on its proposals for recognizing a higher level of practice within post-registration education (UKCC, 1998). The definitive document is scheduled for release towards the end of 1999.

The term 'a higher level of practice' applies to those nurses, midwives and health visitors who are working at a higher level of practice than initial registration. The core principles are: a higher level of practice based on clinical competence, a UK-wide standard, and regulation of a higher level of practice.

A higher level of practice is discussed in Chapter 22.

The UKCC Continuing Professional Development (CPD) Standard

The UKCC issued the new PREP (CPD) standard in 1999, and it consists of three requirements (UKCC, 1999d):

PREP is discussed in Chapter 22

1. a requirement to undertake at least five days (35 hours) of learning activity relevant to the nurse, midwife or health visitor's work during the three years prior to renewal of registration;
2. maintenance of a personal professional profile (PPP) that records the learning activities;

3. compliance with any request for auditing of the practitioner's profile by the UKCC.

UKCC Framework of Standards for the Preparation of Teachers of Nursing, Midwifery and Health Visiting

In 1997 the UKCC published its framework for the standards, which describes four clearly identified roles and functions (UKCC, 1997):

1. *Mentors and mentorship.* Mentors provide support, guidance and role-modelling for students in practice settings, and is based on several core components:
   - communication and working relationships;
   - facilitation of learning;
   - assessment;
   - role modelling;
   - environment for learning;
   - improving practice;
   - knowledge base;
   - course development.

   Mentors must have effective UKCC registration, and at least twelve months full time experience.

2. *Practice educators and practice education.* Practice educators are experienced practitioners who make a significant contribution to education of students and practitioners, and lead practice developments within their setting. The core components are the same ones listed for mentors above. Practice educators must have effective UKCC registration, and at least three years full time experience (or part time equivalent) within the last ten years.

3. *Preceptors.* Preceptors provide support for newly-registered practitioners. The core components are:
   - communications and relationships;
   - facilitate learning;
   - professional development.

   Preceptors are first level nurses, midwives or health visitors with normally twelve months experience within the same or associated fields as the practitioner they are supporting.

4. *Lecturers and education.* Lecturers undertake their main teaching role in a higher education institution, and also contribute to teaching in practice settings. The core components are:
   - communication and working relationships;
   - facilitation of learning;
   - assessment;
   - evaluation;
   - environment for learning;
   - context of education;
   - knowledge base;
   - course development.

Lecturers have effective UKCC registration, a minimum of three years full time experience (or part-time equivalent) in relevant professional practice in the last ten years. Their additional professional knowledge must be no less than first degree level; their teaching qualification must be at postgraduate level and contain the equivalent of twelve weeks of full time teaching practice.

At the time of writing this book, the framework of standards has not yet been implemented.

ENB Standards for Approval of Higher Education Institutions and Programmes

In October 1997 the English National Board for Nursing, Midwifery and Health Visiting published its standards for approval of higher education institutions and programmes (ENB, 1977). There are 18 standards, each having several criteria that further elaborate them, and are measurable, achievable, and research-based or evidence-based where possible. ENB Education Officers will use the standards for validation, monitoring and review of educational programmes.

The standards are discussed in Chapter 12.

DEVELOPMENTS IN THE NHS SECTOR

Three recent Government documents have implications for nurse education, the White Paper *The New NHS – Modern, Dependable* (DoH, 1997), the consultation document *A First Class Service* (NHS Executive, 1998),, and the White Paper *Saving Lives: Our Healthier Nation* (DoH, 1999c).

The New NHS – Modern, Dependable and *A First Class Service*

A First Class Service builds upon the changes outlined in the White Paper *The New NHS – Modern, Dependable*. These documents contain a number of initiatives, including:

- establishing primary care groups in the NHS with responsibility for commissioning primary health care;
- establishing clinical governance as a framework for assuring clinical standards and continuous improvement;
- incorporating clinical effectiveness into the clinical governance framework, i.e. evidence-based practice, and review and evaluation;
- establishing a National Institute for Clinical Excellence (NICE), a nation-wide appraisal body for new and existing treatments, and for disseminating advice;
- establishing a Commission for Health Improvement to offer an independent guarantee that local monitoring systems are in place to ensure and improve the quality of clinical services;
- establishing NHS Direct, a 24-hour telephone advice line, staffed by nurses to provide information and advice, to ease overcrowding in GP surgeries and accident and emergency departments;

These developments are discussed in Chapters 21 and 22.

work with the professions to reach a shared understanding of the principles of lifelong learning and continuing professional development, to ensure treatment and skills are up to date and effective.

Saving Lives: Our Healthier Nation (Government White Paper)

This public health White Paper builds upon the Green Paper *Our Healthier Nation* published in 1998, and contains new Government health targets for coronary heart disease and stroke, cancer, accidents, and suicide. The White Paper is underpinned by a philosophy of mobilization of the public to meet the Government targets, and includes an expansion of training in first aid and other health skills. New roles for health visitors and school nurses are envisaged.

The White Paper and its forerunner, the Green Paper *Our Healthier Nation*, are discussed in Chapter 17

DEVELOPMENTS IN HIGHER EDUCATION

The Dearing Report, and the Government response

The Report of the National Committee of Inquiry into Higher Education *Higher Education in the Learning Society* was published in 1997, and made 93 recommendations (Dearing, 1997). The Government response was *Higher Education for the 21st Century* (DfEE, 1998), and some of the key outcomes are outlined below.

The Institute for Learning and Teaching

The establishment of the Institute for Learning and Teaching (ILT) was endorsed by the Government, and its functions include the accreditation of programmes of training for HE teachers, the commissioning of research and development into *effective* teaching and learning practice, and stimulating innovation. Its aims are:

The ILT is discussed in Chapters 12 and 21.

- enhance status of teaching in H.E.;
- monitor and improve quality of learning and teaching in H.E.;
- set standards of good professional practice for members, and in due course, all those with teaching and learning responsibilities.

The Quality Assurance Agency for Higher Education

Another recommendation that was accepted by the Government is the establishment of the Quality Assurance Agency (QAA) which has taken over the functions of the now-defunct Higher Education Quality Council (HEQC). The Agency will provide independent verification of the quality of programmes of study throughout higher education, by a process of scrutiny of institutions and review of subject units.

The QAA is discussed in Chapter 12.

RESEARCH ASSESSMENT EXERCISE

The Research Assessment Exercise (RAE) is a mechanism for allocating research funding to institutions based upon the quality of their research, and is conducted by the four UK Higher Education Funding Councils every four to five years. The process involves peer review of an institution's research active staff. In order to be considered research active, a member of academic staff must have had a minimum of four books, book chapters, or papers published in refereed journals within the four years preceding a given RAE.

The RAE is discussed in Chapter 21.

REFERENCES

Dearing, R. (1997) *Higher Education in the Learning Society*, The Report of the National Committee of Inquiry into Higher Education, HMSO, Norwich.
Department of Health (1997) *The New NHS – Modern, Dependable*, London, The Stationery Office.
Department of Health (1999a) *Health Service Circular 1999/030* Wetherby.
Department of Health (1999b) *Making a Difference: Strengthening the Nursing, Midwifery and Health Visiting Contribution to Health and Healthcare*, London, The Stationery Office.
Department of Health (1999c) *Saving Lives: Our Healthier Nation*, London, The Stationery Office.
DfEE (1998) *Higher Education for the 21st Century. Response to the Dearing Report*, HMSO, London.
English National Board for Nursing, Midwifery and Health Visiting (1997) *Standards for Approval of Higher Education Institutions and Programmes*, London, ENB.
NHS Executive (1998) *A First Class Service* Leeds, NHS Executive.
UKCC (1997) *Framework of Standards for the Preparation of Teachers of Nursing, Midwifery and Health Visiting*, London, UKCC.
UKCC (1998) *A Higher Level of Practice: Consultation Document*, London, UKCC.
UKCC (1999a) *Commission for Education*, http://www.ukcc.org.uk/Submission-%20Education%20Commiss.htm.
UKCC (1999b) *Fitness for Practice: Report of the Commission for Education* London, UKCC.
UKCC (1999c) *Education Commission:Press Statement*, http://www.ukcc.org.uk/2010%20Press%20Statement.htm
UKCC (1999d) *The Continuing Professional Development Standard*, London, UKCC.

PART ONE

THE PSYCHOLOGICAL BASIS OF TEACHING AND LEARNING

Individual psychological differences 2

The practice of teaching relies heavily upon psychology for its theoretical underpinning, and this takes two main forms: explanations about general psychological characteristics of individuals, and specific explanations about human learning. This chapter focuses on the former by addressing four key Individual Differences: motivation, personality, learning styles and intelligence. Chapters 3, 4 and 5 focus on the latter by addressing a range of approaches to human learning.

Tennant (1997) suggests three main ways in which teachers might apply the psychology of adult education to their everyday practice of teaching:

1. *Control of events in the learning environment*. Teachers may have an expectation that psychology offers an underpinning of principles and rules that can be directly applied to the practice of teaching. However, given the complex and uncertain nature of teaching and learning, it is preferable to consider the contribution of psychology as helping the teacher to interpret events rather than just accepting them, and thus influence events in the teaching and learning environment.

2. *Interpretation and influence*. Tennant suggests that teachers hold a 'world-view' about their practice, based upon their theorizing and reflecting on practice. The literature of psychology can help them to re-evaluate and re-interpret this 'world-view' and hence influence future practice.

3. *Critical understanding*. This implies that the teacher adopts a critical approach to the range of psychological theories in the literature, identifying inconsistencies and contradictions between them, and assessing the quality of evidence supporting each theory and its practical application in adult education. This approach will help to ensure that the teacher is not limited to a single 'world-view' of practice.

The science of psychology

The science of modern psychology has its roots in the discipline of philosophy and this link is very much in evidence when one examines the variety of explanations that psychologists offer in their attempts to make sense of the world. These explanations are influenced by the particular models or metaphors through which psychologists view man and his environment and these have led to a variety of approaches or schools of psychology. One such philosophical metaphor is that of reductionism, which postulates that all things can be reduced to simple, indivisible parts; this atomistic view of the world led to an analytical way of explaining things, i.e. by breaking down wholes into their constituent parts or substages. In biology, these indivisible parts are cells, in physics, they are atoms and in psychology these units of behaviour are called stimuli. Another philosophical concept that has been influential in science is the notion of causal explanation, in which things are explained using only a simple cause–effect relationship. Effects are determined entirely by causes and this approach has been termed deterministic, which implies that everything happens according to physical laws. These philosophical notions of reductionism and cause–effect are inherent in the work of the early psychologists, beginning with the founding of the Leipzig psychology laboratory by Wilhelm Wundt in 1879. Wundt had been impressed by the advances gained in other fields of science by the use of the scientific method, so he attempted to apply this to the field of psychology. His approach was to use a method he termed analytic introspection, in which the subject of the experiment was presented with visual or auditory stimuli and then requested to report the sensations and images he experienced. Wundt carefully controlled the stimuli so that he could generalize the results to other situations, and this belief in the structuring of an individual's mental processes into sensations and images gave rise to the name 'structuralist' for this school of thought.

Schools of psychology

Behaviourism

Behaviourism is a reductionist approach which, whilst denying the value of introspective methods, emphasizes the importance of associations between a stimulus and a response. The concept of mind was rejected as being unnecessary for explaining behaviour. J.B. Watson envisaged the mind as a 'black box', concentrating instead on observable stimulus–response connections. The behaviourist position was further developed by Pavlov (1927), Thorndike (1931) and Skinner (1971) to become the main paradigm in psychology until the 1950s.

Cognitive psychology

During the time Watson was describing behaviourism, a group of German psychologists were propounding an alternative approach called Gestalt psychology, which emphasized the organizational processes in the mind. They rejected reductionist views, arguing that the whole was greater than the sum of its parts. This early approach was cognitive, in that it emphasized internal mental processes rather than observable, measurable behaviour. However, it was largely overshadowed as an approach until the advent of the digital computer in the late 1950s, when interest was revived in the study of mental processes. This new cognitive psychology represents a paradigm shift away from behaviourism towards expansionism and systems thinking (Ackoff, 1973). Expansionism is the opposite of reductionism, in that it sees a whole as made up of interrelated systems that are interdependent upon each

Behaviourist	Cognitive
Reductionism: all things reducible to indivisible parts	Expansionism: focuses on wholes
Analytic thinking: breaking down into constituent parts	Synthetic thinking: role of parts in relation to whole system
Causes and effect explanation: effects determined entirely by causes	Teleological explanation: uses purposes and goals to explain things
Determinism: everything happens according to physical laws	Free-will: man is free to make choices

Table 2.1

Philosophical comparison of behaviourist and cognitive psychology

other. It uses a synthetic mode of thinking, where components are explained in terms of their contribution to the total system. Table 2.1 draws together some of these key differences between cognitive and behaviourist psychology.

Humanistic psychology

This approach involves the study of man as a human being, with his thoughts, feelings and experiences. This is in direct contrast to behaviourism which studies man from the point of view of his overt behaviour, disregarding his inner feelings and experiences. The humanistic approach differs from cognitive theory also, in that the latter is concerned with the thinking aspects of man's behaviour, with little emphasis on the affective components. Exponents of humanistic theory claim that the other two theories omit some of the most significant aspects of human existence, namely feelings, attitudes and values.

INDIVIDUAL DIFFERENCES

Learning theories have attempted to provide explanations about learning that apply to people in general, but in reality, there are no 'people in general' because every individual is unique. At best, the general approaches can provide insight into some of the phenomena that are likely to be associated with learning, but any given individual will differ in the degree to which such phenomena manifest themselves. It is of little practical use to consider theories of learning in isolation from the individual who is the consumer of education and indeed, from the environmental context within which he or she operates. Students are likely to exhibit marked differences in a number of characteristics such as motivation, personality, cognitive style and intelligence, and these individual differences will inevitably impact in some measure on students' learning.

HUMAN MOTIVATION

Theories of motivation attempt to explain the processes by which human actions are directed; there is an implicit assumption here that human actions are purposeful as opposed to random, and are therefore directed towards some goal or another. Motivation is considered an important factor in the learning process, and one of the key aims of teaching is to increase students' motivation to learn.

Explanations of human motivation inevitably reflect the standpoints of the different schools of psychology. For example, the *behaviourist* approach sees motivation as being due to factors in the environment, rather than arising within an individual. In this approach, a person's current actions are determined by the success or otherwise of past actions, i.e. whether or not these were reinforced by past environmental events. In this approach, an individual's motivation to attend a concert is determined by the fact that her previous visits to concerts were pleasurable, and therefore her concert-going behaviour was reinforced.

The *mediationist* approach adopts the opposite stance to behaviourism, i.e. whilst not ignoring the role of the environment in motivation, it emphasises the importance of an individual's perceptions, attitudes, beliefs, etc., in mediating their behaviour (Mook, 1996). The following sections highlight some of the most influential theories of human motivation.

Motivation as instinct

Instincts are aspects of animal behaviour that are innate and untaught, and which govern much of their total repertoire of behaviour.

Ethology

Ethology is a branch of psychology concerned with the study of animals in their natural settings rather than in the artificial surroundings of the laboratory, and one of the founders of this school was Konrad Lorenz. He demonstrated that animals possess instinctive behaviours called fixed-action patterns (FAP), which can be triggered off by innate releasing mechanisms (IRM). Nikko Tinbergen has described these in relation to the male stickleback; fixed-action patterns of attack or courtship are released by the red underside of another male, or the swollen abdomen of the female respectively. Another example of a fixed-action pattern, according to Lorenz, is imprinting. This occurs in young animals within two days of birth or hatching, and consists of the animal following the first moving object it encounters. This is normally the parent and the process has survival value to the species, in that the young animal follows, and remains close to, the parent. Lorenz demonstrated that imprinting will occur on the first moving object, even if this is a human being or an inanimate object, but that it is difficult or impossible after two days, when fear of strange objects has developed.

Some psychologists believe that certain aspects of human behaviour are instinctual; Eibl-Eibesfeldt has summarized the innate releasing mechanisms in man, citing examples such as the cues in an infant's appearance, which trigger off caring behaviour in adults. Bowlby (1970) considered that the attachment behaviour of the newborn infant towards a preferred figure is a form of imprinting.

Freudian psychoanalytic theory

Another theory that utilizes the concept of instinct is that of Sigmund Freud. His psychoanalytic theory sees man as being motivated by two basic instincts or drives, Eros and Thanatos. The former are life drives and are divided into ego drives, which are concerned with self-preservation, and libido, which is concerned with sexual drive and preservation of the species. Thanatos is composed of self-destructive drives and aggressive drives, and constraints imposed on these by self or society result in their repression below the level of consciousness. According to Freud, such repressed drives function as powerful unconscious motivators of behaviour.

Motivation as needs and drives

Drives are internal states of arousal of an organism that arise as a consequence of some form of need, either biological or non-biological. Biological needs are homeostatic needs such as hunger, thirst and body temperature control, which work on the principle of negative feedback. A negative feedback loop operates as follows: when a given level of production output is detected by sensors within the organism, mechanisms come into play that 'switch off' further production, allowing the output level to fall. When the output falls below a given level, the negative feedback loop is inhibited, allowing output production to resume.

To clarify the process of negative feedback, let us take the example of maintenance of body temperature. The hypothalamus controls the sympathetic and parasympathetic nerves supplying the smooth muscle of blood vessels, and hence controls vasoconstriction and vasodilatation; it also contains a 'thermostat' i.e. a collection of cells that detect the body temperature. When the thermostat detects a rise in body temperature, the negative feedback loop operates to 'switch off' vasoconstriction and thereby allowing vasodilatation to increase the blood flow to the skin, where heat loss occurs by sweating and evaporation.

One interesting example of a homeostatic approach to the acquisition of motives is the Opponent–Process theory, and this is outlined below.

The opponent–process theory

The opponent–process theory (Solomon and Corbit, 1974; Solomon 1980) focuses on emotional states and their role in motivating individuals' behaviour. The basis of the theory is similar to the concept of homeostasis, i.e. the tendency of an organism to counter any changes from the normal state by producing a counter-effect to that change, as in the example of temperature regulation However, the theory focuses on emotional states such as pain and pleasure, rather than physiological ones.

The basic principle is as follows: when some circumstance or other generates an emotional reaction within an individual, this will in turn generate the opposite emotional state, e.g. a visit to the theatre may

Figure 2.1

The opponent–process theory

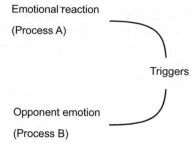

Emotional reaction

(Process A)

Triggers

Opponent emotion

(Process B)

generate a feeling of happiness, but this in turn generates the opposite emotion, i.e. unhappiness. Similarly, an unpleasant experience will generate displeasure, and this will trigger off the opponent emotion, i.e. pleasure. In other words, the processes are pulling in opposite directions, resulting in modification of the initial emotional state and a consequent reduction in the level of intensity. The process is illustrated in Figure 2.1

One of the most important characteristics of the opponent–process is that, whilst the initial emotional reaction (Process A) does not change when experienced frequently, the opponent–process (Process B) increases in intensity each time. An imbalance therefore develops between them, with the original emotional reaction (Process A) getting smaller and the opponent–process (Process B) getting stronger and stronger. The theory has been used to explain the development of drug tolerance in addictive behaviour; with each dose of the drug, the unpleasant opponent–process emotions (Process B) become more powerful at the expense of the initial pleasurable emotions (Process A), so that bigger and bigger doses of the drug are required to produce the pleasurable emotional reaction. When the drug is withdrawn completely, there is no longer any Process A emotional state, so the Process B opponent emotions (withdrawal symptoms) are left free to wreak their havoc.

The theory has been criticised for being overly-general, in that it can be applied to a very wide range of situations. For example, it is quite usual for a student teacher to experience a degree of anxiety when she delivers her first few lectures. This unpleasant emotional state (Process A) triggers off the opposite or opponent process, i.e. a relaxed emotional state (Process B). As her exposure to lecturing increases, this relaxed state grows progressively bigger at the expense of the anxious emotional state, until this relaxed state becomes her normal reaction to lecturing.

Apart from homeostatic needs, human beings have other forms of need including cognitive, emotional and social needs. Abraham Maslow's influential theory of human motivation incorporates this wide range of human needs, and is outlined below.

Maslow's theory of human motivation: the hierarchy of needs

Abraham Maslow was one of seven children and he was a rather shy and nervous child. His father was a rather colourful character who liked to drink and fight. Maslow began by studying the law but then changed to study psychology, eventually becoming a trained therapist. He published his 'theory of human motivation', in which there are five classes of need arranged in hierarchical order, from the most basic up to the highest level (Maslow, 1971). Each class of need is stronger than the one above it in the hierarchy, in that it motivates the individual more powerfully when both needs are lacking. Gratification of needs is a key concept in this theory; when a need is gratified at one particular level, the next higher need emerges. The needs are arranged in a hierarchy as shown in Figure 2.2

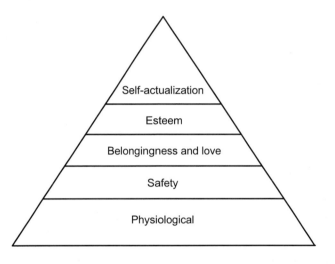

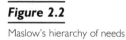

Figure 2.2

Maslow's hierarchy of needs

Physiological needs are the most basic and include hunger, thirst, sleep, maternal needs, etc. An individual dominated by these needs sees everything else to be of secondary importance and this can occur to such an extent that he or she no longer sees anything beyond the gratification of them. The next class is the safety needs, which include security, stability, protection, the need for order and structure, etc., and above this come the belongingness and love needs, including affection, friendship and sexual needs, although the latter can be classified with physiological needs also.

Esteem needs are concerned with strength, achievement, mastery and competence and also include reputation, prestige and dignity. Self-actualization is the highest class of needs and is concerned with the fulfilment of one's potential. This will vary greatly from person to person, according to how he or she perceives that potential. There are two further classes of need that Maslow originally included in the hierarchy – the need to know and understand and the aesthetic needs. These are now seen to be interrelated to the basic needs, rather than to separate classes. The order of these remains fixed for most people, but there are exceptions. For example, some people prefer assertive self-esteem more than love. There are examples in life where lack of basic needs seems to be subjugated to the attainment of self-actualization, as with monks who fast for lengthy periods.

Characteristics of self-actualizing individuals

Maslow examined the lives of well-known public figures and came up with a list of shared characteristics, which are hallmarks of self-actualizing individuals:

- more efficient perception of reality;
- acceptance of 'self' and others;
- spontaneity, simplicity and naturalness;
- problem-centring;
- quality of detachment, a need for privacy;
- autonomy, independence of culture and environment;
- continued freshness of appreciation;
- peak experiences;
- deeper, more profound interpersonal relations;
- democratic character;
- philosophical, non-hostile sense of humour;
- creativeness;
- transcendence of any culture.

Maslow's theory is open to criticism on a number of counts. The imperative to satisfy basic needs before becoming motivated at the next level does not accord with the facts. There are many documented incidents of individuals becoming highly creative despite a lack of basic needs; for example, in concentration camps during World War II. Martyrdom is another example which conflicts with the theory; some individuals embrace the prospect of certain death as the ultimate fulfilment of their purpose on earth. There is no convincing evidence for the hierarchy of needs, but despite this the theory has influenced many curricula in nurse education.

One of the major problems with conceptualizing motivation as needs and drives is that it does not explain why animals or people try to achieve things that are not associated with biological deficits, such as watching television and reading books. It is likely that most real-life situations are characterized by multiple motivation, where the individual is motivated by a number of different motives. These may be in harmony, thereby increasing the strength of motivation or they may be in conflict, with some producing a positive incentive and others a negative incentive. This has been described as 'approach–avoidance conflict' and there are three types (Bourne and Ekstrand, 1985):

1. approach–approach conflict, i.e. conflict between two equally desirable courses of action;
2. avoidance–avoidance conflict, i.e. the choice is between two negative motivators, neither of which is desirable;
3. approach–avoidance conflict, i.e. incentives have both positive and negative components, such as eating and weight gain.

McClelland and Atkinson's achievement motivation

Achievement motivation was first explored by McClelland and Atkinson in the mid-1950s using the 'thematic apperception test' (TAT) (McClelland *et al.*, 1949). The subject's *need for achievement* (n ach) is tested by showing a series of ambiguous pictures about which the subject has to make up a story. The assumption is that the subject's own wishes and thoughts are projected into the picture and are thus a measure of achievement motivation

There are at least two factors involved in achievement – the *need for success* and the *fear of failure* – and both are present in everyone. The resultant motivation depends upon the relative strength of the two aspects. If an individual is motivated predominantly by the need for success, he is likely to keep trying in the event of initial failure. If, on the other hand, he is motivated predominantly by fear of failure he will be put off by initial failure, but encouraged by initial success. The balance between these two aspects will influence the choice of problems that students select. Students motivated by fear of failure tend to select either very difficult or very easy problems, whereas those motivated by need for success select moderately difficult ones. Achievement motivation appears to be a relatively stable phenomenon over time and there are a number of studies that show that subjects with high 'n ach' do better on tests of problem-solving and mathematics and that, in school and in business, the high 'n ach' individual performs better (Atkinson, 1958)

In teaching students, it is likely that high 'n ach' (need for success) individuals will benefit from more challenging assignments, stricter marking and feedback; whereas low 'n ach' (fear of failure) individuals will respond to less challenging assignments, more flexible marking and avoidance of failure in public.

Weiner's attribution theory of motivation

A closely related theory to achievement motivation is that of Weiner (1979). His attribution theory of motivation puts the emphasis on an individual's search for understanding as the key factor in motivation. In social settings, people are continually trying to understand both their own and other people's behaviour and they do this by making attributions about such behaviour. With regard to his or her own successes and failures in learning, each individual attributes this to a number of factors and Weiner identifies eight of these major causes, as outlined in Table 2.2

The stable/unstable dimension is related to future expectations; if the student perceives success or failure as related to stable factors, this will confer a degree of predictability for future outcomes. The internal/external dimension is related to student's feelings; if outcomes are seen to have external causes then likely feelings are gratitude and perhaps surprise if the outcome is successful, whereas unsuccessful outcomes may lead to anger and surprise. Internal causes, on the other hand, may

Table 2.2

Weiner's attribution theory of
motivation

	Internal to individual		External to individual	
	Stable	Unstable	Stable	Unstable
Controllable	Typical effort	Immediate effort	Teacher bias	Unusual help from others
Uncontrollable	Ability	Mood	Task difficulty	Luck

lead to feelings of guilt or incompetence if outcomes are unsuccessful and to pleasure and contentment if successful. The controllable/uncontrollable dimension is closely associated with motivation to perform tasks; students are less likely to undertake tasks when they feel that such a task is uncontrollable by their own efforts. Conversely, they are more likely to attempt tasks that are seen to be under the control of their own actions. The greatest problems of motivation arise when students attribute their lack of success to internal, stable, uncontrollable factors such as their own ability, which is perceived as being beyond their power to change.

PERSONALITY

Personality is a particularly difficult concept to define since any definition reflects the individual stance of the person defining it. Krahe (1992) suggests three basic components of the term 'personality' that are generally accepted by researchers regardless of their theoretical orientation:

1. personality is the reflection of individual uniqueness;
2. personality is enduring and stable;
3. personality and its reflection in behaviour are determined by forces or dispositions assumed to reside within the individual.

This definition shows the difference between idiographic and nomothetic approaches to the study of personality: the former looks at an individual, the latter seeks laws that can be generally applied.

Freudian psychoanalytic theory

Sigmund Freud was born in Austria in 1856, the son of a cloth merchant. His father was almost 30 years older than his mother, who was his third wife and doted on Sigmund, her first-born child. Sigmund studied medicine at the University of Vienna and researched into physiology and cerebral anatomy. He was influenced by Charcot's use of hypnotism and became interested in neurotic disorders, developing his theory of psychoanalysis that was to achieve world-wide fame.

The three components of personality

Freud considered that there were two observable aspects of mental life or psyche – the brain and consciousness. In 1923, he developed a formal model of the structures that fill the gap between these, identifying them as the id, the ego and the super-ego (Freud, 1923). The id is the source of psychic energy that resides in the inherited instincts of Eros (life drive) and Thanatos (death drive); the energy of the former is called the libido and the latter comprises self-destructive drives and aggression. The id operates on the 'pleasure principle', which involves the pursuit of pleasure, the avoidance of pain and is irrational, impulsive and demanding. The ego, in contrast, operates according to the 'reality principle' and its function is to express the demands of the id in accordance with the demands of society, blocking or delaying gratification until an appropriate time for its release. The superego is somewhat equivalent to conscience and is an internalized sense of right or wrong that judges actions.

In the Freudian system, then, personality is seen as consisting of three components:

1. the id, an inherited instinctual component that comprises sexual and aggressive impulses;
2. the ego, which serves to find ways of gratifying id impulses within the context of external reality; and
3. the super-ego, which acts as an internalized system of values derived from society.

Stages of personality development

Psychoanalytic theory lays great emphasis on the development of the libido, whose energy focuses on the regions of the body called the erogenous zones. The first of these to develop is the mouth, from which the infant derives satisfaction by sucking and feeding – the oral stage. The second stage of development is the anal stage, which occurs at about the age of two to three, with pleasure being derived from the expulsion of faeces. The third stage is termed the phallic stage, in which sensation is focused on the genitals. Male infants sustain erections, which draw their attention to their genitals, leading to the awareness that females do not possess a penis. The child fears that he may lose his penis also, a phenomenon termed 'castration anxiety' by Freud. His father is seen as a rival for his mother's affection and the fantasy that the child will kill his father and possess his mother is termed the 'Oedipus complex'. These conflicts are normally resolved slowly by the identification of the male child with the father. Female children develop somewhat differently during the phallic stage, with the concept of 'penis envy' being paramount. The father becomes the 'love object' and antipathy develops towards the mother, a term called the 'Electra complex'. Again, these conflicts are gradually resolved by identification with the parent of the same sex.

Following these three stages, there is a period of latency until puberty, when the genital stage occurs. Here, sensation remains in the genitals, but assumes its adult nature through intercourse rather than auto-eroticism.

Freud developed the concepts of fixation and regression in relation to these stages of development; the former implies remaining at a particular level when seeking satisfaction at a later stage of development, such as when a person who is fixated at the oral stage continues to seek satisfaction by chewing gum or smoking. Regression implies the return to an earlier stage of development, such as overeating when under stress.

Levels of consciousness

There is a further aspect of Freudian theory called consciousness, which has three levels: the preconscious, the conscious and the unconscious. The first relates to things that we are aware of, the second, to the things we are able to become aware of if we attend to them and the third, to the things that we are not normally aware of. The three aspects of personality, the id, the ego and the super-ego, operate below conscious level, although the ego and super-ego are partially in the conscious level.

Freudian defence mechanisms

These three components are in a constant state of conflict with each other with the ego serving to prevent unacceptable id impulses from entering consciousness. It does this by a number of defence mechanisms:

- repression means that the unacceptable desires are prevented from gaining access to the conscious;
- denial occurs when the individual behaves as if nothing has happened, even after serious occurrences such as the death of a loved one;
- reaction formation is the adopting of behaviours diametrically opposite to those of the unconscious impulse, such as disguising hostility by extreme politeness;
- projection involves the attribution to other people of the unacceptable impulses;
- rationalization consists of finding plausible reasons for the unacceptable impulses without being aware of the real unconscious reasons;
- displacement is commonly thought of as 'kicking the cat', where hostility is displaced to a weaker or more acceptable object;
- sublimation is the channelling of unacceptable impulses into other forms of expression such as art.

Hence, these defence mechanisms serve to protect the individual from anxiety, but if they break down, the person is likely to regress to earlier forms of behaviour.

A number of variations grew out of Freud's theory as a result of several of his colleagues developing their own psychoanalytic theories. These included Carl Jung, Alfred Adler and the neo-Freudians Karen Horney and Erich Fromm.

Psychoanalytic theory has always been controversial and has been criticized on a number of grounds. In a most telling critique, Eysenck (1985, p. 208) condemns the non-scientific approach adopted by Freud and his followers:

> *'Psychoanalysis is at best a premature crystallization of spurious orthodoxies; at worst a pseudo-scientific doctrine that has done untold harm to psychology and psychiatry alike, and that has been equally harmful to the hopes and aspirations of countless patients who trusted its siren call. The time has come to treat it as a historical curiosity and to turn to the great task of building up a truly scientific psychology.'*

Eysenck's criticisms are summarized in his four rules, which he suggests should be followed by anyone wishing to understand psychoanalysis.

1. Do not believe anything written about Freud or psychoanalysis, particularly when it is written by Freud or other psychoanalysts, without looking at the relevant evidence.
2. Do not believe anything said by Freud and his followers about the success of psychoanalytic treatment.
3. Do not accept claims of originality, but look at the work of Freud's predecessors.
4. Be careful about accepting alleged evidence about the correctness of Freudian theories; the evidence often proves exactly the opposite.

Trait (dispositional) theories

Traits are relatively permanent aspects of personality that affect people's behaviour and are seen as points lying along a continuum between poles. The work of two influential trait theorists will be considered here – R.B. Cattell and Hans Eysenck.

Cattell's personality factors

Cattell used a multivariate approach to personality in that he attempted to examine the interrelationships between a number of variables at the same time, a technique termed factor analysis. He first identified all the words in the dictionary that described behaviour and then used a sample of subjects who were rated for these trait elements. Cluster analysis revealed 50 surface traits, which were factor-analysed to reveal 16 source traits – the basis of the 16PF personality test (Cattell, 1966). Cattell used data from observers, questionnaires and objective measures to arrive at his 16PF test and it is possible to construct a profile of personality based upon the individual's performance in the test. The categories for the 16PF test are given in Table 2.3.

Cattell drew a number of conclusions about the application of his work to education:

- outgoing and adaptable students who are warmly related to the teacher learn more quickly;
- students who are more emotionally balanced and less easily upset learn more easily;

Table 2.3

Cattell's 16PF personality factors

Reserved	——	Outgoing
Less intelligent	——	More intelligent
Affected by feelings	——	Emotionally stable
Humble	——	Assertive
Sober	——	Happy-go-lucky
Expedient	——	Conscientious
Shy	——	Venturesome
Tough-minded	——	Tender-minded
Trusting	——	Suspicious
Practical	——	Imaginative
Forthright	——	Shrewd
Self-assured	——	Apprehensive
Conservative	——	Experimenting
Group-dependent	——	Self-sufficient
Undisciplined self-conflict	——	Controlled
Relaxed	——	Tense

- those with greater conscientiousness will make more progress for the same degree of intelligence;
- more dominant students learn more slowly;
- introverts show more vocabulary and grammatical skills than extroverts; and
- docility is associated with passing examinations.

Cattell's work has been criticized because of the inability of other researchers to replicate his findings.

Eysenck's dimensions of personality

Hans Eysenck's theory of personality, like Cattell's, utilizes factor analysis as a statistical technique to isolate the dimensions of personality (Eysenck, 1981). His work has isolated three unrelated (orthogonal) dimensions of personality:

- introversion/extroversion;
- neuroticism/stability;
- psychoticism/stability.

A typical extrovert is sociable and outgoing, whereas an introvert is quiet and inward looking. Eysenck views personality as being biologically inherited but arising out of interaction with the environment, pointing out the similarities between the traits identified by factor analysis and the typologies of body humours identified by Galen. The Eysenck Personality Questionnaire is used to measure personality and reveals scores on each of the dimensions, which can be then compared with published norms. The educational implications of Eysenck's theory are not clear cut, but the following are suggested:

- students withdrawing from college for academic reasons tend to be extroverts, whereas those withdrawing for psychiatric reasons tend to be introverts;
- introverts tend to become bored and fatigued more easily than extroverts;

- excitement tends to interfere with an introvert's performance whilst it enhances that of an extrovert;
- stability is related to academic success; and
- there is a correlation between attainment and extroversion in school children.

Trait theories have been criticized on the grounds that behaviour is much more variable from situation to situation than trait theorists accept (Mischel, 1968). Despite these criticisms, however, trait theories are still very important in personality psychology, and the 1990s have seen the further development of trait theory in the form of 'the big five'.

The big five personality domains

As we have seen earlier, trait theorists differ in the number of dimensions or factors that comprise personality, and the 'big five' approach suggests there are five broad domains of personality, each with desirable and undesirable traits (Hampson, 1999):

Domain	Desirable traits	Undesirable traits
Extroversion (I)	Sociable and outgoing	Reserved and introverted
Agreeableness (II)	Trusting and kind	Selfish and hostile
Conscientiousness (III)	Organized and tidy	Careless and unreliable
Emotional stability (IV)	Even-tempered and calm	Moody and temperamental
Intellect or openness (V)	Intelligent and creative	Shallow and imperceptive

Hampson suggests that other traits, such as Eysenck's dimensions of extroversion, neuroticism and psychoticism, can be incorporated into the 'big five'. It is therefore a useful approach for organizing the wide range of traits in other theories.

Carl Rogers' self theory

Carl Rogers, one of six children in a close family, was originally destined to become a religious leader. However, after three years at theological college, he transferred to psychology, spending several years with delinquent children before moving into counselling and psychotherapy.

Internal frame of reference

His approach belongs to the humanistic school of psychology and focuses on the subjective nature of the self-concept. This approach emphasizes that people should be seen in terms of how they see themselves and the world around them – their phenomenal field. This is termed the 'internal frame of reference' and this is the best point from which to understand a person's personality; empathy is the relating to another person's internal frame of reference (Rogers, 1959).

The self-concept

Rogers views the person as having a self-actualizing motive, which is a basic tendency to achieve one's full potential and reach fulfilment. The self-concept begins to develop when the infant can distinguish its 'self' from other aspects of the environment and self is often divided into two components – actual self and ideal self. The former is self as it is and the latter, self as one would like it to be, and Rogers suggests that the individual strives for consistency between self and experience. Individuals attempt to behave in ways that are consistent with their self-concept, but discrepancies result in states of incongruence, leading to psychological maladjustment.

Rogers distinguishes between internal and external locus of evaluation; internal locus implies that the individual relies on his own values to make choices in life, whereas an external locus implies that he uses other people's values. Increasing maturity and growth leads to a move from an external locus of evaluation to an internal one, with the individual becoming responsible for himself. Self-acceptance is a necessary prerequisite for accepting other people and Rogers uses the term 'fully functioning person' to describe the individual who has become what he truly is.

Teacher–student relationships

Rogers' theory has several applications to education – the quality of the relationships between teacher and student is paramount and empathic relationships will foster genuine learning. He has formulated a 'law of interpersonal relationships' for two people willing to be in communication – the greater the communicated congruence of experience, awareness and behaviour of one of them, the greater will it be for the other. This law emphasizes the importance of reciprocal congruence and is the keystone for much of Rogers' psychotherapy. In Rogerian psychotherapy, the therapist must not be the expert, since this implies an external locus of control. Rather, he functions as a facilitator who uses unconditional positive regard for the client, helping him to use his own resources. There is, however, growing disillusionment with this approach, as studies fail to support the claimed relationship between therapist conditions and outcome, i.e. facilitators' skills are not related to outcome.

George Kelly's personal construct theory

George Kelly, the son of a Presbyterian minister, graduated in mathematics and physics before studying educational sociology. He became interested in psychotherapy and developed his theory of personal constructs.

The nature of constructs

Personal construct theory is an unusual personality theory in that it is neither traditional philosophy nor traditional psychology in orientation. Kelly proposes that each individual views the universe in his own unique way and that he actually creates these ways of seeing by the use of constructs (Kelly, 1955). A construct can be likened to a pattern or template with which the individual attempts to match the realities of the universe. Kelly maintains that because the universe is constantly changing, it follows that these constructs must be continually altered over a period of time – no construct can ever be right and therefore man is always trying to make better constructs with which to view the world. He can extend his repertoire of constructs in order to view the world more clearly, or he can modify his existing ones to match reality. Constructs are bipolar, possessing similarity and contrast dimensions. For example, hot and cold, wet and dry, and constructs may be subsumed under super-ordinate constructs. The process of creating new constructs may be psychologically painful, especially if there is much personal investment in existing ones. It may take prolonged psychotherapy to assist an individual to restructure his constructs, since it is these that determine his ways of relating to other people and his adjustment to the environment.

Constructive alternativism

Personal construct theory has a very clear underlying philosophy called 'constructive alternativism', which states that everything in the universe is open to a number of alternative interpretations, rather than some fixed immutable truth. Man views the universe through his own unique system of constructs and is best studied in the context of his time on earth. Kelly always resisted attempts to classify his theory under one of the schools of psychology, but it deals with essentially cognitive aspects of perception. He emphasized the nature of man as the scientist, who attempts to predict and control events in the same way that scientists do, by his use of constructs. The whole purpose of constructs is to anticipate events and each individual attempts to expand his construct system so that he can better anticipate events. An individual's personality is thus seen as his personal constructs plus his feelings and actions.

Repertory grid technique

Personal construct theory forms the basis of the 'repertory grid technique', which is designed to elicit an individual's constructs and their interrelationships. Subjects are asked to indicate from a list of roles or titles the way in which two people on the list are alike, but different from a third. This gives the similarity and contrast dimensions, and over the course of the test, the subjects' own constructs are elicited without contamination by the views of the experimenter. This aspect of the repertory grid technique is important, since it differs markedly from other forms of test which are generated by the experimenter; subjects are free to reveal their own constructs. Kelly's repertory grid technique has had wide application in education, particularly in eliciting the ways in which teachers view their students.

However, Kelly's theory has been criticized for its lack of emphasis on feelings and for its vagueness on how an individual knows which constructs to use to make the best predictions.

Myers–Briggs 16 personality types

This approach to personality is based upon Carl Jung's theory of psychological types, and was devised by Katherine Cook Briggs and Isabel Briggs Myers. The individual's personality type is measured using a self-report questionnaire called the Myers–Briggs Type Indicator (MBTI). There are 16 personality types identified, based upon the individual's preferences on four scales (Kirby and Myers, 1993).

Extraversion–introversion (IE) scale

This scale reflects the individual's preferred focus of attention. Individuals at the 'extroversion' end of the scale prefer to focus on the outer world of things, people and experiences, whereas those at the 'introversion' end prefer to focus on their inner world of mental processes and reflections.

Sensing–intuition (SI) scale

This scale reflects the individual's preference for taking in information. Individuals at the 'sensing' end of the scale prefer to focus on concrete information obtained by the use of their five senses to find out what's going on. Those at the 'intuition' end prefer to see the whole picture and the pattern of relationship between facts.

Thinking–feeling (TF) scale

This scale reflects the individual's preference for making decisions. Individuals at the 'thinking' end of the scale prefer to analyse choices in a logical fashion. Those at the 'feeling' end prefer to adopt an empathic approach to decisions, putting themselves in the other person's shoes, and deciding what is important to themselves and others.

Judging–perceiving (JP) scale

This scale reflects the individual's preferred orientation to the outside world. Individuals at the 'judging' end of the scale prefer to live a planned and organized way of life. Those at the 'perceiving' end prefer to live a more spontaneous, flexible way of life, keeping their options open.

It can be seen that a given individual will have a preference for one or other end of each of the four scales. The four letters corresponding to the preferred end of each scale are then used to classify the individual's personality type, and there are sixteen possible combinations of letters and hence sixteen personality types, e.g. ISFP, ESTJ, etc.

Individuals in each of the personality types share common characteristics to a greater or lesser extent, and are classified into sensing types or intuitive types, and introverts or extroverts. For example, ENTJ means the individual has preferences for Extroversion, Intuition, Thinking and Judging, and the combination of characteristics associated with these preferences are 'frank, decisive leaders in activities. Develop and implement comprehensive systems to solve organizational problems. Good in anything that requires reasoning and intelligent talk, such as public speaking. Are usually well-informed and enjoy adding to their fund of knowledge' (Kirby and Myers, 1993, page 9).

It is important to acknowledge that these personality types simply identify individual differences on a number of parameters; there is no type that is better or worse than another. It should also be noted that each of the terms used in the scales has a specific meaning that is unique to the scale, and should not be confused with the same term when used in other theories. For example, 'extrovert' in Eysenck's personality dimensions means outgoing and sociable.

Type A personality and coronary heart disease

One very specific approach to personality is that of Friedman and Rosenman (1974), who identified a range of personality characteristics (Type A personality) that were typical of patients who had suffered from coronary heart disease. These individuals were typically extremely competitive, highly achievement-oriented, rushed, aggressive, angry or hostile, hasty, impatient and restless. They tended to talk fast and to interrupt others, and appeared self-confident on the outside, but self-doubting on the inside. These characteristics were classified as 'Type A' personality.

A second type of personality was identified, Type B, with almost diametrically opposite characteristics. Individuals with Type B personality characteristics were much more 'laid back', less competitive, and less hostile. Studies revealed that individuals with Type A personality were twice as likely to suffer from coronary heart disease in comparison to those with Type B personality (Rosenman *et al.*, 1964). Evidence from clinical trials suggests that interventions to change Type A behaviour can reduce morbidity and mortality from coronary heart disease (Brack and Thoreson, 1996).

Locus of control theory

Locus of Control Theory (LOC) was formulated by Rotter (1954, 1966) and is concerned with the degree to which individuals perceive themselves to have control over events in their lives. This control may be perceived as being either under the control of the individual, i.e. an *internal locus of control*, or outside the individual's control, i.e. an *external locus of control*. Hence, individuals with an external locus of control believe that they have little or no control over events in life, whereas those with an internal locus of control believe that they control their own destiny.

Locus of control theory appears at first glance to be similar to Carl Rogers' notion of *internal and external locus of evaluation*, which was outlined earlier in this section. However, Rogers' approach is centred on the individual's values as a basis for life choices.

Rotter devised a test that measures locus of control, the internal–

external locus of control scale (I–E scale). A number of important claims are made for locus of control theory in a variety of social applications. Lefcourt (1982) suggests that an internal locus of control may well serve as a defence against unquestioning obedience to authority, by enabling an individual to maintain a sense of responsibility. Individuals with an external locus of control may experience greater levels of stress, which in turn may have an adverse effect upon health. With regard to learning, internals may be more efficient at processing information, more inquisitive and receptive to their surroundings.

Learned helplessness

A phenomenon related to locus of control is that of learned helplessness (Seligman and Maier, 1967). This was discovered in a series of experiments on the effects of inescapable shock on the subsequent escaping behaviour of dogs. In the first experimental procedure, dogs were placed in a harness that limited their movements and were then given aversive electric shocks through the hind feet, the dogs being unable to prevent or escape from the shocks. In the second procedure, dogs were placed in a two-way shuttlebox that had a grid floor through which electric shocks could be administered. In this case, though, the animals could escape the stimulus by crossing to the other side of the box; indeed, they could escape the stimulus altogether if they responded to a prior warning signal by crossing to the other side. Seligman compared the effects of the shuttlebox on dogs that had previously received no shock treatment and also on dogs who had been in the harness and had received inescapable shocks. The results were strikingly different; the previously untreated dogs reacted by barking and running until they escaped the shock, whereas the dogs who had been subjected to inescapable shock previously, made a very passive response to the shock. The conclusion of the experimenters was that these dogs had learned helplessness from their experience of inescapable shock in the previous experiment.

The concept of learned helplessness has been applied to the study of human behaviour in a number of contexts. Seligman proposes that depressed patients demonstrate the same passivity and apathy as that shown by the animals in the experiments, and that the cause is the same, i.e. powerlessness over events such as bereavement, illness, etc. Many nurses will recollect caring for patients who seemed to have lost the will to fight their illness, and just give up hope. The theory may also shed light on such diverse phenomena as 'battered wife syndrome' and the effects of long-term unemployment. It has also been suggested that learned helplessness may affect the immune system, leading to serious illness such as cancer.

LEARNING STYLES (COGNITIVE STYLES)

We have already seen that there are differences in motivation and personality between individuals, but there are also differences in their preferred ways of learning or processing information. In other words, individuals differ in their learning styles (also termed cognitive styles). An outline of the main categories of learning styles is given below.

Field dependence and field independence

These terms refer to ways in which individuals perceive and order the world around them; some people tend to see patterns as wholes, whereas others focus on particular parts. Witkin and his colleagues (Witkin, 1977) carried out extensive research into this phenomenon using tests that involve the separation of figure from background or context. Individuals who are higher on one dimension than another are not better or worse because of it, since field dependence or field independence are not value-laden. Table 2.4 shows the main differences between the two types of cognitive style.

Field dependent	Field independent
Need structured materials	Impose own structure on material
May have difficulty reorganizing material already organized in another way	Can break down material and reorganize it
May need clear instructions on how to solve problems	Likely to solve problems without specific guidance
May need to learn to use mnemonics	
Are better at learning and remembering social information	May need assistance with materials containing social information
Are likely to work in social careers such as psychiatric nursing or social work	Are likely to work in science or practical things like mechanics or surgical nursing

Table 2.4

Characteristics of field dependent and field independent students

Reflective and impulsive styles

These styles refer to an individual's tendency to either produce an answer to a problem very quickly, or to spend some time in reflection before giving an answer. The kind of test used in this situation is called the 'matching familiar figures test' (Kagan, 1965) and consists of a number of pictures of familiar objects that the individual has to match with another picture. There are two styles of answering the problem; some people answer very quickly and others take time to answer. Kagan considers the former to be impulsive and the latter reflective, taking only the speed variable into account. Thus, whether or not a person is accurate is not relevant to the test. Students can be taught to become more reflective by the use of self-instruction and scanning strategies.

Kolb's learning style inventory

Another approach to cognitive style is Kolb's learning style inventory (LSI, Kolb, 1976). Kolb's experiential learning theory is discussed in Chapter 3, and the learning styles inventory utilizes concepts from the theory. There are two dimensions measured by this approach, concrete to abstract, and action to reflection, and four types of learning styles are identified.

1. *Converger*. The converger is so-called because they tend to do best in situations requiring a single correct answer or solution. Convergers excel in the application of ideas to practical situations, and their dominant learning abilities are abstract conceptualization (AC) and active experimentation (AE). Persons with this style tend to prefer things to people, and often work in engineering and other physical sciences.

2. *Diverger*. Divergers, as the name implies, are the opposite of convergers. They tend to do best in situations requiring generation of ideas, and they tend to excel in the use of imagination and the organization of concrete situations into meaningful wholes. Their dominant learning abilities are concrete experience (CE) and reflective observation (RO). Kolb suggests this style is characteristic of people with humanities and liberal arts backgrounds, and also counsellors and personnel managers.

3. *Assimilator*. Assimilators tend to do best at creating theoretical models and inductive reasoning, and are less interested in practical applications. Their dominant learning abilities are abstract conceptualization (AC) and reflective observation (RO). People with this style tend to be found in basic maths and science, and in research and planning departments.

4. *Accommodator*. Accommodators tend to do best at carrying out plans and experiments. They tend to be risk-takers more than the other styles, and they excel in situations where they need to accommodate and adapt to the specific circumstances. Their dominant learning abilities are concrete experience (CE) and active experimentation (AE). People with this style tend to be found in action-oriented positions such as marketing or sales.

Serialist and holist strategies

In a series of experiments (Pask and Scott, 1972; Pask, 1975, 1976) on learning strategies, Pask and his co-workers found that subjects could be classified into two categories, serialist and holist. He used a system of classification for imaginary Martian animals as the learning task and found that subjects approached the problem in very different ways. Those subjects using a serialist strategy tended to proceed in a step-by-step manner, whereas the holists adopted a more global approach to what was to be learned. Pask suggests that these strategies reflect basic learning styles; holist strategies reflect a comprehension learning style and serialist strategies an operation learning style. Some students are able to employ both serialist and holist strategies as appropriate and this learning style is referred to as versatile. Pask has related specific learning pathologies to the two strategies. The holist is prone to the pathology called 'globe-trotting', which involves a tendency to overgeneralize from insufficient evidence and to use inappropriate analogy. Serialists, on the other hand, are prone to improvidence, which means that they may not build up an Overview of how the sub-components of the topic interrelate, nor utilize important analogies. In an experiment that matched and mismatched holist and serialist students with holist and serialist teaching styles, there was a clear superiority for students whose learning style matched the teaching style, but the sample size was small.

Deep approach and surface approach

Marton and his co-workers at Gothenburg focused on how students read academic articles (Marton and Saljo, 1976). Students were given an academic article to read and were then interviewed afterwards to ascertain their approach to the article. These interviews were recorded and the audiotapes transcribed and analysed in terms of level of under-standing and approach to learning. The latter showed a clear-cut distinction between deep approaches and surface approaches. Those adopting a deep approach commenced with the intention of understanding the article, relating it to their own experience and evaluating the author's evidence. Those adopting a surface approach concentrated on memor-izing the important points and were guided by the type of questions they anticipated being subsequently asked. The researchers suggest that these approaches are indicators of the students' normal approach to study. Sutherland (1999) undertook a study of nurse tutors taking a professional qualification using a semi-structured interview. He reported a general rejection of the surface approach in favour of the deep approach as subjects' dominant approach to learning.

Lancaster inventory of study strategies

Entwistle and his colleagues at Lancaster also studied how students read academic articles (Entwistle *et al.*, 1979; Entwistle, 1981) and this culminated in the development of the Lancaster Inventory of Study Stra-tegies. The inventory contained the following scales:

1. *Achieving* relates to competitiveness and organized methods;
2. *Reproducing* relates to surface approach and the syllabus-bound concept;
3. *Meaning* relates to deep approaches and intrinsic motivation;
4. *Comprehension* reflects a holist strategy;
5. *Operation* reflects a serialist strategy;
6. *Versatile* indicates a versatile approach to learning;
7. *Pathological* indicates pathological symptoms in learning;
8. *Overall academic success* prediction for success.

Shorter versions of the inventory have subsequently been developed.

Honey's learning styles

Honey (1982) developed a scheme of learning styles involving a ques-tionnaire of 80 items. Learning styles are classified under four headings – activists, reflectors, theorists and pragmatists – and the questionnaire data reveals the subject's scores on each of these variables.

1. *Activists* are characterized by openness to new experiences and a sociable nature, albeit rather egocentric and impulsive.
2. *Reflectors*, on the other hand, tend to be cautious people who like

to explore things carefully before coming to a decision. They are observers rather than participants.

3. *Theorists* are logical, rational people who like theories and systems; they are unhappy about subjective impressions and ambiguity.

4. *Pragmatists* like very much to apply things in practice and to experiment with ideas; they tend to be impatient and like to get going with new ideas.

Syllabus-bound and syllabus-free students

Malcolm Parlett (1970) classifies students into two types, syllabus-bound (sylbs) and syllabus-free (sylfs). The terms are largely self-explanatory. Sylbs tend to accept the system and are very much examination-oriented and like to know exactly what is required of them in assignments. Sylfs, on the other hand, find the confines of the syllabus very limiting and wish to explore much more widely than that. They are happy to find things out for themselves and take responsibility for learning.

Dunn and Dunn's four learning styles

Dunn and Dunn (1978), and Dunn *et al.* (1984) have identified four preferred learning styles of students, as outlined in Table 2.5.

Table 2.5

Dunn and Dunn's four learning styles

Environmental conditions		
Needs quiet	——	Tolerate sound
Needs bright light	——	Needs dim light
Needs cool environment	——	Needs warm environment
Needs formal design of furniture	——	Needs informal design
Emotional and motivational states		
Self-motivated	——	Unmotivated
Persistent	——	Not persistent
Responsible	——	Not very responsible
Needs structured learning	——	Needs little structure
Sociological preferences		
Prefers learning		Alone / With one peer / With two peers / With several peers / With adults / Through several ways
Physical characteristics and needs		
Prefers		Auditory / Visual / Tactile / Kinaesthetic
Requires food intake	——	Does not require food
Functions best in:		Morning / Late morning / Afternoon / Evening
Needs mobility	——	Does not need mobility

An inventory based on these learning styles has been devised, which enables teachers to arrange the environment so that students' preferences are catered for.

Problems with the concept of learning styles

The validity of attempting to match teaching styles with learning styles is criticized by Tennant (1988) on the grounds that it would produce harmonious viewpoints between teacher and student, but that educational growth is more likely to occur when the student has to move outside the confines of his or her own learning style. In other words, a degree of challenge or conflict may well result in more creative learning. Tennant goes on to suggest that teachers should use the theories of learning styles to assist students to understand how they may approach learning, to facilitate expansion of their learning styles, and to provide a learning climate in which diversity is encouraged.

INTELLIGENCE

Intelligence is not something that is achieved or attained, rather, it is a cognitive ability that enables an individual to learn and to adapt to his environment. It is that capacity of people commonly referred to as 'native wit' and needs to be distinguished from the concept called 'education'. A person can be highly intelligent, yet uneducated, since education and knowledge are attainments rather than abilities. Of course, intelligence is important in education and it may transpire that many well-educated people are also highly intelligent, but the two concepts need to be seen as interrelated rather than identical. Another point of difficulty lies in the nature of intelligence – whether it is some sort of overall, global ability or a multidimensional concept. The following sections outline a range of approaches to intelligence.

Wechsler's approach

Wechsler (1958) defines intelligence as 'the aggregate or global capacity of the individual to act purposefully, to think rationally, and to deal effectively with his environment' and this definition falls into the global category.

Spearman's approach

Spearman (1927) believed that there were two factors that constitute intelligence – a general factor called 'g' and a number of specific factors termed 's'; the general factor 'g' accounts for the correlation between scores on intelligence tests and the specific factors 's' are specific to a given test.

Cattell's approach

Cattell (1966) proposed two kinds of intelligence – fluid and crystallized. Fluid intelligence is genetically determined and corresponds to Spearman's 'g', whereas crystallized intelligence is determined by the environment and learning. Fluid intelligence reaches its maximum in individuals by their mid-twenties, but crystallized intelligence continues to increase throughout life. Cattell believes that the quality of an individual's fluid intelligence will influence the development of crystallized abilities such as vocabulary.

Thurstone's approach

Using factor-analytic techniques, Thurstone (1938) identified seven primary mental abilities:

1. verbal comprehension,;
2. memory;
3. word fluency;
4. number;
5. perceptual speed;
6. spatial;
7. reasoning.

These mental abilities show wide variation between individuals and to some extent, contradict the notion of a general factor of intelligence.

Guilford's approach

Guilford (1967) developed a model of intelligence that envisages ability as consisting of three components – the 'faces of intellect': mental operations, contents and products. Mental operations are processes used by the individual to deal with information, and the combination of operations, content and products are given 120 cognitive abilities. Table 2.6 shows the categories of these three 'faces'.

Table 2.6

Guilford's model of intellect

1.0 Mental operations	
1.1 Cognition	Understanding of information
1.2 Memory	Storage and retrieval of information
1.3 Divergent production (thinking)	Creativity and conformity
1.4 Convergent production (thinking)	Correctness or conformity
1.5 Evaluation	Making judgements
2.0 Contents	
2.1 Figural	Information in form of sensory representations
2.2 Symbolic	Letters and numbers, music, etc.
2.3 Semantic	Information in forms of meanings
2.4 Behavioural	Interpersonal perception
3.0 Products	
3.1 Units	Smallest items of information
3.2 Classes	Concepts
3.3 Relations	Principles and rules
3.4 Systems	Larger combinations of principles and rules
3.5 Transformations	Changes in existing information
3.6 Implications	Expectations or predictions

Gardner's approach

This approach takes the view that there are multiple intelligences rather than a single concept. Gardner identifies six kinds of intelligence that are independent of each other (Gardner, 1983):

1. linguistic;
2. logical-mathematical;
3. spatial;
4. musical;
5. bodily-kinesthetic;
6. personal.

The first three are included in most other intelligence tests, but the remaining three are more controversial. Musical intelligence underlies the ability to understand and perform music; bodily-kinesthetic intelligence refers to the motor control of the body as in performing complex movements; personal intelligence is the ability to understand and monitor our feelings, and also to appreciate the needs and feelings of other people. Gardner's contribution has helped to focus attention on abilities that are not normally considered important in educational systems.

Sternberg's approach

This approach focuses on practical intelligence, i.e. intelligence that operates in the real world as opposed to the laboratory. This is the kind of intelligence that underlies success in the world of work, and bears little relationship to the kind of intelligence measured by conventional intelligence tests (Sternberg and Wagner, 1993). The basis for practical intelligence appears to be tacit knowledge, i.e. the kind of knowledge that is not learned in any formal way, but 'absorbed' during the day to day activities of living and working. Traditional measures of intelligence are poor predictors of success in the world of work.

The artificial intelligence approach

Artificial intelligence (AI) is defined as 'the use of computer programs and programming techniques to cast light on the principles of intelligence in general and human thought in particular' (Boden, 1977). This involves the use of computer simulation to develop theories about human cognitive processes such as language or problem-solving and the approach has been termed 'theory development' by Miller (1978) to contrast with the standard approach in psychology, which is 'theory demonstration'. Theory demonstration involves a written explanation of some specific aspect of cognitive performance and the subsequent experimental testing of it. Theory development or AI, on the other hand, are explanations stated in the form of computer programs, which address more general aspects of cognition by attempting to model human cognitive processes prior to experimental testing.

One of the advantages of this approach is that great clarity is required in the formulation of the program, otherwise it will not work. The main differences between the two approaches is that theory demonstration emphasizes parsimony as a criterion for a theory, i.e. an explanation that explains the phenomenon more economically is better than one which is more complex. With the AI approach, sufficiency of the theory is the main criterion and there is more tolerance of alternative theories. There are many computer programs in existence that can simulate aspects of human cognition and this artificial intelligence is demonstrated in their ability to translate language, to play chess and to solve complex problems with great speed.

Testing intelligence

Intelligence tests are a source of great controversy among both psychologists and the lay public and this stems largely from the social and racial implications of their use in educational testing. Three main tests have been developed over the years: the Binet–Simon test, the Stanford–Binet test, and the Wechsler tests.

The Binet–Simon test

This test was developed in France to identify children who needed special education and consisted of a scale of test items for children aged between three and thirteen years. The underlying assumption is that there is an average mental level for each age and test items were devised to measure this. If a child could answer items from a higher age-bracket than his own, he was said to have a mental age higher than his chronological age. If, on the other hand, he could only answer items from a lower age-bracket than his own, his mental age would be less than his chronological age. This notion was developed by Stern to produce a ratio that is called the 'intelligence quotient' (IQ). It utilizes the concepts of mental age (MA) and chronological age (CA) to calculate an individual's intelligence relative to the average, using the formula:

$$IQ = \frac{MA}{CA} \times 100$$

Thus, if a child is aged eight years, but can only answer test items that an average five-year-old could answer, then his IQ is:

$$\frac{5}{8} \times 100 = 62.5$$

Since the average IQ is 100 (MA = CA), this child would be considered mentally retarded. Another child may have a mental age of ten and a chronological age of eight, giving an IQ of 125, which indicates superior intelligence.

The Stanford–Binet test

This was developed in America by Terman, to give a standardized test for use in that culture and consisted of a series of revisions of the Binet–Simon test, including the first use of the concept of IQ.

Wechsler tests

There are three tests used here and each is designed to measure both verbal and non-verbal intelligence.

1. WAIS-R: Wechsler adult intelligence scale (revised version);
2. WISC-R: Wechsler intelligence scale for children (revised version);
3. WPPSI: Wechsler preschool and primary scale of intelligence.

Wechsler developed his adult scale because of the problems of measuring the IQ of adults using the Stanford–Binet test. The concept of mental age depends upon the notion that intelligence increases along with chronological age in children, but there is no evidence that this continues beyond adolescence; this would result in an adult's chronological age increasing steadily, whereas his or her mental age may remain the same, leading to a progressively declining IQ. Wechsler overcame this by introducing the deviation IQ, which compares the individual's score with standardized norms for his age group and is expressed in standard deviation units. It is clear that, in considering the usefulness of intelligence tests, we must be sure that the test is measuring ability rather than attainment, since the latter is very much influenced by environmental factors. In practice, however, this is very difficult to ensure and many criticisms are levelled at the cultural bias of tests. In any test, the two main criteria are its validity and reliability, i.e. does the test measure what it is supposed to measure and does it measure this consistently. Intelligence tests do correlate highly with each other, so reliability is high, but this does not prove that validity is equally high. It may well be that these tests are measuring something consistently, but that 'something' is not intelligence. All the tests rely on teachers' opinions about students' ability and this can be unreliable; also, the tests assume a normal distribution of intelligence within the population and this may not be the case.

IQ: fixed or changeable?

One important issue concerning intelligence is whether or not an individual's IQ remains unchangeable throughout life, or whether it can be improved by educational interventions. This question is of fundamental importance for education, since it has profound practical implications. For example, if a child's IQ is considered to be fixed, then there would be no point in the Government spending money on measures to improve it. On the other hand, if improvements to IQ following interventions could be demonstrated, then appropriate interventions could be initiated to help children improve their low IQ scores.

Howe (1998) reviews the evidence for IQ changes from a number of sources; for example, the average IQ scores of adopted children can be some 20 points higher than those of siblings and biological parents. He also cites a range of studies that demonstrate evidence of gains in IQ scores in children on intervention programmes funded by the Head Start initiatives. He summarizes his position in the following statement: 'there is massive evidence that IQ is far from being immutable. The objections that have been raised in relation to that evidence are not at all convincing. There are no clear reasons for insisting that it is qualitatively more difficult to change the mental capacities that determine a person's score at an IQ test than it is to alter those mental capabilities that are acknowledged to be acquired as a result of a person's experiences. The empirical findings provide no support for the pessimistic conclusion that low intelligence and the problems associated with it are inevitable and unalterable.'

Heredity environment and IQ

One of the major issues in the field of intelligence concerns the relative contribution of genetic and environmental factors to intelligence. Indeed, intelligence tests have been the focus of severe controversy for more than two decades between hereditarian and environmentalist psychologists.

The hereditarian viewpoint

The hereditarian viewpoint considers that intelligence is genetically-determined, although it does acknowledge that some contribution is made by environmental factors. One of the main hereditarians, Arthur Jenson, argues that a genetic viewpoint must be considered for two pressing reasons. He claims that, first, environmentalist approaches have failed to provide satisfactory explanations for the results of IQ tests and second, that it is common sense to suppose that mental traits are genetically determined because so many physical characteristics are so determined. The main support for his arguments lies in the concept of heritability (H2) estimates, which attempt to measure the extent to which genetic and environmental factors explain differing performance in IQ tests. The higher the H2 estimate, the more genetic influence. For example, Jensen claims that the H2 estimate for intelligence is 0.80 for white Americans, which implies that 80% of the variance in IQ is attributable to genetic factors, the rest being environmental. This is a population statistic, however, and no conclusions can be drawn about any particular individual within that population. Jensen also claims to be able to falsify every argument put forward by environmentalists to explain the gap between IQ scores of black and white Americans.

Another proponent of the hereditarian view was Hans Eysenck, who used results from studies with twins to support his points. Twins are classified into monozygotic (identical) or dizygotic (fraternal); the former are produced from the same ovum that has split into two and thus share the same genetic material; the latter are from different ova and are therefore no more alike than ordinary siblings. In twin studies, the amount of resemblance on a given trait between identical over fraternal twins is taken as evidence of genetic influence. There are numerous studies (e.g. Bouchard and McGue, 1981) in which a high positive correlation is found between the IQs of identical twins, but not for fraternal twins, whose scores are much the same as ordinary siblings. Of course, this may be due to environmental influences such as having identical twins dress the same, or by people treating them in the same way.

Further evidence for the hereditarian viewpoint comes from studies of identical twins who were reared apart; these show high positive correlations between the IQs of identical twins who have been raised apart, and also a high correlation with the IQs of their natural parents. Studies of adopted children also show that there is a higher correlation between their IQs and those of their biological mothers, than there is between those of their adoptive mothers.

The environmentalist viewpoint
The environmentalist viewpoint emphasizes the importance of social and physical surroundings and events in determining the intelligence of an individual. Evidence for this viewpoint comes from a variety of sources, such as studies of enriched environments. Children from impoverished backgrounds show average gains in IQ when they are adopted into a better home background. Leon Kamin argues against the hereditarian viewpoint of intelligence, quoting the terrible effects of eugenics movement on such things as immigration quotas and the American sterilization laws (Eysenck and Kamin, 1981). A genetic explanation of intelligence has led to the consigning of many students to the 'educational scrap heap' and he maintains that the genetic arguments can all be explained in terms of environmental effects, or of poor or fraudulent data. He does not actually state an environmentalist theory as such, but relies chiefly on criticizing the arguments of the genetic viewpoint.

REFERENCES

Ackoff, R. (1973) Science in the systems age: beyond IE, OR and MS, *Operational Research*, **21**, 661–71.
Atkinson, J.W. (1958) *Motives in Fantasy, Action and Society*, Van Nostrand, Princeton.
Boden, M. (1977) *Artificial Intelligence and Natural Man*, Harvester Press, Brighton.
Bouchard, T.J. Jr and McGue, M. (1981) Familial Studies of Intelligence: A Review. *Science*, **2212**, 105–59.
Bourne, L. and Ekstrand, B. (1985) *Psychology: Its Principles and Meanings*, Holt, Rinehart and Winston, New York.
Bowlby, J. (1970) *Attachment*, Penguin, Harmondsworth.
Brack, P.E. and Thoreson, C.E. (1996) Reducing type A behaviour patterns: a structured-group approach, in R. Allen and S. Scheidt (eds) *Heart and Mind*, American Psychological Association, Washington, DC.
Cattell, R.B. (1966) *The Scientific Analysis of Personality*, Aldine, Chicago.
Cattell, R. (1971) *Abilities: Their Structure, Growth and Action*, Houghton Mifflin, Boston.
Dunn, R. and Dunn, K. (1978) *Teaching Students through their Individual Learning Styles: A Practical Approach*, Reston Publishing Co, Reston Va.
Dunn, R., Dunn, K. and Price, G. (1984) *Learning Style Inventory Research Manual*, Lawrence, PO Box 3271, Kansas.
Entwistle, N. (1981) *Styles of Learning and Teaching*, Wiley, Chichester.
Entwistle, N., Hanley, M. and Hounsell, D. (1979) Identifying distinctive approaches to studying, *Higher Education*, 8, 365–80.
Eysenck, H. (1981) (ed.) *A Model for Personality*, Springer-Verlag, New York.

Eysenck, H. (1985) *Decline and Fall of the Freudian Empire*, Penguin, Harmondsworth.

Eysenck, H. and Kamin, L. (1981) *Intelligence: The Battle for The Mind*, Pan, London.

Freud, S. (1923) *The Ego and the Id* Translated by J. Riviere, Norton, New York, 1962,

Friedman, M. and Rosenman, R.H. (1974) *Type A Behaviour and Your Heart*, Knopf, New York.

Gardner, H. (1983) *Frames of Mind: The Theory of Multiple Intelligences*, Paladin, London.

Guilford, J. (1967) *The Nature of Human Intelligence*, McGraw Hill, New York.

Hampson, S. (1999) Personality: state of the art, *The Psychologist*, **12**(6), 284–8

Honey, P. (1982) *The Manual of Learning Styles*, Honey and Mumford, Maidenhead.

Howe, M.J.A. (1998) Can IQ change?, *The Psychologist*, February 1998, 69–71.

Kagan, J. (1965) Reflection-impulsivity and reading ability in primary grade children, *Child Development*, **36**(3), 188–90.

Kelly, G. (1955) *The Psychology of Personal Constructs*, Vol. 1, Norton, New York.

Kirby, L.K. and Myers, K.D. (1993) *Introduction to Type*, Consulting Psychologists Press Inc., Palo Alta.

Kolb, D. (1976) *The Learning Style Inventory: Technical Manual*, McBer and Co, Boston.

Krahe, B. (1992) *Personality and Social Psychology: Towards a Synthesis*, Sage, London.

Lefcourt, H. (1982) *Locus of Control: Current Trends in Theory and Research*, 2nd edn, Erlbaum, New Jersey.

Marton, F. and Saljo, R. (1976) On qualitative differences in learning. 1.outcome and process, *British Journal of Educational Psychology*, **46**, 4–11.

Maslow, A. (1971) *The Farther Reaches of Human Nature*, Penguin, Harmondsworth.

McClelland, D., Clark, R., Roby, T. and Atkinson, J. (1949) The effect of need for achievement on thematic apperception, *Journal of Experimental Psychology*, 37, 242–55.

Miller, L. (1978) Has artificial intelligence contributed to an understanding of the human mind? *Cognitive Science*, 2, 11–128.

Mischel, W. (1968) *Personality and Assessment*, Wiley, New York.

Mook, D.G. (1996) *Motivation: The Organisation of Action*, Norton and Co., London.

Parlett, M. (1970) The syllabus-bound student, in *The Ecology of Human Intelligence* (ed. Hudson), Penguin, Harmondsworth.

Pask, G. (1975) *The Cybernetics of Human Learning and Performance*, Hutchinson, London.

Pask, G. (1976) Styles and strategies of learning, *British Journal of Educational Psychology*, **46**, 128–48.

Pask, G. and Scott, B. (1972) Learning strategies and individual competence, *International Journal of Man-Machine Studies*, **4**, 217–53.

Pavlov, I. (1927) *Conditioned Reflexes*, Oxford University Press, Oxford.

Rogers, C.R. (1959) A theory of therapy, personality, and interpersonal relationships as developed in the client-centred therapy framework, in Koch, S. (ed.) *Psychology: A Study of Science*, Vol. 3, McGraw Hill, New York.

Rosenman, R., Friedman, M. and Straus, R. (1964) A predictive study of CHD, *Journal of the American Medical Association*, **189**, 15–22.

Rotter, J. (1954) *Social Learning and Clinical Psychology*, Prentice-Hall, New Jersey.

Rotter, J. (1966) Generalised expectancies for internal v external control of reinforcement, *Psychological Monographs*, **80**, 1.

Seligman, M. and Maier, S. (1967) Failure to escape traumatic shock, *Journal of Experimental Psychology*, **74**, 1–9.

Skinner, B.F. (1971) *Beyond Freedom and Dignity*, Alfred Knopf, New York.

Solomon, R.L. (1980) The opponent process theory of acquired motivation: the costs of pleasure and the benefits of pain, *American Psychologist*, **35**, 691–712.

Solomon, R.L. and Corbit, J.D. (1974) An opponent process theory of acquired motivation, *American Psychologist*, **35**, 119–41

Spearman, C. (1927) *The Abilities of Man: Their Nature and Measurement*, MacMillan, New York.

Sternberg, R.J. and Wagner, R.K. (1993) The egocentric view of intelligence and job performance is wrong, *Current Directions in Psychological Science*, **2**, 1–5.

Sutherland, P. (1999) A study of the learning of mature adult students on a professional course, *Journal of Further and Higher Education*, **23**(3), 381–9.

Tennant, M. (1988) *Psychology and Adult Learning*, Routledge, New York.

Tennant, M. (1997) *Psychology and Adult Learning*, 2nd edn, Routledge, London.

Thorndike, E. (1931) *Human Learning*, Appleton Century Crofts, New York.

Thurstone, L. (1938) Primary mental abilities, *Psychometric Monographs*, No 1.

Wechsler, D. (1958) *The Measurement and Appraisal of Adult Intelligence*, 4th edn, Williams and Wilkins, Baltimore.

Weiner, B. (1979) A theory of motivation for some classroom experiences, *Journal of Educational Psychology*, **71**, 3–25.

Witkin, H. (1977) Field dependent and field independent cognitive styles and their educational implications, *Review of Educational Research*, **47**, 1–64.

3 Adult learning theory

Like all members of the human race, adult learners in nursing, midwifery and health visiting differ widely from one another in their personal characteristics. These individual differences encompass physical characteristics such as age and gender, and psychological characteristics including motivation, personality, intelligence, learning styles, and expectations. The literature of adult education points out that adult learners do, however, have one thing in common, i.e. they are all voluntary participants. Whilst this is true at face value, it ignores the pressures that employers and the professional nursing bodies exert upon individuals to undertake continuing education.

This chapter begins with a review of human development across the life-span, and then focuses on the main theoretical underpinnings of adult learning, namely humanistic approaches exemplified by Abraham Maslow and Carl Rogers, the work of Malcolm Knowles on andragogy, and the experiential learning approach exemplified by David Kolb, and finally, Peter Jarvis' typology of learning.

Alan Rogers presents a useful list of the general characteristics of adult learners, as shown in Table 3.1 (Rogers, 1996).

Table 3.1

General characteristics of adult learners

1. They are adult by definition
2. Their process of growth is continuing, rather than starting
3. They come to the learning situation with a set of experiences and values
4. They come to the learning situation with intentions and expectations
5. They have competing interests
6. They have established patterns of learning

Human development across the life-span

Given that an individual's physical development seems to stop once adulthood is attained, one might be forgiven for thinking that human development is therefore complete. On the contrary, it is a continuous process throughout the life-span of an individual, and it is possible to identify a series of broad stages of development, commencing with infancy and progressing through childhood, adolescence, adulthood and finally, old age. The term 'development' is normally taken to mean some form of physical, intellectual or social improvement as an individual progresses through the developmental process, but in the case of ageing the changes may be degenerative. This section focuses on three aspects of human development; the first is concerned with intellectual development, the second with adult development, and the third with ageing.

Piaget's theory of cognitive development

Piaget's work focuses on the intellectual development of the individual and his or her adaptation to the environment (Piaget and Inhelder, 1969). For adaptation to occur there must be some form of organization within the individual, and these two processes work interdependently and in parallel.

Schemas

The internal organization of an individual consists of schemas, which are ways of giving meaning to, and dealing with, aspects of the environment that are encountered. They can be likened to mini-theories that develop as a result of the infant's interactions with the environment. In early infancy, schemas equate to reflexes but as development progresses these schemas become more complex, and this occurs through two processes: assimilation and accommodation. When children encounter a new situation they try to assimilate it into their existing familiar schemas but if the latter are inadequate then their schemas have to be modified to accommodate the new situation. For example, a child's schema for 'dog' may include all smallish, four-legged animals such as cats and foxes, but as accommodation progresses these become schemas in their own right. Hence, the child's knowledge of the world is modified and extended by the processes of assimilation and accommodation, and these processes are in balance with one another; Piaget calls this balancing process equilibration – a dynamic process that prepares the child for new learning. In Piagetian theory, motivation is intrinsic and arises from the application of schemas to the environment.

Stages of cognitive development

Cognitive development is seen by Piaget as consisting of four stages:

1. sensorimotor (birth–2 years);
2. pre-operational (2–7 years);
3. concrete operational (7–11 years);
4. formal operational (12 years and up).

Sensorimotor stage (birth–2 years)

At birth, the infant is equipped only with basic reflexes and these serve as the first schemas, hence thinking equates with doing. Gradually 'self' becomes differentiated from objects, and intentional behaviour begins at eight months or so. The infant begins to understand that objects exist even when they cannot be seen; this object permanence is an important characteristic at this stage since it demonstrates that a mental representation of the object must be present. It also indicates the beginnings of a move away from the egocentric focus of early infancy.

Pre-operational stage (2–7 years)

This stage is called pre-operational because the child is unable to use mental rules or operations for transforming information. He or she is still egocentric – focusing on general aspects instead of on the individual aspects of a situation. This is strikingly demonstrated in the child's lack of conservation; for example, if presented with two balls of clay of equal size, the child will indicate that they are the same size. If one ball is then rolled into a cylindrical shape, the child will say it has more clay. Lack of conservation also applies to numbers: if two rows of coins are evenly spaced-out, and then in one row the coins are spaced closely together, the child will indicate that the original row contains more coins. Thus, the child lacks reversibility, i.e. the ability to understand that if an operation is reversed it reverts back to its original state.

Concrete operational stage (7–11 years)
In this stage, the child develops conservation, and the ability to undertake mental operations. However, these operations are limited to the here-and-now; in other words, the child cannot reason hypothetically.

Formal operational stage (12 years and up)
This final stage is characterized by the ability of the child to reason hypothetically, i.e. he or she can focus on the form of a problem without being limited to the concrete aspects as in the previous stage.

Implications for teaching and learning
Piaget's work does not consider individuals beyond the age of adolescence, but Tennant (1997) suggests that it is relevant to adult learning because:

1. it emphasizes qualitative rather than quantitative development;
2. it emphasizes the active role of individuals in constructing their own knowledge;
3. the concept of formal operations as representing adult thinking.

It is possible to extrapolate from Piaget's approach some implications for the teaching of adults; for example, the active involvement of adult students in their own learning might assist them in their own knowledge construction. When teaching difficult abstract concepts to adult students, the teacher could initially try to frame his/her explanations at Piaget's concrete operational level, and once this had been understood could then adopt a more abstract approach.

Piaget's work has been subject to criticism on a number of grounds, including criticism of his experimental methodology. Some researchers reject his claim that the stage of formal operations marks the end of any further structural change, and also that his approach fails to consider affective or emotional aspects of development.

Levinson's adult development model
Levinson (1986) has developed a model of adult development which identifies four major periods or eras as shown in Table 3.2.

The eras are relatively stable periods, but the periods of transition

1. Era of pre-adulthood	Age 0–22
2. Era of early adulthood	Age 17–45
(a) Early adult transition	Age 17–22
(b) Entry life structure	
for early adulthood	Age 22–28
(c) Age 30 transition	Age 26–33
(d) Culminating life structure	
for early adulthood	Age 33–40
3. Era of middle adulthood	Age 40–65
(a) Midlife transition	Age 40–45
(b) Entry life structure	
for middle adulthood	Age 45–50
(c) Age 50 transition	Age 50–55
(d) Culminating life structure	
for middle adulthood	Age 55–60
4. Era of late adulthood	Age 60–?
(a) Late adult transition	Age 60–65

Table 3.2

Levinson's adult development model

between stages are characterized by turmoil. The era of early-adulthood marks the adolescent's entry to the adult world. It is a time for exploring possibilities and for the beginnings of stability in life. The age-30 transition is a period of settling down, of taking a more serious approach to life and work. The transition stage into middle adulthood or midlife has become synonymous with the term 'midlife crisis'. For some 80% of Levinson's sample this transition period was extremely stressful and characterized by self-doubt and a realization that their career progression had probably reached its limit. In the midlife era, there are added pressures such as elderly parents to worry about, the beginnings of physical decline such as the need to wear spectacles, and children becoming independent young adults. There is a positive side to midlife, though, such as being financially more secure, and enjoying life as a couple again after children have left home.

Implications for teaching and learning

Levinson's model may help teachers to gain greater insight into the developmental stage of their adult students and an appreciation of the factors that might help or hinder such students in their studies. For example, the midlife crisis may provide a useful explanation for some of the difficulties adult students may experience whilst undertaking studies in middle age. Although Levinson's methodology was sound, the model has yet to gain universal acceptance.

The ageing process and the adult learner

Technically speaking, ageing begins at birth but the accompanying decline in human performance does not significantly manifest itself until the onset of old age between approximately 60 and 65 years of age. A number of sub-categories of old age can be found in the literature; the term 'young elderly' applies to those aged between 65 and 75, and the old elderly to those over 75. Another classification is that of the 'third

age' and the 'fourth age', the former referring to those elderly individuals who are independent and active, the latter to those who are
dependent upon others for activities of living.

General effects of ageing

There are many theories that attempt to explain why the human body
ages but the general effects of the process are well-documented, the
usual classification being physiological and psychological ageing.

Physiological ageing

The ageing process involves a decline in the effectiveness of many
bodily functions, including breathing, circulation, digestion and elimination but the most obvious deterioration is in eyesight and hearing. The
main eyesight problem in the elderly is concerned with their ability to
focus correctly, leading to long-sightedness or, more seriously, loss of
acuity or sharpness of vision. Hearing loss of varying degrees is
common in the elderly and can be attributed to a range of factors such
as wax blocking the auditory canal, degeneration of the small bones that
conduct sound in the middle ear, and degeneration of the nerves of the
inner ear. Perception of high frequency sounds sustains greater loss than
that for low frequency sounds, and the ability to discriminate pitch may
be affected (Stuart-Hamilton, 1996).

Psychological ageing

In considering the effects of ageing upon psychological functioning, it is
useful to distinguish between two types of intelligence, crystallized intelligence, which indicates the knowledge acquired by an individual
throughout the life-span, and fluid intelligence, which is concerned with
information-processing and problem-solving, and which is much less
dependent upon acquired knowledge. Crystallized intelligence is often
equated with wisdom, i.e. the accumulated knowledge gained over a
lifetime, whereas fluid intelligence equates with wit, i.e. the ability to
deal with novel or abstract problems. Research studies indicate that
there is a decline in fluid intelligence in old age, but that crystallized
intelligence is largely unaffected. Many elderly people feel that their
memory has declined as they have grown older, and research findings
support the fact that memory does indeed decline with ageing.

Implications for teaching and learning

From the foregoing outline of ageing, it is apparent that no significant
deterioration in intellectual abilities is likely to be present in those adult
learners in nursing, midwifery and health visiting who are below the age
of 60–65. However, the teacher may be able to assist the adult learner
to compensate for the gradual decline in some aspects of functioning
which occurs progressively during adulthood. With regard to eyesight
problems, the teacher can ensure adequate lighting is provided by
simply switching on the classroom lights at the commencement of the
lesson, and can advise older students to sit closer to the front of the

classroom so that visual materials can be more easily seen. It may also be helpful to furnish such students with photocopies of any transparencies or slides used in the lesson. The teacher can help students with hearing problems by suggesting that such students sit at the front of the class, and by ensuring that the volume of his/her voice is sufficiently audible and the speed of delivery is not too fast. Also, particular attention needs to be given to the volume and tone settings of audiotape and video presentations.

Given the comments about the decline in fluid intelligence with ageing, when setting problem-solving activities in the classroom the teacher may need to allocate extra time for older students to complete the activities. Similarly, in the light of the decline in memory with ageing, when asking questions the teacher should allow older students a little longer to structure their reply, as they may be slower to recall the information they require to answer.

In addition to these specific aspects of ageing, older students may lack confidence in their academic and study ability, especially if they have not been engaged in formal study for some considerable time. If older students are in the minority within a group, they may feel marginalized or isolated from the younger students. It is not always easy to bridge the 'generation gap' and mix freely with a younger group, so teachers may need to offer additional support to older students if they become isolated. On the other hand, the younger students may benefit enormously from the experience and stability of the older students.

THE HUMANISTIC BASIS OF ADULT LEARNING THEORY

Adult learning theory has been strongly influenced by humanistic psychology, although there is no single theory that represents the humanistic approach. However, all theories share a common view that this approach involves the study of man as a human being, with his thoughts, feelings and experiences. This is in direct contrast to the stimulus–response theorists, who study man from the point of view of his overt behaviour, disregarding his inner feelings and experiences. Humanistic differs from cognitive theory also, in that the latter is concerned with the thinking aspects of man's behaviour, with little emphasis on the affective components.

Exponents of humanistic theory claim that the other two theories omit some of the most significant aspects of human existence, namely feelings, attitudes and values. Humanistic theory is closely related to the philosophical approach called phenomenology, which asserts that reality lies in a person's perception of an event and not in the event itself. The humanistic viewpoint has never been better crystallized that in Hamachek's (1978) definition:

'It is a psychological stance that focuses not so much on a person's biological drives, but on their goals; not so much on stimuli impinging on them, but on their desires to be or to do something; not

*so much on their past experiences, but on their current circum-
stances; not so much on life conditions per se, but on the subjective
qualities of human experience, the personal meaning of an experience to persons, rather than on their objective, observable responses.'*

Humanistic theory, then, is concerned with human growth, individual
fulfilment and self-actualization and it is claimed that this approach is
'intuitively right', as it agrees with the ideas most people have about
what is uniquely human. However, the behaviourist approach is not
considered to be wrong; rather, humanistic theory prefers to emphasize
the affective aspects of man as being of equal importance to the
cognitive and psychomotor elements. There are two main principles that
apply to the humanistic approach to learning and teaching, namely
teacher–student relationships and the classroom climate. The former
stresses the importance of the interpersonal relationship between learner
and teacher as a major variable affecting learning and this in turn affects
the climate of the classroom. The presence or absence of conflict and
tension will depend largely on the quality of relationships within the
classroom setting.

Self-direction, empowerment and autonomy

Humanism's emphasis on the importance of the Self is reflected in three
of its key tenets, i.e. self-direction, empowerment, and learner
autonomy. The term 'self-direction' is used in three different senses
within the literature of adult learning (Cafarella, 1993, cited in
Tennant, 1997):

1. the ability of adult students to plan and manage their own
   learning;
2. a personal characteristic of adult learners associated with personal
   autonomy;
3. a way of organizing teaching that allows greater student control
   over the learning process.

The basic underlying concept in each of these is the belief that adults
are naturally self-directing and autonomous with regard to learning, if
given the opportunity to be so. Autonomy is one of the basic values of
Western society; its literal meaning is 'self-governing', which implies
independence and a sense of control over external forces. Hence,
learner autonomy is really about the re-distribution of power; self-
directed learning aims to shift the power base away from the educational organization (teachers, curriculum, etc.) and towards the adult
learners themselves. Autonomy is not an all-or-nothing phenomenon,
but a continuum from lesser to greater autonomy; it is also a characteristic that can be developed (McNair, 1996).

Humanistic psychology: Abraham H. Maslow's approach

Abraham H. Maslow (1908–1970) was a major exponent of the humanistic approach to psychology, and has also made a significant contribu-

tion to motivation theory with his theory of a hierarchy of needs (see Chapter 2, p. 18). He coined the term 'third force' psychology because he considered the first force to be Freudian psychotherapy and the second to be the stimulus–response school. The latter school, he felt, had little relevance to the human personality: 'these extensive books on the psychology of learning are of no consequence, at least to the human centre, to the human soul, to the human essence' (Maslow, 1971). One of the key concepts he defined was that of 'self-actualization' and he studied the behaviour of people whom he classified as self-actualizers. Maslow stated eight ways in which an individual self-actualizes, and these include 'experiencing fully, vividly, selflessly, with full concentration and total absorption' (p. 44). He mentions the 'peak experience', which is an ecstatic moment that can be brought on by such experiences as classical music and religious experiences. For the humanist, the goal of education is to assist the individual to achieve self-actualization, or, as Maslow puts it, 'to help the person to become the best that he is able to become' (p. 163). This intrinsic approach is in contrast to the extrinsic educational ethic, in which the transmission of factual knowledge is seen to be more important than the development of an individual. The ideal college, according to Maslow, would be one in which the main objectives would be the discovery of one's identity and the destiny or vocation for each person.

Humanistic psychology: Carl R. Rogers' approach

Carl R. Rogers made his reputation as a psychotherapist, developing a new approach that he called client-centred therapy (Rogers, 1951). This involves the therapist in a non-directive role in which the client is encouraged to develop a deeper understanding of his or her 'self'. The role of the therapist is to provide a non-critical atmosphere, in which there is no attempt to interpret for the client, but simply a reflecting back of the statements made in order to assist him or her in developing self-awareness. This concept of client-centred therapy led Rogers to formulate his student-centred approach to learning, which is contained in his most important work on the subject (Rogers, 1969; Rogers and Freiberg, 1994). In this work, he stated ten principles of learning, and these are shown in Table 3.3.

These principles illustrate Rogers' approach to learning and his emphasis on relevance, student participation and involvement, self-evaluation and the absence of threat in the classroom. Rogers saw the teacher as a facilitator of learning, a provider of resources for learning, and someone who shares feelings as well as knowledge with their students.

Rogers further articulated his approach to education in his book *Freedom to Learn for the 80s* (Rogers, 1983). He saw learning as being a continuum, with much meaningless material at one end and significant or experiential learning at the other. The former could describe many curricula, which are seen as virtually meaningless by the student for whom they are intended.

Table 3.3

Carl Rogers' principles of learning

1. Human beings have a natural potentiality for learning.
2. Significant learning takes place when the subject-matter is perceived by the student as having relevance for his own purposes.
3. Learning which involves a change in self-organization is threatening and tends to be resisted.
4. Those elements of learning which are threatening to the self are more easily perceived and assimilated when external threats are at a minimum.
5. When threat to the self is low, experience can be perceived in differentiated fashion, and learning can proceed.
6. Much significant learning is acquired through doing.
7. Learning is facilitated when the student participates responsibly in the learning process.
8. Self-initiated learning, which involves the whole person of the learner, feelings as well as intellect, is the most lasting and pervasive.
9. Independence, creativity and self-reliance are all facilitated when self-criticism and self-evaluation are basic and evaluation by others is of secondary importance.
10. The most socially useful learning in the modern world is the learning of the process of learning, a continuing openness to experience and incorporation into oneself of the process of change.

Experiential learning, on the other hand, has a number of qualities such as personal involvement, self-initiation, persuasiveness, self-evaluation and meaningfulness. Rogers contrasts the kind of learning that is concerned solely with cognitive functioning with that involving the whole person.

Teaching, according to Rogers, is a highly overrated activity, in contrast to the notion of facilitation. Teaching by giving knowledge does not meet the requirements of today's changing world; what is required is the facilitation of learning and change and this calls for a different set of qualities in the facilitator.

Qualities required in a facilitator

The most important factor is the relationship that exists between facilitator and learner and Rogers suggests a number of qualities that are required for this: genuineness, trust and acceptance, and empathetic understanding.

1. *Genuineness*. The facilitator should come across as a real person rather than as some kind of ideal model. Hence it is important that facilitators show 'normal' reactions to their students.
2. *Trust and acceptance*. The facilitator should demonstrate acceptance of the student as a person in his or her own right as a person worthy of their respect and care.
3. *Empathic understanding*. Facilitators need to put themselves in the students' shoes in order to see and understand things from their students' perspective.

Rogers suggests that it is possible for the teacher to build into a programme the freedom to learn, which students require. This can be done by using students' own experiences and problems so that relevance is obvious and by providing resources for the students in the form of both material and human resources. The goal of education is that of the student becoming a fully functioning person.

Implications for teaching and learning

Rogers' ten principles of learning can be used as a basis for planning the educational experiences of adult learners. Their natural potentiality for learning can be exploited by strategies that arouse curiosity and present problems or challenges. The importance of relevance cannot be over-emphasized; theoretical concepts should be framed in the context of the real world of adult students, e.g. applied to the workplace, or to wider society. Rogers sees the psychological environment of the classroom as being of paramount importance to learning; by their very nature, classrooms can be perceived by students as places where their ignorance or lack of ability may be exposed to ridicule by both teachers and peers. The first step in creating a psychologically-safe atmosphere in the classroom is for the teacher to state clearly from the outset the ground rules of the teaching and learning interaction. These will include the expectation that students will actively participate in the learning process, that learning is a partnership between teacher and students, that students' contributions will be accepted with respect by other students and the teacher, and that challenge and debate will be part of the agenda.

The development of a facilitative learning environment can take some time to come to fruition, given that it depends on the establishment of trust and respect between all parties in the teaching and learning situation. It should be an environment where psychological safety exists and where the students feel at ease. Some of the barriers between teacher and learner may be lessened by the rearrangement of the seating and the use of small-group techniques. These also facilitate the discussion of feelings and values, an aspect that is considered crucial in the humanistic approach. The humanistic approach to education centres on the relationships between teachers and students, each learner being considered as an individual. The use of forenames between teacher and learner can increase the feeling of identity for the learner and help to reduce barriers to communication.

Involvement in decision-making is a further step in helping the students develop a sense of personal value and worth. While it is impossible to involve each learner in major planning decisions, it is useful to have student representatives on course and pathway committees to contribute ideas and suggestions from their peer group or cohort. Most teachers are aware of the individual differences between students prior to commencing an educational programme, but they also need to be sensitive to the fact that they will still have differences at the end of the course. It is important to remain aware that the students are individuals, even though they have been exposed to a common educational programme and to encourage them to maintain their unique attitudes and values, rather than aiming for a conformist, homogeneous end product.

The role of the teacher is seen by the humanistic approach as being that of helper and facilitator, rather than a conveyor of information. In other words, the teacher becomes another learning resource for the learner. In order to perform their role satisfactorily, teachers must fully understand themselves, and be flexible in their approach to teaching. Rogers' approach encourages active involvement by the student in learning, and this can be achieved by the inclusion of strategies such as project work, practicals and field-based studies. It is also important that students be encouraged to follow-up topics or issues that have particular interest for them, although it is often difficult in practice to make provision for this in a prescribed curriculum. Adult students should be encouraged to engage in self-evaluation of their learning, so that they do not become reliant on external feedback from the teacher. Lastly, Rogers emphasizes the importance of students knowing how to learn, so study skills advice should be made available, usually in the form of study skills workshops or learning packages.

One of the specific applications of humanistic psychology is in the use of learning contracts, which give the students the opportunity to take responsibility for their own learning. Learning contracts are discussed below in the section on Andragogy.

Critique of the humanistic approach

One of the most serious criticisms of the humanistic approach is that it is lacking in empirical evidence to support its claims, relying upon observations and assumptions of human behaviour. Humanistic psychology's emphasis on the *self* and on *feelings* may be seen as devaluing intellectual aspects of learning; the acquisition of knowledge and facts is a quite legitimate educational aim. It could also be argued that the emphasis on personal growth and self-exploration in humanistic theories makes them less useful for some types of vocational education and training.

The writings of Carl Rogers are about the education of children in schools, and the application of his ideas to the teaching of adult professionals, whilst attractive, may have little or no validity. Sigman (1995), in a telling critique, points out that humanistic psychology originated in the USA, a different culture from the UK, and suggests that the principles may not easily translate to the UK culture. He argues that it began as a psychological therapy for illness, but has now become a general approach for the pursuit of self-fulfilment through change. According to Sigman, contentment has been replaced by the need for personal growth and fulfilment, and to illustrate this he contrasts the sayings of a generation ago, such as 'count your blessings', with society's current motto 'go for it'. He claims that the constant emphasis on self-improvement may lead to self-disapproval and rejection of one's own identity, which may be made worse by failure to achieve the desired changes.

ANDRAGOGY: THE TEACHING AND TRAINING OF ADULTS

In recent years, 'andragogy' has become the preferred term in the literature for describing the teaching and training of adults. One of the foremost contributors to this area is the American educationalist Malcolm S. Knowles (Knowles, 1990). The term andragogy is used in the literature as a contrast to pedagogy, literally a leader of children, and Knowles' approach is based upon the differences he perceives between the teaching of adults and children. He maintains that educational systems, including those for adult students, are based on a pedagogical model. Indeed, the dictionary definition of pedagogy reinforces this view: 'the art, science, and profession of teaching'. He notes that all the great teachers in history, such as Socrates and Confucius, were teachers of adults and uses the term andragogy, i.e. a leader of man (adults) to describe his approach. He points out that the term 'adult' has a number of meanings:

1. biological adulthood is the ability to reproduce;
2. legal adulthood is defined by the law;
3. social adulthood is the stage at which adult roles are performed; and
4. psychological adulthood is when self-direction is assumed.

The two models are based on different assumptions about the learner on six dimensions:

1. the learner's need to know;
2. the learner's self-concept;
3. the role of the learner's experience;
4. the learner's readiness to learn;
5. the learner's orientation to learning; and
6. the learner's motivation.

The different assumptions for pedagogy and andragogy are outlined in Table 3.4.

Knowles argues that traditional education conditions the learner to react to teacher stimuli, and this reactive learning does not equip the learner with the skills for lifelong learning. Andragogy encourages a proactive approach to learning in which enquiry and autonomy feature predominantly. However, pedagogy and andragogy should be seen as parallel, rather than as opposing, models and Knowles acknowledges that both may be appropriate for children and adults depending upon the given circumstances. For example, it might be that a pedagogical or dependent approach involving didactic teaching would be more appropriate when the learner first encounters new or unusual learning situations, provided that an andragogical approach is used overall. Similarly, Knowles believes that andragogy can be appropriate for children, with its emphasis on a classroom climate conducive to learning, and the concept of increasing self-direction and autonomy.

Two aspects of Knowles' work have had a particularly strong influence on nurse education curricula, his process model for human resources development, and the use of learning contracts.

Process model for human resources development

Knowles uses the term 'human resources development' to cover the whole range of continuing education and training in a wide variety of

Table 3.4

The different assumptions of pedagogy and andragogy

Assumptions	Pedagogy	Andragogy
Learner's need to know	Students must learn what they are taught in order to pass their tests	Adults need to know why they must learn something
Learner's self-concept	Dependency: decisions about learning are controlled by teacher	Self-direction: adults take responsibility for their own learning
Role of learner's experience	It is the teacher's experience that is seen as important. The learner's experience is seen as of little use as a learning resource	Adults have greater, and more varied experience which serves as a rich resource for learning
Learner's readiness to learn	Learner's readiness is dependent upon what the teacher wants them to learn	Adult's readiness relates to the things he or she needs to know and do in real life
Student's orientation to learning	Learning equates with the subject-matter content of the curriculum	Adults have a life-centred orientation to learning involving problem-solving and task-centred approaches
Student's motivation	Student's motivation is from external sources such as teacher approval, grades and parental pressures	Adult's motivation is largely internal such as self-esteem, quality of life and job satisfaction

contexts, and the implementation of the andragogical model involves a 'process model' as opposed to the pedagogical one of a 'content model'. There are seven elements to the process model.

1. *Establishing a climate conducive to learning.* This involves both the physical, and the human and interpersonal environment; the former takes account of the seating arrangements, decor, ventilation and lighting, and the latter such things as the organizational climate, mutual respect, collaboration, mutual trust and supportiveness, openness and authenticity and a climate of pleasure and humanness.
2. *Creating a mechanism for mutual planning.* This is one of the cardinal principles of andragogy; all those concerned with the educational enterprise should be involved in its planning.
3. *Diagnosing the needs for learning.* According to Knowles, a learning need is a gap between the specified learning outcomes of a programme and the existing state of the learner in relation to these. Andragogy emphasizes the importance of the learner's own perception of this gap, but there may be tension between the needs of participants and the needs of the organization, and this conflict must be negotiated with care.
4. *Formulating programme objectives.* Knowles acknowledges the widely differing viewpoints on the nature of objectives, and

cautiously suggests that behavioural objectives might be more appropriate for training, and more process-orientated outcomes for education.

5. *Designing a pattern of learning experiences*. Self-directed learning is central to andragogical design models and involves a choice of learning methods that are appropriate to the learner's objectives.

6. *Operating the programme*. This involves the administration of the learning programme, and the quality of learning resources is a crucial factor.

7. *Evaluating the programme*. Knowles favours a five-step approach to evaluation:

    (a) reaction evaluation is on-going evaluation during the programme;

    (b) learning evaluation is the gathering of data about the learning outcomes achieved;

    (c) behaviour evaluation takes a wider view of the changes in behaviour, culled from supervisors' reports, etc.;

    (d) results evaluation is organizational data such as costs, efficiency, absence, etc.;

    (e) rediagnosis of learning needs is really a repeat of step 3 above, and involves helping students to re-evaluate where they are in relation to programme objectives.

Learning contracts

As Knowles points out, individuals have a need to be self-directing in their learning, yet traditional curricula were largely controlled by the educational institution. Learning contracts are a means of reconciling the learning needs of the student and those of other interested parties such as educators and employers. The focus of nurse education is the promotion and maintenance of professional competence; what constitutes such competence is decided not only by the individual nurse but also employers and professional bodies. The needs of each of these key players may well conflict on occasions, and learning contracts provide a useful way of negotiating an acceptable compromise. Knowles offers the following stages for developing a learning contract.

Step 1: Diagnosis of learning needs

This involves the students in assessing the difference between their present state of knowledge or skill in relation to an area of learning and the state they aim to achieve in that area. In nursing, this often requires the help of tutors and clinical colleagues.

Step 2: Specifying learning objectives

The learning needs, identified in Step 1, are then written as learning objectives such as acquisition of certain knowledge or skills.

Step 3: Specifying learning resources and strategies

In this step, the students take each learning objective and identify how they are planning to achieve it, e.g. reviewing the relevant literature.

Step 4: Specifying evidence of accomplishment

For each learning objective, the students describe the evidence which they will produce to indicate their achievement, e.g. an essay can provide evidence about knowledge of a topic.

Step 5: Specifying how the evidence can be validated

Here the students state the criteria by which the evidence can be judged, and who will do the judging, e.g. an essay might be judged according to level of analysis and synthesis of arguments by a member of the teaching staff of the institution.

Step 6: Reviewing the contract with consultants

Once the first draft of the contract is complete, each student should seek the opinions of colleagues such as fellow students, supervisors or teachers about the clarity and relevance of the contract.

Step 7: Carrying out the contract

This step involves implementing the contract, and adapting it as necessary as learning proceeds.

Step 8: Evaluating learning

In this final step the evidence presented by the student is judged by the person named in Step 5.

Although extensively used as a model in nurse education curricula, Knowles' approach has been criticized on a number of grounds. Given the humanistic value basis of andragogy, the assumptions of andragogy should apply as equally to children as to adults, e.g. the importance of self-direction and autonomy. The self-directing characteristic of adults is a cornerstone of Knowles' theory, yet experiences with open learning programmes indicate that many adult students find it difficult to unlearn their dependence on tutors and take considerable time to develop self-direction in their learning. This voluntary relinquishing of self-direction is particularly noticeable when students have to learn something new; it does not mean that they are adopting a child-like approach to their learning.

It has been pointed out (Tennant, 1997) that Knowles' work draws upon two opposing (and mutually incompatible) psychological theories, humanistic psychology, and behaviourism, thus weakening the validity of his approach. The superiority of experience in adult learning has also been questioned. Although adults, by virtue of having lived longer than children, have more quantity of experience, they do not automatically bring a better quality of experience to their learning. Indeed, previous experiences may serve to interfere with learning, particularly if stressful or upsetting. There is inconsistency in the fact that Knowles is opposed to teachers prescribing the content of what is to be learned, yet he actually prescribed the process by which learning should occur.

Perhaps the most telling criticism of Knowles' approach is that his focus on the centrality of the individual in learning leads him to ignore the power of social forces in education. In reality, the individual has relatively little power in comparison with the power of the educational system to determine the organization of learning. For example, although choice may be offered within educational programmes, it is almost invariably within a prescribed framework of options imposed by the award regulations. Many commentators on andragogy highlight the conflict between the interests of the educational institution and those of the individual student, e.g. the restriction placed upon self-directed learning by the use of learning outcomes and award requirements. There is also the danger that adult students' expectations of adult education will be raised unduly by the rhetoric of self-directed learning. They may enter adult education expecting something completely different from what they experienced at school, an expectation all too commonly disappointed.

Tennant's reconstructed charter for andragogy

Tennant (1997) offers a useful generic guide for practising teachers in the form of a 'reconstructed charter for andragogy'. He identifies eight characteristics of critical adult education practice that can be considered generic to all forms of teaching, and these are outlined below.

1. *Valuing the experiences of learners.* Learners' life-worlds should be included in all aspects of the teaching and learning enterprise; it is not sufficient merely to have a positive attitude towards them.
2. *Engaging in reflection on experiences.* This involves both the students' existing experiences and the new experiences introduced as part of the teaching. The latter encourages students to progress beyond their own experiences, which in turn helps them to generalize their experiential learning.
3. *Establishing collaborative learning relationships.* Tennant points out the necessity for collaborative group learning, where students' experiences and learning can be shared and enriched from multiple perspectives.
4. *Addressing issues of identity and power relationships between teachers and learners.* This will depend to some extent on the context of learning, but it is important that these issues are addressed.
5. *Promoting judgements about learning which are developmental and which allow scope for success for all learners.* All judgements about students' learning should encourage further development, and should not be framed with reference to other students' success or failure.
6. *Negotiating conflicts over claims to knowledge and pedagogical processes.* It is important that students should feel able to express differences of opinion with regard to educational knowledge, and that this is accepted as an important aspect of the teaching process.

7. *Identifying the historical and cultural locatedness of experiences.* Students should be aware of the social and cultural context of their experiences, and be encouraged to question the assumptions arising from this.

8. *Transforming actions and practices.* This relates to 7 above, and refers to new actions and practices adopted by students as a result of their recognition of the social and cultural context of their experiences.

THE EXPERIENTIAL LEARNING APPROACH TO ADULT LEARNING

Within the past twenty years, experiential learning has become firmly established in nursing, midwifery and health visiting curricula. At its simplest, experiential learning is learning that results from experience, but since almost everything in life constitutes experience, this becomes an impossibly global notion. Essentially, experiential learning is learning by doing, rather than by listening to other people or reading about it. This active involvement of the student is one of the key characteristics of this form of learning, together with student-centredness, a degree of interaction, some measure of autonomy and flexibility and a high degree of relevance.

Kolb: the theory of experiential learning

David Kolb is a major exponent of experiential learning theory:

> 'Experiential learning theory offers a fundamentally different view of the learning process from that of the behavioural theories of learning based on an empirical epistemology or the more implicit theories of learning that underlie traditional educational methods, methods that for the most part are based on a rational idealist epistemology. This perspective on learning is called "experiential" for two reasons. The first is to tie it clearly to its intellectual origins in the work of Dewey, Lewin and Piaget. The second reason is to emphasize the central role that experience plays in the learning process' (Kolb 1984, page 20).

Kolb sees learning as a core process of human development, and makes a distinction between development and simple readjustment to change.

Development results from learning that is gained through experience, and this is the basis of the 'experiential learning model' (or 'experiential learning cycle'). The cycle has become known as 'Kolb's Cycle', but it is interesting to note that Kolb himself refers to it as 'The Lewinian Experiential Learning Model'.

The cycle, as shown in Figure 3.1, begins with some kind of concrete experience, professional or personal, that the student considers interesting or problematic. Observations and information are gathered about the experience and then the student reflects upon it, replaying it over again and analysing it until certain insights begin to emerge in the shape of a 'theory' about the experience. The implications arising from this

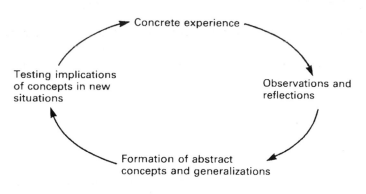

Figure 3.1

Experiental learning model (Kolb, 1984)

conceptualization can then be utilized to modify existing nursing or midwifery practice or to generate new approaches to it.

Generic adaptive abilities

There are four generic adaptive abilities required for effective learning:

1. *Concrete experience (CE)*. The students must immerse themselves fully and openly in new experiences.
2. *Reflective observation (RO)*. The students must observe and reflect on concrete experiences from a variety of perspectives.
3. *Abstract conceptualization (AC)*. The students must create concepts that integrate their observations into logical theories.
4. *Active experimentation (AE)*. The students must apply these theories in decision-making and problem-solving.

Primary dimensions of learning process

These four generic adaptive abilities consist of two pairs of opposites, forming two primary dimensions of learning:

1. concrete experience – abstract conceptualization; and
2. active experimentation – reflective observation.

During a learning situation, the student moves from action to observation to a varying extent according to the nature of the situation, both dimensions being important aspects of the learning process. This approach is compatible with other theories of cognitive development such as those of Piaget and Bruner.

Implications for teaching and learning

Kolb's work has provided a theoretical basis for the implementation of experiential learning in adult education; experiential learning is discussed in Chapter 14 in the context of small-group teaching, and also forms a very useful theoretical basis for the Accreditation of Prior Experiential Learning (APEL), discussed in Chapter 6 (p. 160). Experiential learning theory can be applied to individual differences; for example, Kolb (1976) identifies four learning styles based upon the theory of experiential learning, and these are outlined in Chapter 2 (p. 33).

The experiential learning cycle has been influential in curricula for nursing and midwifery, However, the model does not have a great deal of empirical support, and it is unlikely that every single learning situation will demand an integrated approach using the four general adaptive abilities.

Jarvis' typology of learning

Peter Jarvis has proposed a typology of learning based upon three forms of learning response to experience: non-learning, non-reflective learning, and reflective learning (Jarvis and Gibson, 1997).

Non-learning

Jarvis points out that individuals do not necessarily learn from any given experience, and he identifies three types of non-learning. The first is presumption, i.e. the tendency for individuals to rely uncritically on their past experiences as a basis for their behaviour. Non-consideration is the term Jarvis gives to an individual's failure to respond to a potential learning situation. The third type is rejection, where the individual rejects the possibility of learning from the experience; bigots would come under this category.

Non-reflective learning

As the name implies, this is learning that does not involve a reflective process, and includes memorization, skills learning, and preconscious learning. The latter is also called incidental learning, i.e. the learning that occurs without the individual being aware of it.

Reflective learning

In contrast to the two previous forms of learning, this involves a process of reflection. Jarvis' research identified different types within this category, contemplation, reflective skills learning, and experimental learning.

Implications for teaching and learning

Jarvis' typology is useful in that it expands our view of what constitutes learning; it also emphasizes the importance of the reflective process in learning.

REFLECTION AND ADULT LEARNING

Although reflection as a concept had been established in education since the turn of the century, it was the work of Donald Schon (Schon, 1983, 1987) in the mid-1980s that put it well and truly on the agenda of professional practice in both the teaching and the nursing professions. The significance of reflection in nursing lies in its close relationship to learning in professional practice settings, and the concept of reflective practice in nursing is discussed in detail in Chapter 22 (p. 567).

Hamachek, D. (1978) Humanistic psychology: theoretical – philosophical framework and implications for teaching, in D. Treffinger, J. Kent Davis and R. Ripple (eds), *Handbook on Teaching Educational Psychology*, Academic Press, New York.

Jarvis, P. and Gibson, S. (1997) *The Teacher Practitioner and Mentor in Nursing, Midwifery, Health Visiting and The Social Services*, Stanley Thornes, Cheltenham.

Knowles, M. (1990) *The Adult Learner: A Neglected Species*, 4th edn, Gulf Publishing, Houston.

Kolb, D.A. (1976) *The Learning Style Inventory: Technical Manual*, McBer and Co., Boston.

Kolb, D.A. (1984) *Experiential Learning: Experience as the Source of Learning and Development*, Prentice Hall, Englewood Cliffs, NJ.

Levinson, D. (1986) A conception of adult development, *American Psychologist*, **41**, 3–13.

Maslow, A. (1971) *The Farther Reaches of Human Nature*, Penguin, Harmondsworth.

McNair, S. (1996) Learner autonomy in a changing world, in R. Edwards, S. Hanson and P. Raggatt (eds), *Boundaries of Adult Learning*, Routledge, London.

Piaget, J. and Inhelder, B. (1969) *The Psychology of the Child*, Basic Books, New York.

Rogers, A. (1996) *Teaching Adults*, 2nd edn, Open University Press, Milton Keynes.

Rogers, C. (1951) *Client Centred Therapy*, Houghton Mifflin, Boston.

Rogers, C. (1969) *Freedom to Learn*, Merriill, Ohio.

Rogers, C. (1983) *Freedom to Learn for the 80s*, Merrill, Ohio.

Rogers, C. and Freiberg, H.J. (1994) *Freedom to Learn*, 3rd edn, Macmillan, New York.

Schon, D. (1983) *The Reflective Practitioner: How Professionals Think in Action*, Basic Books, New York.

Schon, D. (1987) *Educating the Reflective Practitioner: Towards a New Design for Teaching and Learning in the Professions*, Jossey Bass, San Francisco.

Sigman, A. (1995) *New, Improved? Exposing the Misuse of Popular Psychology*, Simon and Schuster, London.

Stuart-Hamilton, I. (1996) *The Psychology of Ageing*, 2nd edn, Jessica Kingsley, London.

Tennant, M. (1997) *Psychology and Adult Learning*, 2nd edn, Routledge, London.

4 Cognitive perspectives on teaching and learning

The term *cognition* refers to the internal mental processes of human beings, and encompasses the domains of memory, perception and thinking. These are of fundamental importance to education, given that learning involves all three domains. The first part of this chapter deals with these three domains of cognition, and the remainder is devoted to specific cognitive perspectives on teaching and learning by David Ausubel, Jerome Bruner and Robert Gagne.

MEMORY

Memory is the process that allows human beings to store experiences from the past, and to use these in the present. There are three basic aspects of memory function: encoding, storage and retrieval, and three stages of memory: sensory, short-term and long-term.

Encoding, storage and retrieval

These first of these basic aspects is *encoding*, i.e. putting information into the memory in some form of code such as acoustic or visual coding. *Storage* is also known as the memory trace, and this is kept until it needs to be remembered. *Retrieval* is the bringing up of stored, coded information to mind when required. For example, on first being introduced to a stranger, we encode the person's name into our memory in the form of an acoustic (sound) code, where it is then *stored*. When we meet that person again we try to remember (retrieve) her/his name.

The three types of memory

One of the most influential models of memory is that of Atkinson and Shiffrin (1971). The three types of memory, sensory, short-term and long-term, may indeed be separate systems within the brain or merely different kinds of storage within the same system. Nonetheless, each of the three memory systems has distinctive characteristics outlined below.

Sensory memory
The sensory memory registers incoming stimuli for a very brief period. It is a high-capacity system that registers all sensory inputs in their original form – visual stimuli as images or icons, and auditory stimuli as echoes of the sounds. Visual stimuli last for about one second and auditory stimuli for about four seconds, and we are unaware of these stimuli. However, when a stimulus is registered in sensory memory, contact is made with long-term memory to check whether there is an existing pattern for that stimulus. The role of sensory memory is to

prolong stimuli just long enough to allow for selective attention to important ones. This aspect of memory also features in the section on perception later in this chapter.

Short-term memory (working memory)

This is also called working memory, primary memory and short-term store, and its main purpose is summed up nicely by Logie (1999):

> *'In its broadest sense, working memory can be thought of as the desktop of the brain. It is a cognitive function that helps us keep track of what we are doing or where we are moment to moment, that holds information long enough to make a decision, dial a telephone number, or repeat a strange foreign word that we have just heard.'*

Short-term memory is characterized by a limited capacity for storage, of about seven chunks of information. The term *chunks* is deliberately vague and applies to any unit that is familiar to an individual (Miller, 1956). Hence a chunk may be a single word or a single letter and it is possible to increase the amount of data in short-term memory at any one time by incorporating more information into each chunk. In addition to this storage function of short-term memory, there are control processes such as rehearsal, which can be divided into maintenance rehearsal and elaborative rehearsal (Craik and Lockhart, 1972). Maintenance rehearsal consists of going over and over the material in short-term memory in order to keep it there; it does not affect the long-term recall of the material. Elaborative rehearsal, on the other hand, processes the material much deeper by relating it to existing material in long-term memory. Short-term memory is also involved in the processes of both thinking and language by providing the working area for these, hence the alternative name, working memory. It is likely that information is coded in the form of both acoustic and articulatory codes in working memory; the former involves the sound of a word and the latter involves the way it is pronounced. Baddeley and Hitch (1974) and Baddeley and Leiberman (1980) describe working memory as having a 'central executive' and two slave systems, the 'phonological (or articulatory) loop' and the 'visuo-spatial sketch pad'. The central executive has an overall co-ordinating and control function; the phonological loop is concerned with speech-based information, and the visuo-spatial sketch pad with spatial information.

Long-term memory

There appears to be no limit to the capacity of long-term memory and information stored here has been subjected to considerable processing. Craik and Lockhart (1972) have suggested a levels-of-processing approach, which states that there is a variety of levels at which information is processed, from the physical characteristics of the stimulus through to the identification of meaning of the stimulus. Deeper-level processing results in better remembering of information, because it allows more elaboration of the stimulus, i.e. more links are made with relevant information already existing in long-term memory. This means that the information has been subjected to considerable top-down processing and is therefore more susceptible to distortion and bias. It seems likely that there are two kinds of information stored in long-term memory – episodic knowledge and semantic knowledge. Episodic knowledge is associated with particular events in time and space, such as the memory of an encounter with a particular student, whereas semantic knowledge consists of general concepts unrelated to specific events or episodes (Tulving, 1972). Autobiographical memory differs from other knowledge structures in the degree of self-reference and the sensory/perceptual nature of the knowledge stored (Conway, 1991).

Representation of knowledge in long-term memory

It is useful to distinguish between declarative knowledge and procedural knowledge; the former is about 'knowing that' and the latter is about 'knowing how'. Declarative knowledge consists of knowledge of factual information and can be transmitted verbally to others. Procedural knowledge, on the other hand, is concerned with knowing how to do something, such as administering an injection, and is often more difficult to explain. Indeed, the most effective way of explaining procedural knowledge to someone is by demonstrating the procedure to them and this is the basic way of teaching a psychomotor skill.

Current research suggests two main theories about the way in which knowledge is represented in long-term memory, the 'propositional code theory' and the 'dual-code theory'.

Propositional code theory

Anderson and Bower (1973) and Pylyshyn (1973) state that information is coded in the form of propositions, i.e. the smallest unit that can be judged true or false. Propositions contain a central relationship called the predicate and a number of arguments, and are thus units of knowledge that can stand as separate assertions. All sentences are composed of propositions, and computers can store information in this form also. According to this theory, information in long-term memory is stored in terms of the meanings of propositions rather than their exact words, hence the term 'semantic' memory. Information is thus organized into a network of propositions that is hierarchically arranged via nodes and connections.

Figure 4.1 shows how a simple two dimensional network hierarchy for 'tissues' in semantic memory might appear. The spatial orientation of the nodes is irrelevant, in that it is the connections that matter not the location. (Propositions can also be represented in three dimensions.) It is claimed that these networks can represent both perceptual and linguistic information in long-term memory and that this single-code explanation is more parsimonious than the dual-code theory.

Network systems have been utilized in several computer models, the earliest being that of Collins and Quillian (1969). This computer model

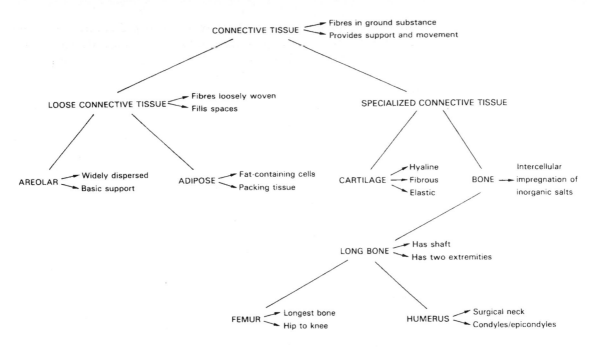

is called the Teachable Language Comprehender (TLC) and it assumes that knowledge is represented in the form of propositional networks. The TLC theory was tested by giving subjects sentences (such as the following) to verify and then measuring their reaction times.

1. A canary is a canary.
2. A canary is a bird.
3. A canary is an animal.

Subjects, according to the theory, should take longer to verify the third sentence because more nodes have to be traversed than in the first or second sentences, and this indeed was the finding. However, later work has shown that this is not always the case; for some concepts, the search is faster for sentences with more nodes to traverse. The sentence 'A dog is a mammal' should be verified faster than 'A dog is an animal', but subjects found the latter more quickly, suggesting that familiarity plays a part in the speed with which propositions are searched.

Dual-code theory
The dual-code theory (Paivio, 1969) states that there are two different kinds of knowledge representations in long-term memory, verbal and imagery. If information is encoded in both modes, there is a much better chance of remembering it; some words are easier than others to encode with imagery, such as words that describe concrete concepts like 'forceps'.

The information-processing approach
The information-processing approach is an important concept in

Figure 4.1

Simple two-dimentional network hierarchy in semantic memory

cognitive psychology, and was developed out of psychologists' interest in the way computers process information. It is claimed that computer programs can provide an analogy for the workings of the human mind, and the interest of cognitive psychologists is more on the 'software' or 'programs' that underlie an individual's thinking, than on the 'hardware' (the physiology of the brain). One branch of psychology, artificial intelligence (AI), involves devising programs that will make computers simulate intelligent behaviours such as reading or translating.

The information-processing model is commonly used to explain a number of human pyschological processes, including memory and perception. Information-processing consists of a flow of information through a system, with this flow taking a finite amount of time. Some parts of the system have a limited capacity for processing information and there are overall control processes that govern the flow. Figure 4.2 shows the basic components of such a system.

Figure 4.2

Basic structures and processes of an information-processing system

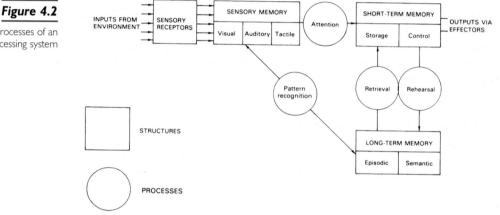

The flow of information begins in the sensory receptors, which detect stimulus inputs from the environment and transfer them to the sensory memory. This records all stimuli encountered in a form similar to the actual stimulus: visual stimuli in iconic form, and auditory stimuli in echoic form, i.e. as an auditory echo. The sensory memory registers stimuli for only about one second and so we are not aware of this process. It does, however, allow time for further processing if the particular stimuli are given attention. When stimuli are attended to, the next stage in information flow is to the short-term memory, which has both storage and control functions, but is very limited in capacity. Information can be transferred to long-term memory by further processing, particularly rehearsal. Information required for outputs must first be retrieved from long-term memory and put back into the short-term memory, from whence it can be used to generate outputs via effector organs. There is one other pathway in the flow of information that connects the sensory registers with long-term memory. This is not a direct pathway for storage of stimuli, but it is hypothesized that whenever a stimulus enters the sensory registers, contact is made with long-term memory to see if the stimulus has been encountered and stored before. This process is called pattern recognition.

So far we have examined the flow of information from the external environment through the system, but information can also arise from within an individual, i.e. from his or her own memory. Thus, people often sit and think about things and their thoughts may trigger off a course of action, with a flow of information through the system. This kind of processing is termed 'knowledge-driven' or 'top-down' processing; the processing of stimuli from the environment is termed 'data-driven' or 'bottom-up' processing.

Remembering

An early pioneer of memory study was Ebbinghaus who used himself as the subject of experiments in which he used nonsense syllables to eliminate any interference from previous knowledge of the words to be remembered. One group of very effective techniques is that called mnemonics. These make the subject think about the item to be remembered by using some kind of scheme. The following offers a selection of these techniques.

Method of loci
In this method, the student first imagines a familiar place such as home or work and chooses a sequence of rooms to remember. He then pictures an item to be remembered in each room until his whole list of items has been used. When he wishes to recall the list, he simply does a mental walkabout through his house to find the items in their locations.

Natural language mediation
This mnemonic is useful for learning unfamiliar words, such as many of those encountered in nursing, and consists of turning the strange word into one that the student already knows and which relates to the new word. For example, if a student is trying to learn the name of the drug streptomycin, he might think of 'strapped the mice in', which implies containment of the spread of the pest.

Key word method
This can be helpful when learning the vocabulary of a foreign language; the student first chooses a French word such as 'pain' (bread) and then makes a visual image of a loaf of French bread 'crying out in pain'.

Acronyms
These are lists of letters arranged vertically to form a word, with each letter itself forming the first letter of a horizontal word. For example, the curriculum components might be remembered thus:

A (aims);
C (content);
M (methods);
E (evaluation).

Forgetting

It was pointed out earlier in this section that there are three stages of memory: encoding, storage and retrieval. Encoding involves putting representations into the memory system, storage is maintaining these in memory, and retrieval is the recovery of memories from the memory system. There are a number of explanations for forgetting, but all of them involve either the original memory trace not being available, or being available but not accessible. The latter is termed 'tip of the tongue' (TOT) phenomenon and is a familiar experience for most people.

Decay theory

Forgetting was originally ascribed to a simple process of fading or decay over a period of time. However, this explanation is insufficient to explain forgetting, as it takes no account of the influence of an individual's experience of forgetting.

Interference

This states that forgetting is due to interference from other memories. Retroactive interference (retroactive inhibition) occurs when new learning material interferes with that previously learned. Student nurses may attend two or three lectures during an afternoon and the first one may be forgotten due to retroactive interference from the ones that followed it. Proactive interference (proactive inhibition) means the opposite; the second lecture of the afternoon is largely forgotten due to interference from the first.

Encoding specificity theory

The key point of this approach is that all forgetting occurs because the cues that were present when the memory was encoded are not present when it is retrieved. It is claimed that the best cues for remembering something are the cues that were present when the memory was encoded. It is well-established that when someone visits a place where they lived as a child, the context cues the recall of memories long thought to have been forgotten.

Consolidation theory

In this theory, the idea is that every experience sets up a trace in the brain and this trace needs to be consolidated if the information is to be remembered. Hence, the trace can be destroyed before it has had time to be consolidated, as in electro-convulsive therapy and retrograde amnesia following head injury.

PERCEPTION

In order to discuss the processes involved in perception, we need to refer again to the diagram of the information-processing system in Figure 4.1. It can be seen that sensory inputs from the environment are first registered in the sensory receptors such as the cells of the retina in the eye. These receptor cells transform the physical stimulus into electrical impulses and transfer it to the brain. *Sensation* is the term given to the initial processes of reception of the stimulus by the sense organ, whereas *perception* is used for the processes that occur centrally in the information-processing model. Perception can be defined as an organized process in which the individual selects cues from the environment and draws inferences from these in order to make sense of his experience. Each of the components of this definition will now be outlined, beginning with the notion of organization.

Organization

When a particular stimulus such as the letter 'T' impinges on the cells of the retina, the information is transmitted to the cells of the visual cortex and it is here that the process of perception begins. These cortical neurones are designed to respond to particular types of stimuli or patterns, with some responding to vertical lines, some to horizontal, others to acute angles and so on.

Pandemonium

Selfridge (1959) constructed a model of perception that he called 'Pandemonium', in which the various detector neurones are envizaged as little demons who do specific jobs inside our heads. These 'demons' are organized hierarchically at different levels, with the most important ones at the top and those doing the least work at the bottom. These bottom-level demons merely record the stimulus and then the next level of demon takes over and looks for evidence of special features such as acute angles, curves and the like. These feature demons then hand over to the cognitive demons that represent each letter of the alphabet and the appropriate ones are activated by the particular stimulus in question. The final demon is called a decision demon and his job is to decide which of the cognitive demons is correct, thus making the final perceptual recognition of a letter 'T'. This is called 'bottom-up' processing, but there is also some 'top-down' processing in the form of prior expectations or set. This predisposes the system to perceive things in a certain way.

Selective attention

The next component of the definition is selectivity and this is concerned with attention. Of the many thousands of stimuli that are registered by the receptors each day, only a certain selection go through to the level of awareness. Take watch straps as an example; normally we are not aware of the presence of the watch, even though the pressure will be registered by the skin receptors. Hence some selecting mechanism must be working that keeps the sensation from being perceived. The criteria for selection will normally include the following:

- new or unusual stimuli;
- changing stimuli;
- very high-intensity stimuli such as bright lights or loud noise;
- motives- or needs-related stimuli, such as the sight of a restaurant sign when you are hungry and searching for somewhere to eat.

The definition also refers to cues from the environment and these cues are used in perception of movement, depth, objects and people.

Perceptual cues

Cues for objects are such things as shape, size, colour, texture, smell and taste. If I saw a large, square, red object coming towards me I would use those cues to make the inference it was a bus, especially as my past experience has led to my being correct on previous occasions when I encountered the stimulus.

Movement cues include the covering and uncovering of background and a change in the shape or sound of the object. Cues for depth perception are both monocular and binocular; the former include nearer objects occluding far ones and convergence of lines. Binocular cues are due to stereoscopic vision, in that each eye sees things from a different angle and when superimposed gives depth cues.

Perception tries to keep things constant, so that when we perceive a bus going along the road, we are not aware of any change, even though its shape and size will alter as it recedes into the distance. This perceptual constancy can lead to illusions if the stimuli are ambiguous.

Gestalt laws of perception

It was mentioned earlier that 'top-down' processing occurs in perception and one of the early descriptions of this was by the group known as the gestalt psychologists. The three main exponents of this school were Max Wertheimer (1880–1943), Kurt Koffka (1881–1941) and Wolfgang Kohler (1887–1967). Their work was originally concerned with the study of perception, but this became closely involved with a theory of learning. Gestalt psychology developed in the opposite direction to stimulus–response theory, its exponents decrying the piecemeal analysis of behaviour as an explanation of learning. The gestalt view was that people see things as unified wholes, not as separate components, the German word 'gestalt' meaning 'pattern' or 'configuration'. These patterns, or 'gestalten', tend to stand out distinctly from the background against which they are seen, giving rise to the concept of figure and ground in perception. The gestalt psychologists formulated laws of perception, which govern whether or not a particular stimulus will be perceived as figure rather than ground. The laws are as follows.

Law of similarity

Stimuli which are similar to one another tend to be grouped together in one's perception. In Figure 4.3, the observer tends to see alternate rows or columns of dots and crosses rather than 25 items in a square.

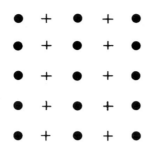

Figure 4.3

Law of similarity

Law of proximity

Stimuli that are closer together tend to be grouped into patterns. The example in Figure 4.4 is seen as four pairs of vertical lines rather than eight separate ones.

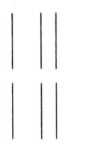

Figure 4.4

Law of proximity

Law of closure

Areas that enclose space tend to form 'gestalten', and thus stand out against the background. In Figure 4.5(a), the four pairs of lines can be made to form a unified whole by adding two incomplete lines to the inner four lines. Closure also occurs with six lines, as in Figure 4.5(b).

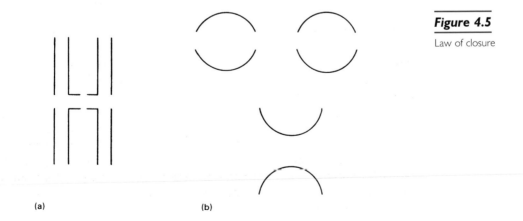

Figure 4.5

Law of closure

(a)　　　　　(b)

Koffka considered that these laws of perception could also be seen as laws of learning, with application to the teaching situation. This is further elaborated in the section on problem-solving later in this chapter.

Perception in practice-based learning

There are a great many implications for nurse education in both teaching and practice-based learning. In practice settings, students need to be taught about the factors that affect their perception of things, particularly the influence of 'top-down' processing, which might make them miss cues that patients might emit. Nurses need to recognize that a patient's perception may be altered by illness and must make the necessary allowance for this by giving more frequent explanations and reassurance, in case the patient may not have perceived the message. Selective attention will operate in clinical areas where patients may be kept awake by jangling drug keys or the sound of a trolley. Some patients may become disoriented and so experience perceptual distortion; the nurse's role in this case is to reduce stimulation by maintaining a quiet, dark environment. In teaching, it is important to use methods that hold the attention of the students with, for example, bright visual aids and changes of activity at frequent intervals. The teacher should maintain a central position as 'figure' separate from the 'ground' of background noise and distractions. The teaching should be for 'insight' rather than just giving factual information, so that students experience 'penny-dropping' when learning concepts.

THINKING

Thinking is a cognitive process consisting of internal mental representations of the world, and it includes a wide range of activities including problem-solving, reflecting and decision-making. Some mental representations are in the form of pictures in the mind, while others are in the form of propositions.

Propositional thought

Propositions are assertions or claims that relate a *subject* and a *predicate*, and they may or may not be true.

For example, the proposition 'nursing is a caring profession' relates the subject (nursing) to the predicate (is a caring profession). Propositional thinking is made up of symbolic building blocks called concepts.

Concepts

Concepts can be defined as 'objects, events, situations or properties that possess common criterial attributes and are designated by some sign or symbol' (Ausubel *et al.*, 1978). A concept is thus a category or class of objects, rather than an individual example, each member of that class sharing one or more common characteristics.

- The word 'cell' represents a concept, in that it stands for a class of things that possess a number of common qualities or attributes, such as a cell membrane, cytoplasm, nucleus and so on.
- The words 'Florence Nightingale' do not represent a concept, since there is only one example of this individual.

The common characteristics that members of a concept share can be either structural or functional attributes or both; for example, the concept 'bandage' contains a wide variety of shapes and sizes, but the functions are largely identified as support, pressure and securing of dressings.

In order to qualify as a member of a particular concept group, an individual example must possess certain key characteristics called critical attributes. Without these, the individual example cannot be classified as one of the concept in question; for example, the concept 'myocardial infarction' is a class of events that includes chest pain, vomiting, pain in the arms, breathlessness and myocardial necrosis.

Individual examples (i.e. patients) exhibit much variation in these features making it difficult to decide the critical attributes of this concept; it is possible to suffer from a myocardial infarction without experiencing pain, vomiting or breathlessness, so it seems that the only critical attribute of the concept is myocardial necrosis. The concept 'angina pectoris' may share the attributes of chest pain and breathlessness, but lacks the critical attribute of myocardial necrosis and hence does not belong to the class of concepts called 'myocardial infarction'.

Concrete and abstract concepts

Concepts that can be observed are termed 'concrete' whereas those that are not observable are termed 'defined' or 'abstract'. 'Liver' is an example of a concrete observable concept, whereas 'intelligence' is an abstract one. Abstract concepts tend to be more difficult to learn than concrete concepts. Concepts form hierarchies, with the most inclusive ones at the top and the more specific ones below and they also cluster together with other related concepts.

Schemata

The work discussed so far has referred largely to simple concepts, whereas in real life, most information-processing involves connected sequences of events such as reading of connected discourse. Schema theory attempts to explain the inferences we make when processing events and was first introduced by Bartlett (1932). Here are two definitions of schemas:

- Mental frameworks or structures which encompass memories, ideas, concepts, and programmes for action which are pertinent to a particular topic (Banyard and Hayes 1994);
- a relatively abstract representation of objects, episodes, actions or

situations which contains slots or variables into which specific instances can be fitted in a particular context (Doyle, 1983).

From these definitions, it can be seen that schemata are larger units of knowledge than propositions. A number of different theorists have adopted schema theory (Minsky, 1975; Rummelhart and Ortony, 1977; Schank and Abelson, 1977). People have schemata for a large range of familiar events and they use these to fill in gaps and make inferences in conversations or stories. Schemata do not represent specific objects, but rather they represent general categories; propositions represent specific things or people.

The work of Elinor Rosch has shed much light on the nature of schemata for natural categories of events in the real world. She has postulated that instances of a category share certain family resemblances and it is these which define whether the instance is a member of the category. Some category members are seen as more typical of the category than others. For example, apples are more typical fruits than rhubarb, since more fruits grow on trees than in the ground. There is often wide disparity in subjects' agreement of category members. Schema theory states that people are aware of which features in the environment tend to go together, and that these features are noticed and remembered. Schemata tend to be incomplete, in that they leave some features unspecified, namely, those features that are considered irrelevant.

Rummelhart and Ortony (1977) suggest that there are four essential characteristics of schemata.

1. Schemata have variables and may have different variables on different occasions, depending on the context of the schema. (For example, the schema for 'take' might have three variables – a recipient, an object and a donor – in one context and only one variable in another, such as in 'taking one's time'.)
2. Schemata can embed into each other, i.e. schemata are represented in terms of other schemata, these others being termed sub-schemata. Only the names of these are represented though, since this avoids the problem of having every piece of knowledge included with every schema.
3. Schemata vary in their levels of abstraction; this is the characteristic that most differentiates schemata from propositions. Schemata can be seen as parcels of information at many different levels of abstraction, from simple concepts to very inclusive aspects of comprehension.
4. Schemata represent knowledge; schemata are not merely dictionary entries, but abstract representations of knowledge. Schemata, then, constitute the 'basic building-blocks of the human information-processing system' and play a key part in the process of comprehension. Understanding of something involves the selection of schemata that will satisfactorily account for the information being processed.

CRITICAL THINKING

Within higher education, the aims of undergraduate programmes tend to be two kinds: the specific aims of the pathway in relation to its subject area, e.g. nursing or midwifery, and the more general educational aims that apply to all undergraduate programmes, e.g. development of skills in communication, problem-solving, evaluation, and critical thinking. At post-graduate or post-registration level, typical learning outcomes require the students to reflect upon and critically evaluate their own professional practice.

The word 'critical' is a very common term in education, but it has a very different connotation from the lay use of the word. In society, the term is equated with 'criticism', which carries negative overtones from childhood and schooldays. In this context, it usually meant hostile or unkind comments about aspects of an individual's behaviour, and this notion may carry through to adult life. Critical thinking is very different from criticism, in that it is basically a positive activity. To question established assumptions may be interpreted as undermining them, but in reality such critical appraisal of situations is a positive and necessary process for growth and development to occur within a society or an organization. Critical thinking is not confined solely to learning in higher education, but permeates all the activities of adult life including interpersonal relationships and work.

The nature of critical thinking

Within the literature there is considerable variation in what is considered to be critical thinking, but it is commonly interpreted as a core concept consisting of a number of abilities such as the ability to:

1. define a problem;
2. select relevant information for problem-solving;
3. draw inferences from observed or supposed facts;
4. recognize assumptions;
5. formulate relevant hypotheses;
6. make deductions, i.e. draw conclusions from premises;
7. make interpretations from data; and
8. evaluate arguments.

However, interpretations like these that equate critical thinking to a set of generic cognitive skills or procedures have been criticized as unhelpful (Bailin *et al.*, 1999a). They point out that these are simply lists of what people must be able to do (e.g. make deductions), and that they shed no light on the psychological processes involved in critical thinking. They also question the view that critical thinking is a generic skill that can be applied to any situation, because this ignores the importance of context. For example, the ability to evaluate arguments is included in the above list of critical thinking abilities, but in order to do this one needs to have specific knowledge of the context in which it takes place. A nurse may be able to evaluate arguments within the field of her nursing specialism, but this would not generalize to the ability to evaluate arguments on the merits or otherwise of a Samuel Beckett play.

Bailin *et al.* (page 287) suggest that there are three features of critical thinking:

1. It is done for the purpose of making up one's mind about what to believe or do.
2. The person engaging in the thinking is trying to fulfil standards of adequacy and accuracy appropriate to the thinking.
3. The thinking fulfils the relevant standards to some threshold level.

Given their antithesis towards lists of abilities, Bailin *et al.* tackle the problem of identifying the characteristics of critical thinkers by suggesting the intellectual resources necessary for critical thinking:

1. *Background knowledge.* The depth of a person's background knowledge in a specific context determines the degree to which they can think critically about that context.
2. *Operational knowledge of the standards of good thinking.* This is acquired by analysis of current critical thinking practices, but judgement must be used in their application to specific contexts.
3. *Knowledge of key critical concepts.* Critical concepts are those that enable the critical thinker to differentiate kinds of intellectual products such as arguments or statements. Examples of critical concepts are *premise* and *conclusion*.
4. *Heuristics (strategies, procedures, etc.).* Critical thinkers require a repertoire of heuristic devices, such as double-checking something before accepting it as fact.
5. *Habits of mind.* This can be summarized as having a 'critical spirit', and refers to attitudes and values to which the critical thinker is committed, e.g. respect for truth, open-mindedness, etc.

An alternative approach by Brookfield (1987) identifies four characteristics of critical thinkers:

1. *Identifying and challenging assumptions.* Critical thinkers ask awkward questions in order to identify and challenge the assumptions which underlie issues and problems.
2. *Challenging the importance of context.* Critical thinkers are aware that beliefs, actions, and established practice reflect the context in which they are set, both cultural and professional. For example, opinions about the standard of appearance for nurses and midwives may be based upon the norms of a generation or more ago, such as a particular view of what constitutes an acceptable hairstyle. Modern hairstyles that are entirely appropriate in a social context may be perceived as being 'unprofessional' in a nursing or midwifery context. The same may be said about so-called 'designer-stubble' in male nursing or medical staff.
3. *Imagining and exploring alternatives.* Critical thinkers have the ability to imagine and explore alternatives to established ways of

thinking or behaving, because they are aware of the assumptions and the context of issues or problems.

4. *Reflective scepticism*. Reflective thinkers take a sceptical view of established dogma and practices, carefully scrutinizing them and questioning their current validity. For example, this approach is encouraged in initial programmes of nurse education, but may be perceived as threatening by qualified nurses whose own professional education did not foster such an approach. Hence, their reflective scepticism needs to be handled with some sensitivity by students if they are to avoid conflict with qualified colleagues.

Assessing critical thinking

There are a number of tests of critical thinking in common use and although these tests contain different sorts of items, there is considerable overlap within them. A classic example is the Watson–Glaser critical thinking appraisal (Watson and Glaser, 1961). This tests the subject's ability on five aspects of critical thinking: inference; assumptions; deduction; interpretation; and evaluation of arguments.

Inference

This is a conclusion based upon facts or observations. For example, by looking at a post-operative patient's facial expression and body posture, a nurse may infer that he or she is in pain. However, there may be other, equally plausible, explanations, such as anxiety about whether their job will still be there when they are well enough to leave hospital.

Assumptions

These are something assumed or taken for granted. For example, a nurse may assume that a post-operative patient will wish to be given analgesia as soon as pain is experienced. However, the patient may have a negative attitude to taking any form of drug, and so reject the offer of analgesia.

Deduction

This consists of drawing conclusions from stated premises. Either the conclusion follows from the statements, or it does not. For example, consider the two statements:

Some nurses look untidy.
Being untidy is unprofessional.

It is possible to deduce the conclusion that 'some nurses are unprofessional'. However, the conclusion that 'unprofessional nurses look untidy' does not follow from the two statements given, since unprofessional nurses may well look tidy, and yet have other shortcomings that contribute to their being considered unprofessional.

Interpretation

This involves judging whether or not a conclusion follows, beyond a reasonable doubt, from the facts given. Let us take a purely hypothetical example; suppose a survey of professional misconduct within the Barsetshire Region found that female nurses were involved in 34 cases of complaints from patients, but male nurses were involved in only 22 cases of complaint. The following conclusions might be drawn.

A: There were more complaints by patients against female nurses than male nurses in Barsetshire.
B: Patients are generally more satisfied with male nurses than female nurses.

Conclusion A follows beyond a reasonable doubt, since it a factual statement supported by the evidence of the numbers involved. However, conclusion B does not follow beyond a reasonable doubt, as it makes unwarranted generalizations from the given data, e.g. its takes no account of the number of male/female nurses – 34 may represent 1% while 22 represents 5%.

Evaluation of arguments

When attempting to make important decisions about an issue or problem, it is necessary to be able to distinguish between strong and weak arguments. Watson and Glaser use two criteria for a strong argument: it must be important, and it must be directly related to the issue or problem. If one of these is absent, then the argument is considered to be weak.

Teaching critical thinking

If critical thinking is considered an important aspect of professional practice in nursing, midwifery and health visiting, then nurse teachers need to be able to facilitate its development.

> *'Teaching critical thinking is best conceptualized not as a matter of teaching isolated abilities and dispositions, but rather as furthering the initiation of students into complex critical practices that embody value-commitments and require the sensitive use of a variety of intellectual resources in the exercise of good judgement.' (Bailin et al., 1999b, page 298).*

The authors go on to suggest that teaching critical thinking involves three components:

1. engaging students in dealing with tasks that call for reasoned judgement or assessment;
2. helping them develop intellectual resources for dealing with these tasks;
3. providing an environment in which critical thinking is valued and students are encouraged and supported in their attempts to think critically and engage in critical discussion.

Brookfield (1987) offers a ten-point checklist for teaching critical thinking:

1. *Affirm critical thinkers' self-worth.* It is important when teaching critical thinking to maintain an atmosphere of psychological safety, whereby students thinking can be challenged, but they are not made to feel threatened or insulted.

2. *Listen attentively to critical thinkers.* During training the teacher must attend carefully to students' verbal and non-verbal signals, so that interventions are both appropriate and sensitive to the situation.

3. *Show that you support critical thinkers' efforts.* Students do not become critical thinkers overnight; their initial efforts need support and encouragement if they are to progress, and there is a delicate balance between this and the necessary degree of challenge and upset that is important for critical thinking skills development.

4. *Reflect and mirror critical thinkers' ideas and actions.* Trainers can foster the development of critical thinking by using reflection techniques that let the student see how their behaviours and attitudes are perceived by others.

5. *Motivate people to think critically.* There is a delicate balance between motivating students to think critically, and helping them to estimate the risks involved in criticizing and destabilizing established practices. It would be naive to think that by simply criticizing the status quo, change will automatically follow. In reality, established organizational practices and systems tend to be relatively entrenched, and critical thinking may result not in change, but only in the loss of the critical thinker's job.

6. *Regularly evaluate progress.* One of the important roles of the trainer is to encourage students to engage regularly in reflective evaluation of their critical thinking skills, so that behaviour patterns are identified and insights gained.

7. *Help critical thinkers to create networks.* Networking is a common educational strategy, and is akin to self-help groups. Students should be encouraged to network with other students who are developing critical thinking skills, so that experiences and insights can be shared and analysed.

8. *Be a critical teacher.* Teachers themselves can adopt a critical thinking approach to their teaching by questioning assumptions, promoting inquiry, and experimenting with new ideas during their teaching.

9. *Make people aware of how they learn critical thinking.* This focuses on helping students to understand their own learning styles in relation to critical thinking, such as how they sustain their motivation, how they integrate new ideas and experience, and how they approach new areas of knowledge.

10. *Model critical thinking.* Observing a good role model can help students to become critical thinkers, so teachers should model these skills during their everyday teaching.

INTUITION

Intuition is an interesting cognitive phenomenon that has been largely neglected in psychology this century (Claxton, 1998). In lay terms, intuition is thought of as some sort of extra-sensory perception or 'sixth-sense', and was at one time thought to be a particularly female character-istic, 'womens' intuition'. The essence of intuition is a sense of knowing something almost unconsciously; it occurs without deliberation and there appears to be no articulated reason for this feeling of certainty.

However, intuitive learning, or learning intuitively, may actually be superior in some cases than rational problem-solving; Claxton cites as an example of this, childrens' ability to solve the Rubic Cube puzzle. The cube is notoriously difficult for adults to solve, yet children seem to be able to solve it more readily, and the explanation may well lie in the different approaches used by each. Adults tend to use a logical, problem-solving approach which is inappropriate for the complexity of the Rubik cube, whereas children rely on intuitive learning rather than thinking about it.

PROBLEM-SOLVING AND DECISION-MAKING

Problem-solving is a good example of the interrelationship of all the components of an information-processing system of cognition. This first section addresses two approaches to problem-solving: Insightful Learning, and an information-processing approach.

Problem-solving and insightful learning

The gestalt school of psychology was described earlier in this chapter in connection with perception. They also identified a type of learning called learning by insight (or insightful learning), in which the student's perception of a situation or problem undergoes a restructuring, and he or she sees the aspects of the situation in a new relationship to one another. This new relationship forms a unified whole, or gestalt, which is meaningful to the student, who is then said to have insight into the problem or situation.

Kohler demonstrated insight learning in the chimpanzee during a series of classic experiments in Tenerife during World War I. In one experiment, the chimpanzee was placed in a cage which had a banana suspended out of reach and several boxes scattered around. It was impossible to reach the banana by standing on only one of the boxes and the animal would manifest trial and error behaviour, including great restlessness. Suddenly it would pile the boxes one on top of the other, and climb up to the banana. Kohler noticed that this sudden activity often followed a period when the animal had been sitting quietly, not attempting to reach the fruit. He interpreted the behaviour of the chim-panzee as that of gaining insight into the problem, by seeing the banana and the boxes in a new relationship that was meaningful and thus perceiving the solution to the problem.

The laws of proximity and closure can be said to be at work in the insightful learning of the chimpanzee, the former being shown by the fact that all the aspects of the problem, namely the banana and the boxes, must be in the animal's visual field at the same time for insight to occur. Closure is suggested by the sudden awareness of the relationship between the boxes as a means of climbing to the banana, bringing the previously unrelated boxes into a complete, closed gestalt.

This sudden insight into the problem or situation applies to human learning also and has been termed the 'aha' phenomenon. Most people have had, at some time, the experience of suddenly grasping or understanding a problem that has previously perplexed them and have uttered the expression, 'Aha, now I understand'. The cognitive restructuring that occurs in insightful learning is said by the gestalt psychologists to occur also in rats who are running in a maze. They achieve insight into the correct path to the food by a series of partial insights, gained by discovering that certain patterns of movement are non-productive, whilst others lead to food.

Problem-solving and information-processing

The other main approach to problem-solving research is information-processing, which seeks to explain the sequence of operations that subjects use in solving problems. The problem situation is termed the 'problem space', and is composed of an 'initial state' in which the individual is currently in, a 'goal state' which is the desired end state, and one or more 'operators' which are a set of operations that transform the initial state into the goal state (Smythe *et al.*, 1987).

Stages of problem-solving

Howard (1983) gives the following stages:

1. encode the problem in the working memory;
2. search the long-term memory for a plan or production system;
3. execute the production system; and
4. evaluate the results.

This sequence may or may not be successful, depending upon the problem.

When individuals carry out problem-solving tasks, they tend to exhibit similar types of phenomena, such as rigidity, incubation and insight, and 'satisficing'. Rigidity implies that subjects tend to become entrenched in one particular way of seeing a problem, which prevents them from finding a solution. They are also influenced by perceptual set, which makes them respond to the problem as they have done in the past, even if this is not appropriate to the current problem. Incubation and insight refer to the lapse in time between tackling the problem initially and going back to it later, if unsuccessful. There is an increased chance of arriving at a solution after incubation; indeed, it very often results in a 'penny-dropping' insight into the problem. 'Satisficing' is a word meaning that people tend to settle for good choices rather than seeking better ones.

Conditions of learning for problem-solving

Gagne (1985) suggests there are both intrinsic and extrinsic conditions for problem-solving. The conditions within the student that must be met are:

1. recall of relevant rules that have been learned previously;
2. possession of verbal information organized in appropriate ways, i.e. schemata; and
3. cognitive strategies previously learned.

The extrinsic conditions in the learning situation are the verbal instructions issued by the teacher to stimulate recall of rules.

Problem-based learning

Gagne (1985) suggests that the most effective problems for student learning are those that are novel to the students and within their capabilities. Barrows and Tamblyn (1980) recommend problem-based learning as a strategy in teaching health studies and define it as learning that results from the process of working towards the understanding or resolution of a problem. Problem-based learning is different from other problem-solving teaching strategies, because the problem is given to the student prior to any form of input; usually, traditional methods involve the giving of information followed by the application of that information by use of clinical problems. Problem-based learning starts with the problem, and students have to find out what they need to know in order to solve it. This approach is very much a discovery-type approach and can be very motivating (Allen and Murrell, 1978).

Problem-based learning lends itself well to computer-assisted learning, with the use of simulation and case method. Students are given basic data about a patient and are then asked to produce a suitable care plan. Having selected a series of interventions, the nurse can check to see whether in the real case, the ones chosen were actually selected for the patient.

Decision-making

Professional practitioners in nursing, midwifery and health visiting spend a significant part of their professional lives making decisions, many are routine and predictable, others are life-or-death decisions.

Decision theory is about how people decide to take one kind of action rather than another. The theory assumes that people choose the action they think will have the most value or *utility* for them. However, given that decisions are made before the outcomes are known, the choice of action is based upon the *probability* that the outcome will have the expected utility.

When faced with a range of possible actions, the decision about which one to take is made by multiplying the utility by the probability, which gives the *expected utility* of that action (Mook, 1996). However, in real life this calculation takes the form of deciding how well we like the outcome of each alternative action, and how likely it is that the outcome will follow that action. Let us take an example relating to student assessments; it is common practice in higher education for tutors to offer formative feedback on drafts of students' assessment assignments. Institutions normally have a policy about what constitutes a draft, and it is considered inappropriate for tutors to comment on almost-final drafts, as this would constitute pre-marking of the assignment. However, the issue is not straightforward, since it is often difficult to specify what is acceptable as a draft; this can range from a simple outline of the structure of the assignment, through to several pages of text. Hence, the teacher's dilemma is how to decide which drafts are appropriate for feedback, and which are virtually the finished article. Decision theory would analyse the dilemma as shown in Table 4.1. In statistics, the range of probability is between zero and 1.0; zero probability means no chance of the event occurring, and 1.0 means absolute certainty that the event will occur. In Table 4.1, the probability of each utility has been estimated at 0.5, i.e. there is a 50/50 chance of the event occurring, or the alternative event occurring.

Choice of action	Utility (value for me)	Probability (likelihood that action will bring about utility)
1. Provide feedback to student on the draft assignment.	Student's gratitude and continuing good relationship.	Probability of utility is 0.5, because if the assessment is failed, the student may claim that the tutor 'said it was OK'.
2. Refuse to provide feedback, as draft is too complete.	Enhanced feelings of professionalism and rigour.	Probability of utility is 0.5, as feelings of guilt may well be the outcome.

Table 4.1

Decision theory: to comment or not on students' draft assessments

MOTOR SKILLS

Earlier in this chapter (p. 68) the difference between declarative knowledge and procedural knowledge was identified, the latter being knowledge about how to do things. This procedural knowledge is an essential part of motor skills, hence the preferred term *psychomotor skills*. Motor skills are an extremely important aspect of the practice of nursing, since nursing science is largely a practical endeavour, but the notion of skill pervades the whole of society; indeed, the concept of social class is very much influenced by the degree of skill of the occupations in each category of the Registrar General's classification. Motor skills are concerned with movements and a skilled person exhibits certain characteristics over a novice as outlined in Table 4.2

Table 4.2

Characteristics of a skilled performance

Accuracy	Skill executed with precision
Speed	Movements swift and confident
Efficiency	Movements economical, leaving spare capacity available
Timing	Accurate timing and correct sequential order
	Consistency Results are consistent
Anticipation	Can anticipate events very quickly and respond accordingly
Adaptability	Can adapt the skill to current circumstances
Perception	Can obtain maximum information from a minimum of cues

Human motor skills can be divided into three broad categories (Oxendine, 1984):

1. *maturation-dependent skills*, such as crawling, walking and speaking;
2. *educational-related skills*, such as writing, reading and observation; and
3. *intrinsic-value skills*, such as recreational and vocational skills.

It might be useful, at this point, to look at some definitions of motor skill:

1. a persistent change in movement-behaviour potentiality as a result of practice or experience (Oxendine, 1984);
2. a learned ability to bring about a predetermined result with maximum certainty and minimum time and effort (Fitts and Posner, 1967).

Table 4.3 gives some of the terms commonly used in relation to motor skills.

Table 4.3

Terminology of motor skills

Procedure	An intellectual skill consisting of rules for sequencing actions
Motor skill	Ability required for the execution of a procedure
Motor performance	Execution of an overt action
Total skill	Total motor performance with characteristics of a procedure
Part skill	Sub-component of a total skill
Ability	Capacity to execute something

Obviously, not all motor performances need to be learned from scratch, as many of the component skills will already have been mastered. Take the example of a nurse learning how to do a drug round; although she will not have done the motor performances before, such as taking a medicine pot to the patient, she will have acquired the skill of picking up and carrying a small container of fluid without spilling since childhood. Hence, the nurse teacher needs to consider the entry behaviours that students bring to the motor-skill learning situation. Three dimensions of motor skills are commonly identified in the literature: fine/gross, continuous/discrete, closed/open looped.

Dimensions of motor skills

Fine versus gross
Gross performance involves the whole body, or large muscles, such as in

lifting a patient. Fine performance involves fingers and wrists, as in removing sutures.

Continuous versus discrete

The former involves continuous adjustment and corrections to stimuli, such as the continuous movements of external cardiac massage, while the latter is a movement made in response to an external stimulus, such as switching off a patient's nurse-call button.

Closed-looped versus open-looped

Closed-looped performance relies entirely on proprioceptive feedback, so could be performed with eyes closed, whereas open-looped is affected by external stimuli. For example, the painless removal of sutures requires some reaction from the patient, which indicates comfort or otherwise.

Learning motor skills

Motor skills, unlike other forms of learning, require practice in order to be learned and practice consists of repetition of a procedure under specific conditions. These conditions are that the students must intend to learn the skill and they must obtain feedback about their performance. The reason why motor skills require practice is because of the importance of kinaesthetic feedback from the students' own body and this takes time to produce skilled, efficient movements. It is useful to distinguish between physical and mental practice; the former means the actual physical repetition of the procedure, whereas the latter involves thinking about the skill in between practice sessions. Mental practice or imagery is not a substitute for physical practice, but evidence suggests that it is a very useful way of encouraging skills learning when used in conjunction with it. Reminiscence is the term used to describe improvements in performance occurring without physical practice and may be due to mental practice.

The acquisition of a motor skill normally follows a smooth curve when plotted against the time and the number of trials. The occurrence of plateaux, in which the student seems to stay at the same level of performance, are fairly rare. There are also no obvious stages, but Fitts and Posner (1967) suggest that there are three processes that occur, in the following order:

1. the cognitive phase, which is really concerned with the learning of the procedure, and the more complex the skill, the longer this period will take;
2. the associative phase, in which the part-skills are taking on the characteristics of skilled performance and interfering responses are eliminated; and
3. the autonomous phase, during which the skill becomes automatic and can occur without the student thinking about it.

The frequency and distribution of practice can affect learning of motor skills; distribution can be divided into massed practice and distributed practice, the former having little or no rest from beginning to end of practice and the latter having practice sessions separated by rest periods or by longer intervals of time. Distributed practice is generally more effective for learning motor skills, possibly because of the avoidance of boredom, fatigue or loss of attention. Simple tasks, however, are better learned in one session, and short practice periods are preferable to long ones. Of course, student motivational level will influence the amount of practice they can accommodate.

One of the key features of practice pointed out earlier was that it must occur with feedback to the students about their performance in order to help them improve. Thorndike (1931), in a classic experiment, asked subjects to draw four-inch lines whilst blindfolded and they were not told how close to four inches their efforts were. There was much variability in line length drawn, but no trend towards improvement over the trials. Feedback can be classified as intrinsic or extrinsic. Intrinsic feedback is feedback arising within the performer and is further subdivided into reactive and operational feedback: reactive feedback consists of the kinaesthetic feedback from the performer's body muscles and joints; and operational feedback is the observation of the effect of the action by the performer, also termed knowledge of results (KOR). Extrinsic feedback is external to the performer and is also termed augmented feedback; it can be done by teachers, peers or coaches and may be done concurrently during the performance, or terminally when it is finished.

When student nurses learn a new skill, it is likely that there will be some element of transfer from previously learned skills; transfer means that a previously learned skill has a positive or negative influence on the new one, and this is termed pro-active transfer. It is also possible for the new skill to influence the old one, a phenomenon called retroactive transfer. Transfer of skill may be specific or non-specific; specific aspects that are transferred in nursing are such things as lifting patients without injuring oneself, whereas general transfer occurs with less obvious things such as problem-solving ability.

Positive transfer of skills is enhanced by similarity between them, and also if well-learned responses can be used in the new skill. On the other hand, well-learned habits may interfere with new responses, as in driving a car with different controls. There is evidence to suggest that an understanding of the underlying principles will enhance transfer to a different activity.

Guidance on the teaching of skills is given in Chapter 16 (p. 437).

COGNITIVE THEORIES OF LEARNING AND INSTRUCTION

A number of influential learning theorists have taken a cognitive approach in an attempt to explain how people learn, and from their theories have derived principles for instruction or teaching.

AUSUBEL: ASSIMILATION THEORY OF MEANINGFUL LEARNING

The psychologist David P. Ausubel is somewhat unusual among educational psychologists in that he focuses very much on presentational methods of teaching and also on the acquisition of subject matter in the curriculum. He draws a distinction between psychology and educational psychology, the former being concerned with problems of learning whilst the latter is an applied science, the function of which is to study those aspects of learning that can be related to ways of effectively bringing about assimilation of organized bodies of knowledge.

Ausubel *et al.* (1978) distinguishes between types of learning by using a model consisting of two orthogonal dimensions of learning; one on the continuum from rote to meaningful learning; and the other on the continuum from reception to discovery learning (Figure 4.6). These dimensions are unrelated and it can be seen that the diagram consists of four quadrants:

1. meaningful reception learning;
2. rote reception learning;
3. meaningful discovery learning; and
4. rote discovery learning.

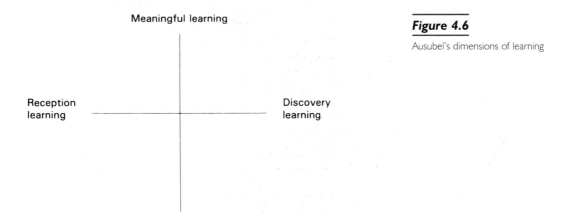

Figure 4.6

Ausubel's dimensions of learning

Ausubel maintains that most classroom learning is of the reception type, in which information is presented in its final form to the student. Discovery learning, on the other hand, consists of allowing students to discover for themselves the principles of content. Discovery learning may fall at any point on the continuum and it is more usual to find a form of guided discovery learning in use in the classroom. Whilst acknowledging the place of discovery learning, Ausubel claims that it is simply not feasible for transmitting large quantities of knowledge, since discovery learning requires greater time and resources. The second, unrelated, dimension is rote/meaningful; rote learning is defined as any learning that does not meet the criteria for meaningfulness.

Types of meaningful learning

There are three types of meaningful learning.

1. *Representational or vocabulary learning.* All other types of learning depend upon this basic form, which consists of the learning of single words or what is represented by them.
2. *Concept learning.* Ausubel defines concepts as 'objects, events, situations or properties that possess common criterial attributes and are designated by some sign or symbol'. He identifies two kinds of concept acquisition, the first occurring in young children, called concept formation, and the second occurring in school children and adults, called concept assimilation.
3. *Propositional learning.* In this form of learning, it is not simply the meaning of single words that is learned, but the meaning of sentences that contain composite ideas. Syntax and grammatical rules must also be understood.

Ausubel takes pains to point out that there is a difference between meaningful learning and the learning of meaningful material. In order for material to be learned meaningfully, it is necessary to meet three criteria:

1. The student must adopt an appropriate learning 'set', which is a disposition to approach a learning task in a particular way. In the case of meaningful learning, the student must adopt a set to learn the task in a meaningful, as opposed to a rote, fashion.
2. The learning task itself must have logical meaning, in that it can be related to the student's own cognitive structure in a sensible way. This cognitive structure is said to provide anchorage for the new information, with both components being modified in the process of assimilation.
3. The student's own cognitive structures must contain specifically relevant ideas with which the new material can interact.

Rote learning, on the other hand, can be considered as any learning in which these conditions are not present. For example, the student may adopt a set to learn the material in a word-for-word fashion, in which case the new material would be linked to the existing structure in a simple, arbitrary way without any real interaction. Such linkage prohibits the direct use of existing knowledge and in addition, the word-for-word nature of learning will place limits on the amount of material that can be learned and retained. Ausubel considers that pure rote learning plays little part in everyday classroom learning beyond elementary school level.

These conditions form an integral part of Ausubel's assimilation theory, which states that most meaningful cognitive learning occurs as a result of interaction between new information that the individual acquires and the specifically relevant cognitive structures that he or she already possesses. This interaction results in the assimilation or incor-

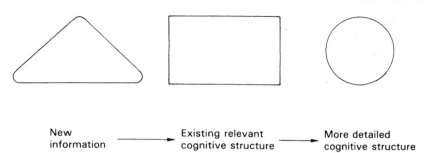

Figure 4.7

The process of assimilation of information

poration of both the new and the existing information to form a more detailed cognitive structure. Figure 4.7 shows this process; the new information is not simply added to the old in a cumulative way – rather, it acts upon the existing information and both are transformed into a new and more detailed cognitive structure.

The pivotal nature of this idea to Ausubel's theory can be seen in his statement (1978, p. 163):

'If I had to reduce all educational psychology to just one principle it would be this: The most important single factor influencing learning is what the student already knows. Ascertain this and teach him accordingly.'

Assimilation theory forms the basis of Ausubel's ideas on the organization of instruction and the main variables affecting learning are outlined below.

1. Cognitive variables:
   (a) the student's previous knowledge of related ideas – seen to be important to the learning of new material, and forms the basis of the notion 'transfer of learning';
   (b) developmental readiness, which is the stage of cognitive development the student has reached;
   (c) intellectual ability of the student;
   (d) practice;
   (e) arrangement of instructional materials in order to facilitate learning.
2. Affective/social variables:
   (f) motivation and attitudes;
   (g) personality;
   (h) group and social factors;
   (i) teacher characteristics.

One of the key strategies for learning advocated by Ausubel is the concept of 'advance organizer', a strategy introduced in advance of any new material in order to provide an anchoring structure for it. This strategy is based on the assimilation theory, which, as we have seen, states that new information is subsumed or incorporated into an anchoring structure already present in the student. Typically, an advance organizer consists of ideas that are similar to the material that is to be learned, but are stated at a higher level of generality and inclusiveness, so that the new material may then assume a subordinate relationship to the advance organizer. The concept is similar to an overview (or summary), except that the latter is presented at the same level of generality or inclusiveness. Advance organizers form the link between the student's previous knowledge and what is needed to be known, before any meaningful learning can take place. A further advantage is that it provides a highly specific anchoring structure because the content is virtually identical to the material that follows, although to be effective, it must obviously be potentially meaningful and capable of being understood.

The process of forgetting meaningfully learned material is also explained by Ausubel in terms of assimilation theory. Learning, as we have seen, consists of the interaction between new information and knowledge already present in the cognitive structure of an individual. During the process of assimilation, this new information gradually loses its discrete identity as it becomes part of the modified anchoring structure; this process is termed obliterative subsumption. This gradual loss of separate identity ends with the meaning being forgotten when the idea falls below the threshold of availability. This threshold forms a level below which an idea cannot be retrieved, but the level is subject to variation, e.g. due to anxiety.

Implications for teaching and learning

How effective are advance organizers in practice? Barnes and Clawson (1975) reviewed 32 students involving the use of advance organizers and found that 12 reported significant effects and 20 were non-significant. They analysed the studies according to selected variables, finding that length of treatment was not critical and that the ability levels of students had no differential effects on learning. Similarly, no clear pattern emerged in relation to the grade level of the students or to the types of organizer. They concluded that the efficacy of advance organizers had not been established. Ausubel, however, states that Barnes and Clawson failed to take into account the fact that most studies did not analyse the students' relevant subsumers nor the conceptual material to be learned. Meena (1980) reports a study in which advance organizers were used prior to information presented in an instructional film; results showed that learning and retention were significantly superior for the organizer groups. Nicholl (1978) studied the effects of advance organizers on a cognitive social-learning group, but the results were not significant.

The most obvious application of assimilation theory is that of advance organizers for lectures. As was pointed out earlier, an advance organizer is a form of introductory material, introduced and taught to the students in advance of the main body of the lecture, and its purpose is to provide the necessary specific anchoring structures for the information presented in the main body of the lecture. In order to do this, the advance organizer must fulfil certain criteria.

1. It must form a bridge between what the student already knows and the new information to be encountered in the lecture.
2. The advance organizer must be more general and inclusive than the material that follows it in the main body of the lecture; it must abstract out from that knowledge the key essence of the lecture.
3. It must be taught and learned just like any other information, either immediately prior to the lecture, or some time in advance of it.

Introduction
good morning and welcome to this lecture on the circulatory system. Before we begin I would like to include some introductory material to help you understand the lecture.

Advance organizer
You are all very familar with the notion of transport systems in society; for example, road, rail, air and sea transport. Any transport system has a number of basic components as follows:

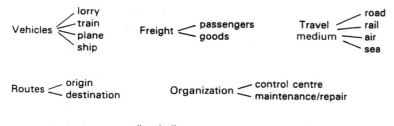

The circulatory system in the body is another example of a transport system with the same basic components. We can usefully examine the system using these components as follows:

Vehicles: In the bloodstream, certain cells act as vehicles for transporting substances, as does the liquid part of the blood, called plasma.

Freight: Many 'goods' are transported in the blood, including foodstuffs, oxygen, chemical messengers and waste products.

Travel medium: The liquid part of the blood is the transport medium.

Routes: There are many routes involved in the circulation. For example, oxygen originates at the lungs (the supplier) and its destination is the tissue cells (the consumer).

Organization: There is a complex organization of circulation, both from central control in the brain to local control in the tissues.

Energy Consumption: Like all other body systems, the circulation burns up glucose to make energy.

Main body of lecture

1. Composition of the blood ⟨ Plasma / Cells ⟨ red / white / platelets
2. Greater and lesser circulation
3. Functions of blood
4. Control of circulation

Figure 4.8

Example of a lesson plan with advance organizer for 'the circulatory system'

One of the difficulties of grasping the concept of an advance organizer is that Ausubel only ever gave one example, because the organizer must relate intimately to the teacher's subject matter and thus cannot be written by anyone else. In order to see how the organizer is structured, it is always necessary to have the subject matter of the lecture available as well. Figure 4.8 shows an example of an advance organizer for a lesson on the circulatory system, including the lesson plan for the main lecture.

The advance organizer is taught at the beginning of the lecture, and is then followed by the main body of information. The advance organizer contains all the elements of the lecture that follows it, but at a much more abstract level. For example, it talks about 'certain cells' rather than giving specific names; the names are introduced later in the lecture. The advance organizer also contains information that the student already knows, i.e. the transport systems of society and so forms a bridge between this prior knowledge and the new information about the circulation.

The principle of meaningful learning can be applied at all levels of nurse education and it is particularly important to ascertain students' prior knowledge when working in the clinical setting. A few minutes spent clarifying what the student understands about the nursing care of a patient will be rewarded by providing a framework upon which further explanation can be hung.

Nurse teachers should try to discourage students from learning material in a rote fashion and instead, encourage them to learn it meaningfully, by asking them to try to explain the material to a fellow student.

BRUNER: DISCOVERY LEARNING

The work of Jerome Bruner (1960) has had a profound influence on educational thinking and he is particularly associated with 'discovery learning'. Bruner sees the learning of a subject as involving three processes.

1. *The acquisition of new information.* This usually builds on something that is already known, albeit tentative or vague.
2. *Transformation of information.* New information is analysed and processed so that it can be used in new situations.
3. *Evaluation.* All aspects of the processing of information are evaluated to check whether they are correct.

Subject matter is usually broken down into a series of units or learning episodes and each episode involves the three processes above.

Structure of a subject

According to Bruner, the purpose of learning is that it should be useful to us in the future and this occurs by the process of transfer. Transfer of learning can occur in two main ways – transfer of specific skills or transfer of general principles. This latter type of transfer is fundamental to the educational process and is dependent upon a thorough under-standing of the structure of subject matter. This concept of structure is explained by Bruner (1960, p.7) as follows:

'Grasping the structure of a subject is understanding it in a way which permits many other things to be related to it meaningfully. To learn structure, in short, is to learn how things are related.'

Structure, then, involves the basic patterns and ideas of the subject, but not the details or specific facts. If students understand the structure, they should be able to work out for themselves much of the fine detail. The structure is made up of concepts or categories and Bruner sees learning as a process of categorization of objects. Classes of objects are seen to be characterized by common properties, and it is these proper-ties that are used as a basis for identifying new objects that are encoun-tered. The new object is compared with the properties of a category, to see if it belongs there. If the object fits a particular category, then we infer that it possesses the characteristics of that category. A category has certain distinguishing properties that differentiate it from other cate-gories and it also has a certain order in which the characteristics are combined. For example, the category 'bed' has the following compo-nents: frame, legs, headboard, footboard, mattress, pillows, blankets and counterpane. These characteristics are assembled in a certain order, such as the legs underneath, the mattress on the frame, the pillows and blankets on top, etc. There are also limits of acceptance for objects to fall within a category. For instance, a bed would still be a bed if there were no headboard, but it would not constitute a bed if there were no frame.

When categorizing an object, an individual tends to follow a sequence of four stages. The first involves isolating the object from its background, a process called primitive categorization. A search for cues then follows, which may be conscious or unconscious, and the indivi-dual attempts to categorize the object using cues available. He or she may employ a conscious cue search by saying, 'I wonder what this can be'. Having made a cue search, the individual makes a tentative categor-ization and this then narrows down the search to those cues that will confirm the tentative categorization. This is termed confirmation check. The fourth stage involves ceasing the search for cues and additional cues are more or less ignored. This stage is called confirmation completion and the object is identified and categorized.

Coding systems for information

The learning of more complex information is explained by Bruner in terms of coding systems. A coding system is a set of general categories that an individual uses to classify and to group information about the world. These systems are hierarchically arranged, with the more specific information in the lowest categories. As one rises in the hierarchy, each category is more general and less specific than the one below, and to recall a specific item, it is necessary to recall the coding system of which

Figure 4.9

Coding system for fractures

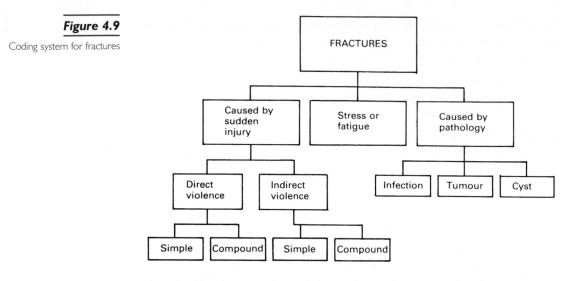

it is a member. Thus, the general principles of a subject are contained in the upper parts of the hierarchy of a category and in transfer of learning, these previously learned coding systems are applied to new events or objects. Figure 4.9 shows a coding system for fractures, with the most general concept at the top, namely fractures and progressively finer subdivisions or subordinate concepts.

Acquisition of coding systems is influenced by a number of factors, including the learning 'set' of an individual towards a learning task, and motivation of the student. In addition, there must be mastery of the specific aspects of a situation before the principles can be combined into a more general or generic coding system, and this acquisition of generic coding systems is enhanced by a variety of learning situations, especially discovery-learning situations.

Discovery learning

Discovery learning involves students in discovering the structure of a subject through active involvement and can be divided into pure discovery and guided discovery. The former is virtually impossible to organize, since it involves no direction whatsoever, so the latter is prefer-able. The role of the teacher is to pose questions or problems that stimulate students to seek answers in an active discovery way. One of the great obstacles to this kind of learning in nurse education is the pressure on students always to produce the correct answers to questions, and this runs counter to the notion of intuitive thinking. Intuition involves making an educated guess about phenomena before one has the complete data, and can be very motivating for students because they then have to check whether their hypothesis was correct or not.

Implications for teaching and learning

The implications of Bruner's ideas on the structure of subject matter are that the nurse teacher must ensure that any new material being taught is first explained in terms of its basic structures and principles. It is not helpful to give lots of fine detail in the early stages of encounter with a new subject and much more sensible to give an outline only. Take the example of microbiology, an important topic for nurses to understand so that they can appreciate the need for asepsis and antibiotics. It would be good practice if the teacher confined the lecture to a general overview of the main principles and concepts of microbiology until the students were well-immersed in them. However, it is not uncommon to find lectures on microbiology given to first-year students that contain very specific detail about the classification of bacteria, a confusing experience for those students who have not encountered the concepts before. Discovery learning can be used to good effect in the context of guided discovery; the nurse teacher can ask students to devise a series of questions or problems related to the topic areas and then to try to find answers to them using whatever resources are available. Another discovery approach is to use practical laboratory sessions to generate activities and then to ask students to try to explain why things happened.

GAGNE:THE CONDITIONS OF LEARNING AND THEORY OF INSTRUCTION

Robert Gagne does not propose a theory of learning *per se*, but focuses on the conditions of learning. Using an information-processing model, he analyses these conditions and develops a theory of instruction based upon them. Learning is defined as 'a change in human disposition or capability that persists over a period of time and is not simply ascribable to processes of growth' (Gagne, 1985). Thus growth is seen very much as being genetically determined, whereas learning is seen as being mainly under the control of environmental influences that interact with the individual. Any learning situation can be seen as having a number of elements, namely the student, the stimulus, the contents of the student's memory and the response or performance outcome. Such a learning situation or occurrence is described by Gagne (1985, p. 4) as follows:

> *'A learning occurrence, then, takes place when the stimulus situation together with the contents of memory affect the student in such a way that his or her performance changes from a time before being in that situation to a time after being in it. The change in performance is what leads to the conclusion that learning has occurred.'*

Learning capabilities

Gagne believes that it is possible to make sense of all the different learning outcomes that people make during a lifetime by organizing them into five performance categories, each representing a different kind of learning capability.

1. Intellectual skills:
   (a) discrimination;
   (b) concrete concepts;
   (c) defined concepts;
   (d) rules;
   (e) higher-order rules.
2. Cognitive strategies.
3. Verbal information.
4. Motor skills.
5. Attitudes.

Prototypes of learning

The five varieties of learning capability include some elements that Gagne terms 'prototypes of learning'; these are commonly identified phenomena of learning that constitute basic forms of learning by association. They include:

1. classical conditioning;
2. operant conditioning;
3. verbal-association learning; and
4. 'chaining'.

These are seen as basic forms because they comprise only parts of specific capabilities and are insufficient to explain all aspects of complex learning. Hence, association is seen as an important aspect, since its various forms constitute some of the components of the five learning capabilities. These prototypes are discussed in Chapter 5 on behaviourism (p. 111).

Having emphasized the importance of association learning as a basic component of all types of learning, we now examine the five varieties of learning capability in more detail.

Intellectual skills

It is useful to think of intellectual skills as forming a hierarchy in which any particular skill requires the prior learning of those skills below it in the hierarchy, as illustrated in Figure 4.10.

The dependence of intellectual skills on the basic prototypes is shown and each level consists of progressively more complex skills. These intellectual skills are what is referred to as 'procedural knowledge' (i.e. knowledge about how to perform such things as mathematical calculations) and are typified by rule-governed behaviour. Rules state relationships between things and are composed of simpler components called concepts, which in turn depend on the ability to discriminate between various characteristics of things.

Discrimination

Young children learn to respond to collections of things by learning the differences between them, a process called discrimination. Discrimination learning involves perceiving differences in size, shape, colour,

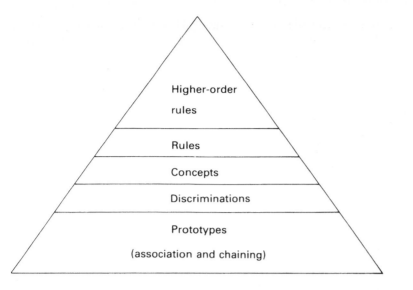

Figure 4.10

Hierarchy of intellectual skillls

texture, etc. and multiple discriminations have to be made when there is more than one stimulus present. Student nurses and midwives may have to learn to discriminate between the various kinds of tissue when using a microscope. This is usually taught by presenting examples and non-examples of a particular tissue, a process called 'contrast practice'. When the student is making multiple discriminations, there is a danger of confusion between stimuli and interference in the learning to discriminations.

Concrete concepts

Discrimination learning is confined to specific stimuli, whereas concept formation allows the student to respond to collections of things by classifying them into categories sharing common abstract properties. Unlike prototypes and discriminations, concepts are capable of being generalized to other situations and hence they free the student from control by specific stimuli. Once a student nurse has acquired the concept of a 'pressure sore', this can be applied to any example on all areas of the body, provided that the concept adequately represents the range of pressure sores possible. It may be that students have inadequate concepts for some classes of phenomena, so these need to be developed and extended by appropriate instruction.

Gagne describes three stages in the learning of a concrete or observable concept: discrimination, generalization and variation in irrelevant dimensions. The first stage involves the student in discriminating between one object and another, e.g. a capsule and a tablet. The next stage involves generalization of the discrimination, in which the student discriminates between the capsule and a variety of tablets of various shapes, sizes and colours. The final stage involves variation in the size, shape and colour of the capsules, as well as the variations in the tablets and if the student can identify all the capsules, then he or she has acquired the concept of a 'capsule'. This attainment can be tested by showing the student nurse a capsule and a tablet, neither of which have been seen before; if the student nurse can identify the capsule, he or she has attained the concept by identifying a novel instance.

The learning of a concept can be made much easier by the use of language, i.e. verbal cues or instructions; indeed, many of the concepts used in nursing are learned verbally by attending lectures or by reading. Concepts learned in this linguistic manner need to have concrete references to the real world if students really are to understand them. Such concrete reference can be made by the use of practical work in laboratories or clinical settings.

Defined concepts

In the previous section, concrete concepts were referred to by Gagne as concepts-by-observation; certain concepts, however, can only be learned as definitions, since they do not actually exist as concrete entities, for example, health or empathy. A definition is a statement that expresses rules for classifying objects or events and consists of 'thing-concepts' and 'relational concepts'. The definition of an object consists of four parts:

1. a thing-concept that is superordinate;
2. a set of characteristics of the above;
3. a relational concept indicating the use of the object; and
4. a thing-concept that is the object of the verb above.

Figure 4.11 illustrates the components of the definition of the concept of a 'syringe'.

Many concepts are themselves relations and the components of these definitions are slightly different:

1. a relational concept that is already known by the student;
2. a thing-concept that is the object of the above; and
3. modifier words that are the characteristics of the relation.

Figure 4.11

Components of the definition of 'syringe'

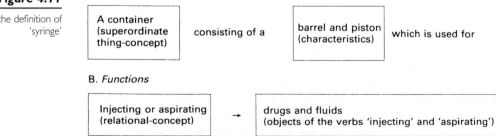

Figure 4.12 illustrates the components of the definition of 'haemolysis'.

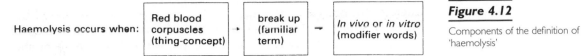

Haemolysis occurs when: | Red blood corpuscles (thing-concept) → break up (familiar term) → *In vivo* or *in vitro* (modifier words)

Figure 4.12

Components of the definition of 'haemolysis'

There is one point of possible confusion between concrete concepts and defined concepts; it is quite common to find that concrete concepts are given definitions, as in the example of syringe, but this does not make them defined concepts. A defined concept cannot be concrete, however, since it is concerned with relations not objects. Defined concepts are taught by pointing out the thing-concepts and the relational concepts to the student and these are then understood, provided the student has already acquired the relevant component concepts of the definition. For example, the term 'diffusion' can be defined as 'the continual intermingling of molecules in liquids or gases', but for the student to understand this concept, he or she must first understand the component concepts of 'intermingling' and 'molecules'.

Rules

A rule is defined by Gagne (1985, p. 118) as 'an inferred capability that enables the individual to respond to any instance of a class of stimulus situations with an appropriate instance of a class of performances'. Rules require as prerequisites, the component concepts and these are then put in the correct sequence, as in the rules of grammar or mathematics. Rules are often thought of as statements in lay terms, e.g. the rule book, but it is important to remember that the rule itself is an inferred capability, which is one of the aspects of intellectual skills. However, verbal statements are very useful for learning rules, as in the 'diffusion' example mentioned earlier. Rules are also termed procedures and may consist of long sequences or steps in a particular sequence. Nursing procedure manuals are published that contains a series of rules about the carrying out of various nursing procedures.

Higher-order rules

We have seen that rules require prerequisite knowledge of the relevant concepts in order to be understood and that such concept attainment is reliant upon the necessary discriminations made by the student, which in turn depends upon associations between stimuli. The increasing complexity of intellectual skill does not stop at rules, but higher-order rules may develop as a result of the student's problem solving, resulting in the combination of several rules into a more complex rule. Much learning can be seen in the form of learning hierarchies, with the simpler rules forming prerequisites for more complex ones and this implies that there is a cumulative process involved in learning. Hence, simpler rules are transferred to more complex rules and these higher-order rules tend to be more generalizable in their application.

Cognitive strategies

These strategies exert control over the internal mental processes of learning such as thinking, memory and problem-solving and are independent of content. They are involved in the learning of intellectual skills and other learning capabilities and are often referred to as meta-cognitive processes or 'learning to learn'. Students use cognitive strategies for attending to stimuli, for encoding and retrieving information in the memory and for thinking and problem-solving, e.g. the use of mnemonics and imagery. Cognitive strategies are easily acquired by students and become better with practice, and there is some evidence to suggest that these skills will transfer to other situations.

Verbal information learning

Verbal learning entails 'declarative knowledge', the kind of knowledge involved in telling or verbalizing, and it utilizes sentences or propositions. There are three forms of verbal learning: names (or labels), facts (or single propositions) and organized verbal knowledge:

1. *Names or labels.* These are normally learned at the same time as the concept is acquired, hence only one or two labels or names are learnt at any one time. On occasions, however, it is necessary to learn several names at one time, such as when a nurse teacher meets a new student group and has to remember each name, which can be very difficult.
2. *Facts or single propositions.* It seems likely that facts are stored in memory as meaningful propositions rather than as verbatim words in some form of semantic network.
3. *Organized verbal knowledge.* This refers to collections of propositions that are organized into connected discourse called prose. It is suggested that a student's previous knowledge is a major influence on the learning of new information from prose texts, due to the previous formation of global schemata for particular situations or events.

Motor skills

Much human learning is to do with movements and a practice discipline like nursing centres around the learning of motor skills and procedures. There are three dimensions of motor skills: fine/gross performance, continuous/discrete movements, and closed/open looped tasks.

Fine versus gross performance

It is possible to distinguish motor skills in terms of the involvement of muscles, gross skills requiring the use of large muscles as in the lifting of patients and fine skills, the use of fingers and wrists, as in the removing of sutures.

Continuous versus discrete

These terms are self-explanatory, the former consisting of continuous movements such as those of external cardiac massage and the latter consisting of single-direction movements, such as the switching off of the nurse call button.

Closed-looped versus open-looped tasks

The former relies entirely on proprioceptive feedback and can be performed with the eyes closed; the latter involves some kind of external stimulus that influences the movement, such as inflating the cuff on a sphygmomanometer according to the level of the column of mercury.

Motor skills often occur as components of procedures, such as giving a blanket bath or changing a dressing; a procedure consists of a series of rules in sequential order, but also requires certain motor skills in order to be executed. It is therefore incorrect to think of procedures as being motor skills alone, rather they involve both intellectual and motor skills. Practice is a basic requirement for the acquisition of motor skills in order to allow the student to learn from the proprioceptive feedback from his or her own body movements; in addition the student receives feedback both from observing the effects of his or her movements and by augmented feedback from someone else: a teacher or a coach. When attempting to learn a procedure, a student combines a series of part-skills into the total procedure in a particular order and these are known as behavioural chains.

Attitudes

According to Gagne (1985, p. 63), an attitude is 'an internal state that influences (moderates) the choices of personal action made by the individual'. Attitudes are learnt as individuals develop during childhood and adult life. Their relationship to behaviour is not clearly identified, but they serve to predispose the individual to act towards things in a particular way. There are three components of an attitude:

1. the cognitive component consists of the beliefs which an individual holds about the attitudinal object;
2. the affective component is concerned with feelings that the individual has about the beliefs that he or she holds about the attitudinal object; and
3. the behavioural aspect – a predisposition to act in some way – although studies have shown poor correlation between attitudes and behaviour.

A nurse may have a positive attitude towards the elderly, believing that they have a right to be treated with respect and dignity and this belief may be very strongly felt. The nurse may endeavour in his or her behaviour towards the elderly to ensure always that they are treated as individuals and made to feel respected.

The conditions of learning

The learning capabilities outlined above form the cornerstone of Gagne's approach to instruction, since this involves identifying the conditions of learning for each of these capabilities, as well as for the prototypes called association. Gagne suggests that in order to infer that learning has taken place, it is necessary to know not only the changes in performance following instruction, but the capabilities that students already possess prior to instruction. These previously learned capabilities are what Gagne refers to as 'internal conditions of learning', in contrast to 'external conditions of learning', which consist of the stimulus situations outside the student. Both are necessary if learning is to take place and Gagne has described the internal and external conditions necessary for learning in each of the learned capabilities and prototypes. These are outlined in Table 4.4.

Gagne's theory of instruction

Gagne points out that there is a difference between theories of learning and theories of instruction in that the latter utilizes a range of theories of learning in order to establish principles of instruction. The events of instruction are different for each of the learning capabilities. Gagne suggests a sequence of instructional events related to internal processes of learning in an information-processing framework:

1. *Gaining attention.* A variety of strategies, including loudness of the voice, gesturing, asking questions, or a practical demonstration of something can be used. Attention-getting devices are applicable to all the learning capabilities.

2. *Informing students of the objective.* If students know the objectives of instruction, they will be motivated to learn, so it is important that such objectives are transmitted to them for whichever type of

Table 4.4

The conditions of learning for prototypes and learning capabilities

Capabilities	Internal conditions (within the learner)	External conditions (the learning situation)
Prototypes Classical conditioning	Presence of a natural reflex in the learner, i.e. unconditioned stimulus results in unconditioned response	(i) Contiguity, i.e. conditioned and unconditioned stimuli must be presented close together (ii) A repetition of the paired stimuli must occur
Operant conditioning	Reinforcement of behaviour is essential	(i) A reinforcement contingency must occur (ii) Contiguity and repetition are also necessary
Chaining	Each stimulus-response association must be previously learned	(i) Learner must state the links of the chain in their correct order (ii) Contiguity, repetition and reinforcement are necessary.
Verbal association	(i) Every link must be previously learned as a stimulus-response association (ii) Mediating connections, i.e. verbal codes, visual and auditory images, must be previously learned	(i) Verbal units must be presented in correct sequence (ii) External cues should be provided, e.g. mnemonics (iii) Student's memory determines the length of the chain he or she is capable of learning at one time (iv) Correct responses must be confirmed to the learner

Capabilities	Internal conditions (within the learner)	External conditions (the learning situation)
Learning capabilities		Selective reinforcement of correct, as opposed to incorrect, responses is required
1. Intellectual skills		
(a) Discrimination	Recall of stimulus–response chains to demonstrate discrimination	Verbal cues should be given, i.e.
(b) Concrete concepts	(i) Discrimination must be previously learned (ii) Verbal labels must have been previously learned if verbal instructions are used (iii) Generalization of basic discrimination	(i) One example and one non-example of concept (ii) Same example plus various non-examples (iii) Variations in both examples and non-examples (iv) Reinforcement of correct responses and contiguity
(c) Defined concepts	(i) Component concepts must be available in memory (ii) Rules of syntax must be previously learned	(i) Definition should be presented verbally or in writing to act as cue for retrieval of concepts (ii) Examples of non-examples of defined concepts should be given
(d) Rules	Knowledge of the concepts involved in the rule	Verbal instruction as follows: (i) Expected performance outcome should be stated (ii) Teacher should evoke recall of the component concepts (iii) Verbal cues should be given for whole rule (iv) Reinforcement and repetition are required
2. Cognitive strategies	(i) Understanding of the meaning of self-instruction strategies (ii) Task-related concepts must be previously learned	Discovery by the learner of strategies for encoding, etc.
3. Verbal learning	(i) Previously learned and organized knowledge in student's memory (ii) Strategies for encoding verbal information	(i) Provision of a meaningful learning context (ii) Making cues for recall as distinctive as possible to avoid interference (iii) Practise retrieving information by review and repetition
4. Motor skills	(i) Part-skills must be recalled (ii) The procedure (executive routine) must be recalled	(i) Verbal instructions should be given (ii) Pictures in the form of diagrams or video to show movements involved (iii) Demonstration of movements by skilled practitioner (iv) Practice must be allowed (v) Feedback about the performance is important for motor-skills learning, i.e. augmented feedback given by instructor
5. Attitudes	(i) Concept to which attitude is related must be previously learned (ii) Certain information is necessary to the establishment of an attitude	(i) Human models for attitudes: model should be credible and appealing; recall of relevant information is encouraged; the desired action is indicated to the learner; the model is seen to receive reinforcement (ii) Alternative forms of modelling can be used, e.g. role-play, reading fiction, television and drama, etc. (iii) Reinforcement is given for choice of desired action

107

capability that might be being taught. These may be stated in the form of behavioural objectives.

3. *Stimulating recall of prior learning.* This is important for all learning capabilities and is commonly done by asking questions of the students.

4. *Presenting the stimulus.* This depends upon what is to be learned and can involve printed materials, the presentation of a problem, a description of a strategy or the demonstration of a motor skill.

5. *Providing learning guidance.* This consists of conveying the meaningfulness of the stimulus by such devices as relating new information to existing knowledge and giving concrete examples of abstract concepts.

6. *Eliciting performance.* Here, the student is asked to demonstrate the application of learning to a novel problem, to ensure that learning has occurred.

7. Providing feedback. Feedback as to the correctness or otherwise of a student's performance is important for his or her further learning and this can be achieved by a teacher giving verbal feedback or written comments. Alternative forms can be given by the use of computers or other technology.

8. *Assessing performance.* This is typically done by means of a test in which the student is given new examples to work on.

9. *Enhancing retention and transfer.* This can be done by giving practice in the relevant capability and by increasing the variety of performance.

Learning is also affected by such variables as the time spent on learning a task and the individual differences in students in terms of motivation, previous knowledge and comprehension.

REFERENCES

Allen, H. and Murrell, J. (1978) *Nurse Training: An Enterprise in Curriculum Development*, Macdonald and Evans, Plymouth.

Anderson, J. and Bower, G. (1973) *Human Associative Memory*, Winston, Washington.

Atkinson, R. and Shiffrin, R. (1971) The control of short term memory, *Scientific American*, **225**, 82–90.

Ausubel, D., Novak, J. and Hanesian, H. (1978) *Educational Psychology; A Cognitive View*, Holt, Rinehart and Winston, New York.

Baddeley, A. and Hitch, G. (1974) Working memory, in G. Bowen (ed.), *The Psychology of Learning and Motivation*, Vol. 2, Academic Press, New York.

Baddeley, A. and Lieberman, K. (1980) Spatial working memory, in R. Nickerson (ed.), *Attention and Performance VIII*, Earlbaum, New Jersey.

Bailin, S., Case, R., Coombs, J.R. and Daniels, L.B. (1999a) Common misconceptions in critical thinking, *Journal of Curriculum Studies*, **31**(3), 269–83.

Bailin, S., Case, R., Coombs, J.R. and Daniels, L.B. (1999b) Conceptualising critical thinking, *Journal of Curriculum Studies,* **31**(3), 285–302

Banyard, P. and Hayes, N. (1994) *Psychology: Theory and Application*, Chapman and Hall, London.

Barnes, B. and Clawson, E. (1975) Do advance organizers facilitate learning? *Review of Educational Research*, **45**, 637–59.

Barrows, H. and Tamblyn, R. (1980) *Problem-based Learning: an Approach to Medical Education*, Springer, California.

Bartlett, F. (1932) *Remembering*, Cambridge University Press, Cambridge.

Brookfield, S. (1987) *Developing Critical Thinkers,* Open University Press, Milton Keynes.

Bruner, J. (1960) *The Process of Education*, Harvard University Press, Cambridge, MA.

Burnard, P. (1989) Developing critical ability in nurse education, *Nurse Education Today*, **9**, 271–5.

Claxton, G. (1998) Knowing without knowing why, *The Psychologist*, May, 1998.

CNAA (Council for National Academic Awards) (1992) *CNAA Handbook*, CNAA, London.

Collins, A. and Quillian, M. (1969) Retrieval time from semantic memory, *Journal of Verbal Learning and Verbal Behaviour*, 8, 2407.

Conway, M. (1991) Cognitive psychology in search of meaning: the study of autobiographical memory, *The Psychologist*, **4**, 301–5.

Craik, F. and Lockhart, R. (1972) Levels of processing: a framework for memory research, *Journal of Experimental Psychology, General*, **104**, 268–94.

Doyle, W. (1983) Academic work, *Review of Educational Research*, 53(2), 159–99.

Edwards, D., Potter, J. and Middleton, D. (1992) Towards a discursive psychology of remembering, *The Psychologist*, 5(10), 441–6.

Fitts, P. and Posner, M. (1967) *Human Performance*, Prentice-Hall, Englewood Cliffs, NJ.

Gagne, R. (1985) *The Conditions of Learning and Theory of Instruction*, 4th edn, Holt, Rinehart and Winston, New York.

Howard, D. (1983) *Cognitive Psychology*, Macmillan, London.

Logie, R. (1999) Working memory, *The Psychologist*, 12(4), 174-8.

Meena, V. (1980) The effect of written and graphic comparative advance organizers upon learning and retention from an audio-visual presentation, *Dissertation Abstracts International*, 40, 3713–14.

Miller, G. (1956) The magical number seven plus or minus two: some limits on our capacity for processing information, *Psychological Review*, 63, 81–97.

Minsky, M. (1975) Artificial intelligence, *Scientific American*, Summer, 1975.

Mook, D.G. (1996) *Motivation: The Organisation of Action*, 2nd edn, Norton and Co., London.

Nicholl, G. (1978) The effect of advance organizers on a cognitive social learning group, *Dissertion Abstracts International*, 38, 4475.

Oxendine, J. (1984) *Psychology of Motor Learning*, 2nd edn, Prentice-Hall, Englewood Cliffs, NJ.

Paivio, A. (1969) Mental imagery in associative learning and memory, *Psychological Review*, 76, 2413.

Piaget, J. and Inhelder, B. (1969) *The Psychology of the Child*, Basic Books, New York.

Pylyshyn, Z. (1973) What the mind's eye tells the mind's brain, *Psychological Bulletin*, 80, 1–24.

Rummelhart, D. and Ortony, A. (1977) The representation of knowledge in memory, in R. Anderson, R. Spiro and W. Montague (eds), *Schooling and the Acquisition of Knowledge*, Erlbaum, New Jersey.

Schank, R. and Ableson, R. (1977) *Scripts, Plans, Goals and Understanding*, Erlbaum, New Jersey.

Schon, D. (1983) *The Reflective Practitioner: How Professionals Think in Action*, Basic Books, New York.

Selfridge, O. (1959) Pandemonium: a paradigm for learning, in *Mechanization of Thought Processes*, HMSO, London.

Smythe, M., Morris P., Levy, P. and Ellis, A. (1987) *Cognition in Action*, Earlbaum, London.

Thorndike, E. (1931) *Human Learning*, Appleton Century Crofts, New York.

Tulving, E. (1972) Episodic and semantic memory, in E. Tulving and W. Donaldson (eds), *Organization of Memory*, Academic Press, New York.

Watson, G. and Glaser, E. (1961) *Watson–Glaser Critical Thinking Appraisal*, Harcourt, Brace and World Inc., New York.

BEHAVIOURIST AND OTHER PERSPECTIVES ON TEACHING AND LEARNING

5

The first section of this chapter discusses behaviourism, one of the most influential approaches to the study of learning, and then considers a closely-related approach called social learning theory. The final section addresses a newer approach called synergogy, which claims to capitalize on the best features of both pedagogy and andragogy.

THE BEHAVIOURIST APPROACH TO LEARNING

John B. Watson is credited with the invention of the term *behaviourism*. The behaviourist approach to learning is often difficult to grasp initially because of the variety of alternative names used, and Table 5.1 gives an explanation of these.

Behaviourism	The central tenet of behaviourism is that explanations of learning must be based solely on observable behaviour.
Stimulus–response (SR) theory	Behaviourism states that learning is a result of an association between a stimulus and a response.
Association theory	Behaviourism states that learning is a result of an association between a stimulus and a response.
Contiguity theory	Behaviourism states that the behaviour and the reinforcement must be contiguous, i.e. reinforcement must occur immediately after the behaviour.

Table 5.1

Alternative terms used for behaviourism

The behaviourist approach identifies two forms of learning; classical conditioning and operant conditioning, the term 'conditioning' meaning the same as 'learning'.

CLASSICAL CONDITIONING: IVAN P. PAVLOV

Ivan P. Pavlov (1849–1936) was a Russian physiologist who, in the course of his work on digestive secretions, observed phenomena that are fundamental to stimulus–response theory (Pavlov, 1927). His main interest was the control of salivary and gastric secretions and by careful experimentation he established that salivation relies upon two kinds of stimulation. With the first kind, salivation was an unlearned, physiological reflex that occurred after food was introduced into the mouth of the animal. With the second type, salivation occurred when the animal merely caught sight of the food, i.e. before the food had actually entered its mouth.

This latter type intrigued Pavlov because he had observed over the course of his work that the dogs had begun to salivate immediately he entered his laboratory. Wondering whether this would occur to other stimuli, he paired a tone on a tuning fork with the immediate delivery of food to the dogs. This pairing was done on a number of occasions and at first the dogs only salivated when food was actually in the mouth, but eventually they salivated after the tone was sounded, but before food had entered the mouth. Pavlov considered that this salivation was a learned response as opposed to an innate reflex and termed the process 'conditioning'. Pavlovian conditioning has since been termed 'classical conditioning' to distinguish it from the other form of conditioning described by Skinner.

The vocabulary of conditioning requires some explanation, as it is fundamental to the behaviourist approach. In the experiments performed by Pavlov the first type of salivation was due to an inherent physiological reflex to the presence of food in the mouth of the dog. This is a natural or unconditioned situation, in which the food is said to be the unconditioned stimulus (US) and salivation the unconditioned response (UR). In the second phase of the experiment, the giving of food to the dog was paired with a tuning fork. After a number of such pairings, the tuning fork, which had previously been a neutral stimulus, now actually functioned as a stimulus for the flow of saliva. This is now a different situation and is called a conditioned situation, as the tuning fork is said to be the conditioned stimulus (CS) and salivation the conditioned response (CR). Although salivation is the response in both unconditioned and conditioned situations, it is considered that the latter response is a new one: hence the term 'conditioned response'. This response is so-called because it is conditional upon the presence of food. If the tuning fork had not been sounded at the same time that food was given to the dog, then the conditioned response of salivation would not occur. In other words, the conditioned stimulus (in this case a tuning fork) serves as a signal to the dog that the unconditioned stimulus (in this case food) is about to occur. Table 5.2 illustrates the sequence of events involved in classical conditioning.

Table 5.2

The process of classical conditioning

Before conditioning	US: presence of food	UR: salivation
During conditioning	US: presence of food in mouth, and CS: tuning fork	UR: salivation
After conditioning	CS: tuning fork (alone)	CR: salivation

US = unconditioned stimulus; UR = unconditioned response; CS = conditioned stimulus; CR = conditioned response.

Four further terms are used in connection with conditioning: extinction, generalization, discrimination and spontaneous recovery.

CLASSICAL CONDITIONING: JOHN B. WATSON

John B. Watson (1878–1958) graduated from the psychology school at the University of Chicago, where he had been trained in the skills of animal experimentation. Such experimentation was used to determine the mental qualities of the animals, but seldom led to much agreement among psychologists. Watson noted that observations on the animals' behaviour yielded far more objective data than did the deliberations concerning the animal's mental state. Watson's position can be summarized in three main statements:

1. Introspective methods have no place in the study of psychology.
2. Observations should be made only on the behaviour of an animal, since this was the object of study in the other scientific disciplines. The emphasis was to be on objective experimentation and replication of results, leaving no place for subjective inquiry.
3. Most behaviour is learned by making an association between a stimulus and a response, hence the term stimulus–response (SR) theory. Experiments in animals can be extrapolated to human beings, as the former differ only in their degree of complexity from man. Watson was convinced that even complex behaviour could be accounted for by this association of stimuli and response, and the publication of Pavlov's work on classical conditioning provided the confirmation he sought.

Watson became famous for his work with Rosalie Rayner on conditioned fear in humans (Watson and Rayner, 1920). By modern day standards their experiments seem ethically dubious although they believed no permanent harm would be done to the child. Their subject was a nine-month-old boy called Albert B. (Little Albert!) who showed no fear when presented with a range of stimuli, including a white rat. He did, however, show a fear reaction to a stimulus consisting of a loud noise which Watson made by striking a metal bar with a hammer behind the child. The conditioning process involved presenting the rat to the child, and when he reached towards it the metal bar was struck loudly behind him, causing him to startle and cry. After repeated pairings of the rat and the noise, presentation of the rat alone caused him to cry immediately and to crawl away rapidly. His fear of the rat showed generalization to other furry objects such as a rabbit and a dog. This demonstrated that the child had learned to be afraid of the rat through the process of classical conditioning; the sequence of events is shown in Table 5.3.

Before conditioning	US: loud noise from hammer striking metal bar	UR: fear response i.e. crying and withdrawal
During conditioning	US: loud noise, plus CS: white rat	UR: fear response
After conditioning	CS: white rat (alone)	CR: fear response

Table 5.3

Classical conditioning of fear in 'little Albert'

Classical conditioning, then, is a basic form of learning that pervades many aspects of daily life, and examples of conditioned reflexes are fear and anxiety.

OPERANT CONDITIONING: EDWARD L. THORNDIKE

The work of Edward L. Thorndike (1874–1949) was concerned with animal learning and in 1898 he formulated his law of effect. This was based on his work with cats in a 'puzzle box'. He confined a hungry cat in a puzzle box and placed food outside the box so that it was clearly visible to the animal. It was possible for the cat to escape from the box by clawing at a cord which released the door. Thorndike observed its behaviour and, in particular, the length of time taken to escape. Initially, the cat made various movements in an apparently random fashion, such as scratching at the door, until it succeeded by chance in escaping. It was allowed to eat the food and was then put back in the puzzle box and Thorndike observed that over a period of trials, the animal's movements became less and less random. It managed to open the door in a successively shorter time in each trial, until it eventually opened the door immediately it was placed inside.

The law of effect states that behaviour that results in success or reward is more likely to be repeated than behaviour that does not. Thorndike explained the importance of what he termed the satisfier in reinforcing behaviour. In the puzzle box, the cat was rewarded for the responses that led to escape (because those responses enabled it to obtain the food), whereas responses which did not lead to escape were gradually phased out.

Thorndike also formulated another law, called the law of exercise which states that knowledge of results must occur before the behaviour can be reinforced.

Thorndike's contribution to learning theory stems from this concept of reinforcement, in which he sees the reward acting as a positive reinforcer for the association between stimulus and response (Thorndike, 1911). This is now seen as a form of conditioning called operant conditioning, which was also developed independently by B.F. Skinner.

OPERANT CONDITIONING: B.F. SKINNER

B.F. Skinner has made an important contribution to the study of learning by his work on another form of conditioning called operant or instrumental conditioning (Skinner, 1938, 1969, 1971). He distinguishes between respondent behaviour and operant behaviour, the former being elicited by specific stimuli and the latter being emitted spontaneously by the organism, such as the random pecking behaviour of pigeons. Classical conditioning involves respondent behaviour, and has only limited relevance for the kinds of academic learning with which education is concerned. This is because the conditioned response can have no effect on the environment; in other words, the animal cannot control the events that occur. For example, the dog in Pavlov's experiments made a conditioned response of salivation, but this response in no way affected the speed of delivery of the food. Operant conditioning, on the other hand, operates on the environment and the learned behaviour is instrumental in controlling events.

The apparatus used for experiments in operant conditioning was the 'Skinner box', a kind of puzzle box containing something that the animal has to manipulate in order to obtain a reward. A great deal of Skinner's work was carried out using pigeons and in a typical experiment the hungry pigeon would be placed in a box containing an illuminated window. In a similar fashion to Thorndike's cat, the hungry bird strutted around in a random manner, pecking here and there until, by chance, it happened to peck at the illuminated window. Immediately, a pellet of food was delivered into a tray beneath the window and this was consumed by the bird. Random behaviour was then resumed until the pigeon happened to peck at the illuminated window again and was reinforced with another food pellet. After a number of trials, the random behaviour would cease, and the pigeon would peck at the window immediately it was put into the box. Skinner described the role of the food pellet as a reinforcer of behaviour, in that the window-pecking behaviour was followed by a food pellet that caused the behaviour to be repeated (to the exclusion of non-reinforced behaviour).

This operant conditioning is clearly different from classical conditioning, in that the pigeon's behaviour actually affects the environment by bringing about delivery of the food pellet. Skinner's view of operant conditioning is that it is not a sequence of stimulus–response connections, but rather that behaviour is spontaneously emitted by the organism. He tends to disregard the role of stimuli. There are four principles in operant conditioning: positive and negative reinforcement, punishment and omission of reinforcement, and these are defined in Table 5.4.

		Table 5.4
Positive reinforcement	This consists of the presentation of some kind of reward following a particular response. The rat is given a food pellet because it presses the lever. This increases the probability of occurrence of the response that precedes it.	Skinner's principles of operant conditioning
Negative reinforcement	In this case, the rat is subjected to an unpleasant stimulus, such as an electric shock, from which it can escape by making a particular response. Pressing the lever of the Skinner box will switch off the current, so the rat will press the lever to escape the unpleasant stimulus. Negative reinforcement increases the probability of occurrence of the response that precedes it.	
Punishment	Punishment differs from negative reinforcement in that the unpleasant stimulus occurs after the animal's response, whereas in the latter it occurs before. If the lever in the Skinner box is wired to deliver an electric shock when pressed, then the rate of the lever-pressing response by the rat will decrease. Punishment decreases the probability of occurrence of the response that precedes it.	
Omission of reinforcement	If the rat presses the lever but receives no reinforcement, the rate of response will diminish. This is similar to the case of classical conditioning, where absence of reinforcement will lead to the extinction of the response.	

Thus, the central tenet of Skinner's theory is the concept of reinforcement, which he considers to be the main factor in learning. He has done considerable research into patterns of reinforcement and their effects upon the response of the animal and this has led to the concept of 'schedules of reinforcement'. Skinner has classified these schedules into two main types, continuous and intermittent. In the former type, every response by the animal is reinforced, whereas in the latter only some of the responses are. Intermittent reinforcement can be subdivided into:

1. ratio schedules, which are determined by the rate of the animal's response; and
2. interval schedules, which are determined by the time factor.

In addition, each of these subdivisions may be fixed or variable, giving four possible schedules of intermittent reinforcement, as shown in Table 5.5.

Table 5.5 Schedules of reinforcement	1. Fixed interval schedule, where the responses are reinforced at a regular interval of time, e.g. every two minutes 2. Variable interval schedule, where reinforcement is given at varying intervals of time, some short, others long 3. Fixed ratio, where reinforcement is given after a set number of responses, such as every tenth response 4. Variable ratio, where reinforcement is given after varying numbers of responses, e.g. ten, and then four, and then one

The importance of these schedules lies in the different rates of response that they produce, ratio schedules giving higher rates than interval ones. This can be explained in terms of the animal's influence over the reinforcement, in that the ratio schedule gives the animal the chance to speed up its response so that reinforcement occurs more often. On an interval schedule, the rate of response has no effect on the delivery because reinforcement is dependent on the passage of time. Variable ratio schedules bring about the consistently highest response rates, and the ones most resistant to extinction.

'Shaping' is another concept that Skinner has developed in relation to animal behaviour. Shaping implies the incorporation of novel behaviours, which are not part of the animal's natural responses, into its behavioural repertoire. He trained pigeons to play table tennis by selective reinforcement of the desired behaviours and this involved, in the first instance, reinforcing the bird when it approached the ball. Reinforcement is then given to successive approximations to the desired table-tennis-playing behaviour, such as pecking at the ball, knocking it over the net and finally, getting it into the opponent's trough.

Animals can be trained to perform complex skills by the use of shaping techniques, but Skinner believes that human behaviour is largely reinforced not by primary reinforcers such as food or drink, but by secondary reinforcers such as money and prestige. The effectiveness of secondary reinforcement is well illustrated by behaviour modification techniques that use a token economy in learning disability nursing. Patients can be helped to become independent by the selective reinforcement of desired behaviours such as washing and dressing, or can be conditioned to modify problem behaviour. Reinforcement in the form of tokens is given for appropriate behaviours, and these can be exchanged for food, cigarettes or other material goods.

IMPLICATIONS FOR TEACHING AND LEARNING

Behavioural objectives

Another educational application of S–R theory is the behavioural objectives approach. This is an approach to curriculum design which emphasizes the detailed prescription of learning objectives by the educational institution. These objectives must be stated in terms of the observable and measurable behaviours of learners, and the model thus enshrines the principles of behaviourism as defined by Watson. Behavioural objectives are discussed in detail in Chapter 6 (p. 137).

Programmed learning (programmed instruction)

Programmed learning is based upon behaviourist psychology and the fundamental notions are those of reinforcement and 'chaining'. Programmed learning requires specially prepared materials, which students use for individual study of particular topics. There are two kinds of programme, linear and branching, which differ in a number of respects from each other.

Linear programmes

This kind of programme was devised by B.F. Skinner and consists of a series of closely linked boxes of information called 'frames'. The students are presented with information in frames and are required to supply a missing word at the end of each frame; they can check whether their answer is correct or not before going on to the next frame. The linear programme thus offers information in very small steps, with immediate reinforcement in the form of feedback of correct answers. Each frame is designed to contain material that overlaps with the previous frame as well as the succeeding one, forming a chain of stimulus–response connections. Since it is correct answers that are reinforcing, errors are reduced to a minimum by careful piloting of the programme prior to production.

Branching programmes

In contrast to linear programmes, these provide the student with a series of choices rather than allowing the student to supply missing words. In this multiple-choice situation, the student is required to select the answer to a question raised in each frame from a choice of answers supplied. When an answer has been selected, the student is directed to a particular frame, depending on whether the student was correct or not; if the answer was incorrect, the student will be directed to a frame that gives remedial information. It can be seen that this kind of programme has a series of branches that the student follows in his or her progress through the programme, the slower students taking in more branches than the brighter ones.

Programmed learning can take the form of printed texts such as books, or electronic machines that contain a window and a series of buttons for choosing responses, or computer programs. Branching programmes are rather cumbersome when used in book form, since the reader has to move backwards and forwards through the book in order to follow the branching frames. Students tend to like the programmed-learning format, particularly for topics with largely factual material; the careful formulation of goals for the student and the small steps in learning make it a useful, if sometimes boring, way of studying.

Mastery learning

Mastery learning is another approach that is based on a behavioural objectives model. The method was devised by Benjamin Bloom (1968) and is premised on the assumption that all tasks can be learned by students provided they are given sufficient time. This key notion of the time taken to learn a task forms the basis for a sequence of instruction called 'mastery learning'. The amount of time taken to learn a task is seen as being dependent on a number of variables:

1. the complexity of the task;
2. the student's aptitude and experience;
3. the ability to understand the material;
4. their perseverance; and
5. the quality of instruction.

Mastery learning takes the view that individual differences in the achievement of students are not inevitable and the sequence is designed to ensure that virtually every student will reach the same level of achievement, i.e. mastery level or grade A. The sequence for mastery learning is given in Table 5.6.

Table 5.6

Sequence for mastery learning

1. The subject or topic is divided up into a number of units, each of one or two weeks duration
2. Learning objectives are prescribed for each of the units
3. The subject-matter of the unit is taught
4. Formative tests are administered at the end of the unit and are used to identify the successful and unsuccessful students
5. If students do not achieve mastery, then remedial teaching is given
6. When a student has completed all the units, a summative test is given to test mastery of the course, which equals a grade A

Mastery learning has spread to a wide range of classes and subjects in education and a number of adaptations have emerged. Mastery learning can be used for competency-based learning, humanities and self-development and it aims to create equality in society by making it possible for all students to attain excellence

There are, however, a number of criticisms of mastery learning, in particular, its use of specific behavioural objectives and the increased amount of time and resources required for its implementation.

General applications of behaviourism

Classical conditioning is confined to lower-order learning such as a conditioned fear response. However, this may still influence adult learning, as in the case of a student nurse who fears written examinations because in the past he or she has been humiliated by school teachers when his or her performance has been poor, thus setting up a conditioned fear of examinations. Even though such an experience may have been long ago, it can still be a very powerful emotion. However, the good news is that conditioned reflexes occur for positive feelings as well as negative, and the learned associations between pleasurable events and feelings can serve to make students enjoy the experience of learning.

One application of classical conditioning that has been used in education is systematic desensitization, a commonly used technique for treating phobias such as fear of spiders or heights. A nurse teacher may encounter a student who has learned a conditioned fear response to participating in small-group discussion or seminar, perhaps due to humiliation in the past. The student could be taught relaxation to counter the effects of anxiety and then the particular stimulus that is causing the fear can be presented in a hierarchy of contact. Having first been taught relaxation, the student would then go through the problem situation in a series of small steps, beginning with discussions with one or two other students only, gradually building up to a full group size. However, such intervention may be considered to be beyond the competence of a nurse teacher, and systematic desensitization may be more appropriately carried out by a behavioural therapist.

Another way in which students may be helped by classical conditioning is by the prevention of negative conditioning situations in the first place. Hence, when student nurses are first introduced to the clinical setting, a concerted effort should be made to make them associate the visit with such positive events as a warm welcome, a sense of *esprit de corps* and a general air of interest and helpfulness.

Operant conditioning offers a greater range of educational applications than classical conditioning. In operant conditioning, reinforcement is a fundamental principle and can be used as feedback on learner performance. Knowledge of success is said to act as a reinforcer of behaviour, so it is important to give immediate feedback on performance, in both clinical and classroom settings. The use of praise may be reinforcing, since it acts as a reward, but it is important to vary the type of reinforcement given, so that the behaviour is maintained. This is more difficult than it sounds, for the teacher may appear insincere if he or she thinks too much about the way to respond, e.g. smiling, nodding, praising and the like.

A variable-ratio type of reinforcement produces the highest response rate, so when learning a new response the student should be given reinforcement at frequent intervals and as performance improves, less frequently, until eventually only really good performances are reinforced.

A fixed-interval schedule of reinforcement may be effective when given following periodic tests, or by feedback during daily ward reports. As indicated earlier, behaviour modification is a well-tried technique in clinical psychology, where selective reinforcement is used to shape acceptable behaviours in patients/clients. It has been suggested that teachers may use it in class to encourage acceptable behaviours and to discourage negative ones. If the nurse teacher wishes to shape student nurses to answer questions in class, he or she may praise the students each time they answer a question, regardless of whether or not their answer is correct. Gradually the teacher will begin to praise the students only when the answer is correct. Extinction can be applied to unwanted behaviour such as dominating a lesson or discussion, or coming into class late. If the teacher ignores these behaviours, they may undergo extinction, rather than being reinforced by having attention drawn to them.

CRITIQUE OF BEHAVIOURISM

Stimulus–response theories of learning have come in for a great deal of criticism over the years. For example, Skinner's laboratory experiments seem to have little ecological validity when generalized to human beings, i.e. they ignore the importance of human relationships and the social context in which behaviours occur. It is also difficult to see how stimulus–response connections can account for the infinitely complex skills of language. Another difficulty arises when attempting to use S–R theory to explain how individuals learn by imitating the behaviour of other people. Humanistic psychologists find S–R theory distasteful, as it makes man merely a puppet, the passive recipient of external forces. In addition, the application of reinforcement theory may lead to a situation where the learner will only consider doing something if there is a reward associated with it, i.e. a 'what's in it for me?' attitude. Another objection concerns the ethical issues surrounding the manipulation of human behaviour, in particular the problem of who has the right to control and manipulate another individual's behaviour.

SOCIAL LEARNING THEORY (OBSERVATIONAL LEARNING THEORY)

Social learning theory has its roots in behaviourism, and while the basic tenets of behaviourism such as reinforcement are still retained in social learning theory, there is an emphasis on cognitive processes and also on social learning. *Social learning* is also termed *observational learning* and *vicarious learning*, and occurs when an individual learns something by observing another person doing it, in other words it is learning by modelling. According to social learning theory, behaviour is seen as a two-way interaction between an individual and his or her environment, that is, both 'people and their environments are reciprocal determinants of each other' (Bandura, 1977, 1986). Exponents of this theory view the behaviourist approach to learning as one that limits the idea of the potential of individuals and their influence over their own behaviour. According to social learning theory, an individual possesses no inherent behaviour patterns at birth other than reflexes, so must learn everything else. Such learning occurs as a result of observing the behaviour of other people, which allows complex patterns to be acquired in a more efficient way than trial and error. Indeed, some behaviours such as language can only be learned, according to Bandura, by observation of human models, as it is highly unlikely that mere reinforcement of random vocalization would lead to the complex use of speech that forms the everyday language of an individual.

Learning, then, is envisaged as behaviour acquired by observation of modelling stimuli, providing the learner with a symbolic image of such behaviour, which may serve as a guide. Bandura identifies four processes involved in the observational learning situation: attention, retention, motor reproduction and motivational processes:

1. *Attentional processes*. These processes are concerned with the characteristics of the model and of the observer. In the former, some of the factors which influence learning are variables such as:
   (a) interpersonal attraction between the model and the observer;
   (b) the usefulness of the observed behaviour; and
   (c) the distinctiveness, complexity and frequency of contact with the modelled stimuli.
   Observer characteristics comprise the level of arousal, capacity to process information, the perceptual set and the amount of previous reinforcement.
2. *Retention processes*. It is obviously important to remember the modelled behaviour if one is to learn from it, so the role of such strategies as rehearsal is crucial. The highest level of learning is achieved when the modelled behaviour is first organized and symbolically rehearsed before actually performing the behaviour.
3. *Motor reproduction processes*. The learner must be capable of actually carrying out the observed behaviour and of evaluating it in terms of accuracy.
4. *Motivational processes*. Modelled stimuli are more likely to be learned if the observer sees some value in them, but the role of reinforcement in social learning theory is one of facilitation rather than necessity. It may take the form of external reward (such as money) or self-reinforcement, where the learners reward themselves with something when a predetermined behaviour has been achieved. For example, a person may set a number of personal objectives to achieve for a course and, having attained them, may choose to go out to dinner as a reward. The likelihood

of the modelled behaviour being learned is increased when the observer sees the model being reinforced for performing that behaviour. This is termed vicarious reinforcement.

Information can be transmitted by the model in a variety of ways, such as an actual physical demonstration, by pictures, words and the mass media. Abstract modelling is the term used for the process whereby the observer elicits the principles of behaviour from a variety of modelled stimuli and applies them to a situation similar to the ones which were observed. Thus, observation of various models performing a nursing procedure would allow the observer to learn the rules of the procedure and these could then be applied to similar situations.

How does social learning theory explain the development of novel or creative responses? Bandura sees the novel response as a utilization of the qualities of many models, to produce a new creative behaviour. There are a number of characteristics of both the model and the observer that make learning more likely. Experiments indicate that persons who possess status, prestige and power are more effective models for those kind of behaviours. Individuals who are lacking in self-esteem and confidence and those who are dependent tend to be more easily influenced by the behaviours of models who are obviously successful. However, one needs to interpret such results with caution, as many confident people readily adopt behaviour of those whose actions are seen to be of value.

IMPLICATIONS FOR TEACHING AND LEARNING

Observational learning is potentially a powerful tool for the nurse teacher in a wide range of applications. One of the important early aspects of nursing which a new student must acquire is that of the professional role and this can be fostered by allowing the student to observe a prestigious trained nurse going about her daily work. The student will be able to observe not only clinical skills, but interactions with patients and other members of the health care team, thus learning about professional attitudes as well as techniques. In an early study of modelling in nurse education, Kramer (1972) took students into the clinical areas and had them work in the vicinity, but not actually attached to her. The students thus had the opportunity to see her inter-acting with patients and giving care, and she acted as a model for their observational learning.

In a British study in an elderly care setting, Raichura and Riley (1985) used modelling as a strategy for teaching trained staff about care of the elderly. The nurse teacher must also act as a professional model when with students, showing enthusiasm about nursing and the ability to do the job skilfully. A good role model must also be a good practi-tioner if students are to learn the correct roles. It is a useful idea when working with student groups to pair the students so that the weaker ones are working with the more able students and learning by observa-tion. The teacher should ensure that the more able students are given responsibility, since these high-status students are more likely to serve as models for the others.

SYNERGOGY

It has been claimed that the traditional model of pedagogy has a number of serious weaknesses when applied to adult students in nursing. It fosters dependence in the learner by its reinforcement of the passive role in learning and it may reduce motivation by causing resentment or hostility among adult students. Andragogy, on the other hand, does rely very much on the students' previous knowledge as well as on the key role of the facilitator. Synergogy attempts to capitalize on the best features of both pedagogy and andragogy by making use of expert knowledge, whilst at the same time, encouraging active involvement of the student. Synergogy is 'a systematic approach to learning in which the members of small teams learn from one another through structured interactions' (Mouton and Blake, 1984). It has four fundamental differences from other approaches:

1. It uses learning materials managed by a learning administrator rather than having a teacher who might be seen as an authority figure.
2. Students have responsibility for their own learning through active involvement with other students.
3. It rests on the premise that learning that arises from teamwork is greater than that done by the individual alone, i.e. the principle of synergy.
4. The planned interaction with colleagues acts as a motivator for learning.

Educational success is promoted by three principles that underpin synergogy. The first involves the use of learning materials that serve to give the students direction without inhibiting their self-development. The second principle is that of teamwork. Synergogy relies on teamwork and the authors emphasize the difference between teamwork and group work, the former involving a learning team with clear goals, learning tasks and outcomes as well as procedures for enhancing team effectiveness. The third principle is that of synergy, in which the whole is greater than the sum of its parts. In contrast to ordinary group discussion, synergogy ensures the systematic sharing of knowledge, with its consequent implications for each student's growth and development.

Synergogy can be applied to the learning of knowledge, skills and attitudes and there are four designs for learning:

- team-effectiveness design (TED);
- team-member teaching design (TMTD);
- performance judging design (PJD); and
- clarifying-attitudes design (CAD).

Each is now considered, in turn.

Team-effectiveness design (TED)

This design is concerned with the domain of knowledge and utilizes teamwork to facilitate learning from each other within a team of students. The team-effectiveness design might be chosen as a revision aid, with the following sequence of segments.

Individual preparation by students

The total group of students is first divided into teams of five or six students. All students are then given the same material to be studied on an individual basis and this may consist of a learning package extract or other material. Each student then completes the test, which is at the end of the study material and is usually a multiple-choice type test.

Teamwork

In this segment, each team must discuss the questions and decide which answers are the best in terms of what the text material contained. A time limit is imposed on this discussion, after which the answer-key is distributed and each team member marks his or her own test. The teams' negotiated answers are also compared with the key and if the teamwork was effective, one would expect that the team score would be better than that of any one individual.

Interpretation of scores

The efficiency of any team's score is decided by checking it against the average individual score, a higher team score is positive and a lower team score is negative.

Critique of teamwork

In this segment, the teams evaluate how well they functioned as a team in relation to the test.

Evaluation of individual progress

Students may take the test or an alternative form of the test at a later date to see how well they have retained the information.

Thus, the team-effectiveness design offers a system in which students can check their understanding of written materials by comparing it and discussing it with their team members.

Team-member teaching design (TMTD)

This design is also concerned with acquisition of knowledge and consists of each member of a team learning a portion of study material and teaching it to the other members. During the teaching presentation, each successive portion is taught by the particular student responsible for it and other students can then see how their portion fits in with the whole. The sequence is as follows.

Individual preparation by students

The selection of material to be learned by each member must be of approximately the same length and capable of being understood on its own, without reference to the other portions.

Team-member teaching

Each team member then teaches their portion of the material, following a logical sequence in the order of presentations. Other team members can take notes or ask questions in order to clarify their understanding of the material. After summarizing the material, each team member takes a test on the whole of the material and the individual scores are calculated using the answer key.

Interpretation of scores

Each team member's score gives an indication of their understanding of each of the portions of the material. The team's average individual score shows how the group as a whole has understood the material and students can see by their own scores for their particular teaching portion how well they prepared for the task.

Critique of teamwork

This involves not only assessing each member's teaching ability, but also the team's use of questions and discussion.

Performance judging design (PJD)

This particular design focuses on the acquisition of psychomotor skills and is therefore of great potential use to nurse teachers. The design gives each team member responsibility for other members' skill development and also for developing criteria by which their own and other students' performances can be evaluated.

Individual performance by students

Students are given a task to work on individually, which will demonstrate their current level of the skill in question. This might take the form of a videotape of each student nurse taking someone's temperature by the oral method, so that there will be approximately five recordings of nurses taking temperatures for each team to consider.

Teamwork

There are two main aspects to this segment of the design. Firstly, the team meets to decide which criteria should be used to judge effectiveness in taking a temperature orally. They are then given external criteria devised by experts to discuss and to compare with their own criteria, and eventually they have to decide upon a series of criteria that will serve as a basis for evaluating the effectiveness of their team members' performances.

Judging performance

Each team member takes one of the examples of performance, i.e. one videotape of another team member and presents it to the rest of the team for comparison with the established criteria. This critique of each member's performance is written down and given to the member in question, so as to have a record of the feedback comments.

Evaluation of progress and upgrading of skills

In this segment, each team member is given something comparable to perform individually and each is required to use the previously agreed criteria when performing the task. It may be that the students are asked to take a temperature by the *axillary* method whilst being videotaped and the same process of team evaluation is repeated. Hence, there is a constant cycle of additional performances that can be used to increase the level of skill amongst the team members in all aspects of nursing.

Critique of teamwork

Here, team members discuss the effectiveness of the teamwork as in previous designs.

Clarifying-attitudes design (CAD)

This final design, as the name implies, is concerned with attitudes, particularly with those in the public domain. In nursing, attitudes are a legitimate area for educational exploration, particularly in such controversial fields as abortion and acquired immune deficiency syndrome (AIDS). This design is used to help individuals to develop awareness of their own attitudes and also to become sensitive to the alternative attitudes that may exist.

Individual preparation by students

In this segment, the individual student first composes a statement of his or her own attitude towards the topic in question and then completes an attitude questionnaire which involves ranking a number of alternative attitude statements. The attitude statement that corresponds most closely to the written statement made by the student at the beginning is noted.

Teamwork

The team then attempts to rank the same items on the basis of which is most sound, or most valid, and to come to a consensus of opinion about the order of ranking. This encourages discussion and questioning of individual reasoning and may well expose the basis for holding such an attitude. The difference between the agreed attitudes and the ranking of the individual members can also be examined and ways in which behaviour may be changed can be explored.

Developing a shared norm of conduct

Each of the team's rankings is shared with other teams within the total group of students and any differences are discussed. It may be necessary to form new teams if the differences persist, until a shared norm exists.

Individual re-ranking of attitudes
Each team member then re-ranks the alternatives, comparing this to the original ranking.

Critique of changes in attitudes
This may be an optional part of the design and involves an exploration of how each member's attitudes have changed as a result of the discussion.

Critique of teamwork
This is the same procedure as in the other designs.

IMPLICATIONS FOR TEACHING AND LEARNING

The four fundamental designs outlined above constitute the system of synergogy, but it is important to look at the role of the learning administrator. This role is very different from that normally seen in education, in that the administrator is neither facilitator nor subject expert. Their function is to carry out four key roles with regard to the organization of synergogy, one of which is to create the teams in which students will work. This requires decisions about the mix of abilities and experience of students, the numbers in any one team and other such aspects of team formation. Another function is to ensure that team interaction is effective, by intervening when procedural difficulties arise; these may be in-fighting, dominance by a single member and other counter-productive behaviours. The learning administrator is also responsible for providing support for individual students in a variety of situations, such as difficulties with materials, presentations, absenteeism and so on. He or she is also responsible for arranging meetings with specific subject-matter consultants, should this be felt to be beneficial for a team.

It is important at this point to address some of the drawbacks associated with its use. As with any type of medium for educational use, the planning and development can be time-consuming and expensive. Teachers may not feel at ease using a method that places responsibility upon the students, particularly one that may seem to reduce the skills of the teacher to those of an administrator of learning. Students themselves may not be happy with a method that makes them take responsibility for their own progress, particularly as it involves openness and honesty in a group setting.

Bandura, A. (1977) *Social Learning Theory*, Prentice Hall, Englewood Cliffs, NJ.
Bandura, A. (1986) *Social Foundations of Thought and Action: A Social-Cognitive Theory*, Prentice Hall, Englewood Cliffs, NJ.
Bloom, B. (1968) Learning for mastery, *Evaluation Comment*, 1(2). Center for

the study of evaluation of instructional programs, University of California, Los Angeles.

Kramer, M. (1972) The concept of modelling as a teaching strategy, *Nursing Forum*, XI, 59.

Mouton, J. and Blake, R. (1984) *Synergogy: A New Strategy for Education, Training and Development*, Jossey Bass, San Francisco.

Pavlov, I. (1927) *Conditioned Reflexes*, Oxford University Press, Oxford.

Raichura, L. and Riley, M. (1985) Introducing nurse preceptors, *Nursing Times*, Nov 20.

Skinner, B.F. (1938) *The Behaviour of Organisms*, Appleton Century Crofts, New York.

Skinner, B.F. (1969) *Contingencies of Reinforcement: A Theoretical Analysis*, Appleton Century Crofts, New York.

Skinner, B.F. (1971) *Beyond Freedom and Dignity*, Alfred Knopf, New York.

Thorndike, E.L. (1911) *Animal Intelligence: Experimental Studies*, Macmillan, New York.

Watson, J. and Rayner, R. (1920) Conditioned emotional reactions, *Journal of Experimental Psychology*, 3, 1–14.

PART TWO

ORGANIZING, DELIVERING AND EVALUATING TEACHING AND LEARNING

CURRICULUM THEORY AND PRACTICE

6

The term *curriculum* is used to describe a plan or design upon which educational provision is based; it is the single most important concept in educational delivery, encompassing all the activities normally included under the umbrella terms *education* and *training* (Quinn, 1994). Educational provision in nursing takes a variety of forms, from short in-house programmes through to longer formal programmes leading to academic awards.

The two main categories in nursing are pre-registration and post-registration education. The former consists of programmes leading to both an academic award, such as a Bachelor of Nursing degree, and entry to the register of nurses. Post-registration provision, on the other hand, is much more diverse and includes the following:

1. in-house study days for qualified staff, e.g. intravenous drug administration;
2. discrete modules (courses) for continuing professional development, e.g. clinical supervision;
3. programmes leading to academic awards such as first degrees and higher degrees.

Within the higher education sector there are a number of terms used to describe the formal process of study undertaken by a student under the auspices of a higher education institution, depending upon the academic information system in use in a given institution. A guide to current terminology of the Banner academic information system used within the University of Greenwich is given in Table 6.1.

Definition	Previous name(s)	Latest name(s)
A period of formal study leading to an academic award	Course; pathway	Programme
A self-contained sub-component of a programme	Module; unit	Course

Table 6.1

Higher education terminology relating to courses

Hence, what the person in the street would call a 'course' is now termed a *programme*, and the sub-components are termed *courses* rather than modules or units. For the sake of consistency, the latest terminology will be used throughout this chapter.

THE NATURE OF CURRICULUM

Curriculum theory is an established field of study within education, but examination of the literature reveals that the concept is by no means straightforward. There is wide variation between definitions and a number of writers – Lewis and Miel (1972), Tanner and Tanner (1980), Saylor *et al.*, (1981) – have attempted to categorize these. Four main interpretations of the concept emerge:

1. *Curriculum as objectives.* '*Any statement of the objectives of the school should be a statement of changes to take place in students' (Tyler, 1949).*
2. *Curriculum as subject-matter.* '*A curriculum is the offering of socially valued knowledge, skills and attitudes made available to students through a variety of arrangements during the time they are at school, college or university' (Bell, 1973).*
3. *Curriculum as student experiences.* '*Curriculum is all the learning which is planned and guided by the school whether it is carried on in groups or individually, inside or outside the school' (Kerr, 1968).*
4. *Curriculum as opportunities for students.* '*A curriculum is all the educational opportunities encountered by students as a direct result of their involvement with an educational institution' (Quinn, 1988).*

Skilbeck's (1984) categorization has considerable overlap with the above, but additionally the aspect of culture is introduced:

1. curriculum as a structure of forms and fields of knowledge;
2. curriculum as a chart or map of the culture;
3. curriculum as a pattern of learning activities;
4. curriculum as a learning technology.

This categorization has been adapted by Beattie (1987) in his fourfold model of curriculum, described later in this chapter. Other writers – Stenhouse (1975), Saylor *et al.*, (1981) – take a more generic view of the concept, seeing it as an overall plan or design for learning:

'*Curriculum is an attempt to communicate the essential principles and features of an educational proposal in such a form that it is open to critical scrutiny and capable of effective translation into practice' (Stenhouse, 1975).*

'*Curriculum is a plan for providing sets of learning opportunities for persons to be educated' (Saylor* et al., *1981).*

'*Curriculum refers to the learning experiences of students, in so far as they are expressed or anticipated in educational goals and objectives, plans and designs for learning and the implementation of these plans and designs in school environments' (Skilbeck, 1984).*

Quinn (1994) offers a definition based upon the principal components of the concept:

'A curriculum is a plan or design for education and training that addresses the following questions:

1. **Who** *is to be taught? Who will learn? This is the* consumer of the curriculum, *i.e. the student, course member, colleague, etc., who will experience the curriculum.*
2. **What** *is to be taught and/or learned? This is about both the* intentions *and the* content of the curriculum. *Intentions may or may not be stated overtly, according to the education ideology underpinning the curriculum. Where outcomes, goals, or objectives are overtly expressed, these statements also indicate to some extent the nature of the curriculum content. If the intentions are covert, then content is usually indicated by a list of topics in a syllabus.*
3. **Why** *is it to be taught and/or learned? This is the* ideology of the curriculum, *i.e. the beliefs and values that underpin the curriculum approach.*
4. **How** *is it to be taught and/or learned? This is the* process of education, *i.e. the teaching, learning and assessment approaches or opportunities available to the consumer.*
5. **Where** *is it to be taught/learned? This is the* context of the curriculum, *i.e. the faculty, department, school, college, campus, rooms, etc. It also refers to the place of a given curriculum within the range of awards of the education provider institution.*
6. **When** *is it to be taught and/or learned? This is the* programming/timetabling *of the curriculum, i.e. the length, pattern of attendance, etc.'*

The concept of curriculum has been further subdivided by some commentators and the more common ones are as follows:

1. *official curriculum*, the curriculum laid down in the policy of the institution;
2. *actual curriculum*, the curriculum as implemented by teachers;
3. *hidden curriculum*, the attitudes and values transmitted by the teachers.

Curriculum terminology

Understanding of curriculum theory is not made any easier by the plethora of terminology used within the literature. Three key concepts in common use are outlined below.

Curriculum theory

The purpose of theory is to try to understand and explain phenomena, and curriculum theory attempts to relate educational scholarship to pragmatic everyday aspects of educational practice. Theories provide a rationale for making decisions about the curriculum and can be thought of as having a basic structure. The basic building blocks are 'concepts' and these can be defined as classes of objects, events or situations that possess common properties. Concepts are not specific entities, rather they are mental constructs with which we make sense of the environment. We are able to classify most things we encounter instantaneously, because we compare the specific stimulus with our concepts to see where it fits most easily. If the specific stimulus fits into a concept category, it can be confidently classified as a member of the concept and this process means that the individual can very quickly make sense of the myriad of stimuli impinging upon his or her senses every day.

Concepts are thus the basic building blocks of theory, and can be developed either deductively or inductively; deduction is the making of inferences from something already known, such as the development of a theory from an existing theory in another discipline. Induction is the making of inferences from data that has been gathered. In curriculum studies, theories are often expressed as models of curriculum, the terms being used interchangeably.

Curriculum model

A model is a physical or conceptual representation of something; physical models are replicas of objects, and may be actual size or built to scale. Curriculum models are conceptual models, i.e. simplified representations of reality in graphic, mathematical or symbolic form. Models of curriculum help to clarify thinking about the nature of curriculum and a number of models have become well established within the literature. These are discussed in detail later in this chapter.

Curriculum ideology

A nurse teacher's concept of the curriculum is shaped by the system of beliefs and values held about education; in other words, the educational ideology to which he or she subscribes.

CURRICULUM IDEOLOGIES

A number of such educational ideologies have been identified (e.g. Davies, 1969; Scrimshaw, 1983), each with its own adherents who share common values and beliefs about the educational enterprise, and whose views may conflict with those of adherents to other ideologies. The essential features of the prevailing curriculum ideologies are outlined below.

Conservative/classical humanism

These ideologies focus on the nation, and view education as the transmission of the cultural heritage of a nation, and key values are stability and a sense of continuity with the past. Curricula are differentiated for the elite and the non-elite and the curriculum is subject-centred and teacher-dominated. Motivation is extrinsic, with an emphasis on discipline.

Democratic/liberal humanism

The emphasis here is on the role of education in the creation of a common democratic culture, with educational opportunity for all. Key values are quality, relevance and lifelong education. Curricula are common core and teacher–pupil negotiation features as a teaching strategy.

Romantic/progressivism

These ideologies see education as meeting the needs, aspirations and personal growth of the individual. They emphasize the process of learning by experience, group discovery, and mutual dialogue between teacher and pupil.

Revisionist/instrumentalism

In these utilitarian ideologies, education must be relevant to the economic and social needs of society by producing a skilled workforce. Vocational relevance is a key principle of curricula and the teaching of science and technology is emphasized. Scrimshaw (1983) further subdivides instrumentalism into traditional and adaptive: the former concerned with the learning of specific vocational skills, while the latter aims to equip the learner to be adaptable to the changing needs of society.

Reconstructionism

This ideology sees education as means of bringing about social change through analysis, discussion and reconstruction of social issues. The key teaching approach is small-group methods. The above review of ideologies portrays them as mutually incompatible, but in practice elements are often combined to meet the needs of a given curriculum design. For example, curricula for health care professionals are by their very nature instrumental in ideology, in that their purpose is to produce a skilled professional workforce. However, they also reflect a progressive ideology in their emphasis on the personal and professional growth of the individual and by the adoption of such strategies as student/teacher negotiation and learning by experience.

COMPONENTS OF CURRICULUM

The term *curriculum* encompasses four main aspects of educational provision, as shown in Figure 6.1. These four components are intimately related to each other and the model adopts a rational stance, in that the curriculum design is seen to begin with the formulating of student learning outcomes, and then progresses to decisions about what outcomes-related subject-matter should be included. Teaching and learning processes are then defined, e.g. lectures, laboratory work, etc., that will help the student to achieve the learning outcomes, and finally,

Figure 6.1

Components of curriculum

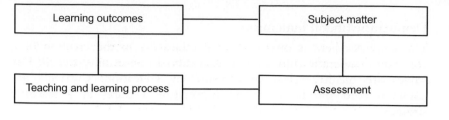

the students achievement of the learning outcomes is assessed using appropriate and relevant assessment methods.

MODELS AND THE CURRICULUM

A model is a physical or conceptual representation of something; physical models are replicas of the things they represent and may be actual size or built to scale. Architects and town planners build scale models of civic developments that aim to show, in miniature, a replica of houses and commercial properties that are to be built. In colleges of nursing, students are encouraged to examine models of the organs of the body so as to understand the structure. Other kinds of model do not represent concrete entities, but concepts. Such conceptual models are usually in graphic or mathematical form and attempt to represent abstract concepts.

The term *model* is used in a variety of ways in relation to curriculum, and there is often confusion between them. There are four main types of model used in curriculum design and development:

1. *Curriculum models.* These attempt to represent the nature of curriculum, and reflect the philosophical stance of the originator, e.g. the behavioural objectives model.
2. *Models of learning.* These attempt to represent the nature of learning, and reflect the philosophical or psychological stance of the originator, e.g. Carl Rogers' humanistic approach.
3. *Models of teaching.* These attempt to represent the nature of teaching, and reflect different philosophical beliefs about the nature of the process, e.g. the transmission model of teaching.
4. *Nursing models.* These attempt to represent the nature of nursing, and reflect the philosophical stance of the originator, e.g. the Roper, Logan, and Tierney model of activities of living.

A given curriculum document may well utilize models from more than one of the above categories. For example, a curriculum for pre-registration nursing might utilize the Stenhouse model of curriculum as an over-arching model, but include Knowles' andragogy approach as a teaching and learning strategy, and the Roper, Logan, Tierney model for nursing theory and practice.

Models of learning are addressed in Part 1 of this book; the other three types of model are discussed below.

CURRICULUM MODELS

A wide range of models exist which attempt to encapsulate the nature of curriculum, each reflecting the particular ideological stance of the author. Four of the better-known models are described below.

Behavioural objectives (product) model of curriculum

Although having its origins in certain writings at the turn of the century, this model is usually ascribed to Ralph Tyler. In his book *Basic Principles of Curriculum and Instruction*, Tyler (1949) articulated a rationale for effective curriculum, viewing education as 'a process of changing the behaviour patterns of people, using behaviour in the broad sense to include thinking and feeling as well as overt action' (Tyler, 1949, p. 5). He identifies four fundamental questions to be answered in developing a curriculum (1949, p.1):

1. What educational purposes should the school seek to attain?
2. How can learning experiences be selected that are likely to be useful in attaining these objectives?
3. How can learning experiences be organized for effective instruction?
4. How can the effectiveness of learning experiences be evaluated?

This notion of rational curriculum planning was taken up by a number of writers and led to the generic model of curriculum as consisting of four main components; objectives, content, method and evaluation. Hence, the emphasis on this model is on the achievement of objectives by the student. In other words, it is an output model. Tyler stressed the importance of stating objectives in terms of student behaviours: 'any statement of the objectives of the school should be a statement of changes to take place in students' (Tyler, 1949, p. 44). This emphasis on student behaviours was taken up by other proponents of the model and led to a move to limit behavioural objectives to observable, measurable changes in behaviour, leaving no room for such things as 'understanding' or 'appreciation'. The behavioural objectives model has influenced education throughout the world; indeed, in 1977 the then General Nursing Council for England and Wales (1977) issued a circular which espoused the behavioural objectives model for nursing curricula and by the early 1980s, such objectives were almost universally applied in both classroom and clinical settings.

Educational goal statements

There is no universally accepted terminology with regard to the formulation of educational goals, but the following guide may serve to clarify the concepts involved.

Educational aim

An aim is a broad, general statement of goal direction, which contains reference to the worthwhileness of achieving it. The educational aim is the most important part of the goal system, since all the other objectives are derived from it. The following is an example of an educational aim in nursing: 'Understands the nature of malignant disease, so that she may perform skilled nursing care of the patient with such disease'. This statement gives a very general indication of the goal to be achieved, namely the understanding of malignant disease. It does not give details as to what this understanding should consist of, but it does stress the value of achieving this goal, which is the skilled care of the patient. Some authorities subdivide these general goals into immediate and long-term goals and in nursing, it is likely that teachers will need to state goals for the learner that apply to practice after qualification and so are long-term goals.

Learning outcome

This is the desired end-state of student learning, and describes the knowledge, skills, attitudes and values that a student should acquire as a result of the educational process. They are derived from the educational aims of a programme, but are stated in terms of the capabilities that students should attain as a result of instruction. There is a very specific type of learning outcome called a behavioural objective, and this is described below.

Specific behavioural objectives

Also termed instructional objectives or terminal objectives, these are highly specific statements that describe the changes in behaviour that constitute learning. They must always contain a verb that indicates exactly what the learner must do in order to achieve the objective and this verb should describe an observable action so that achievement can be measured. Behavioural objectives are derived from the secondary goals, for example: 'List five factors which predispose an individual to malignant disease'. The word 'list' describes an observable action on the learner's part, which can be measured simply by asking them to write down the list on paper.

If the curriculum uses a behavioural objectives approach to the formulation of goals, then the following guidelines may be helpful:

1. Formulate the educational aims, ensuring that there is some indication of the worthwhileness of achieving them.
2. Formulate the secondary-level goals, which will break down the material into manageable sections for study.
3. Formulate specific behavioural objectives from the secondary-level goals.
4. Formulate any experiential objectives from the secondary-level goals.

Components of a behavioural objective

Behavioural objectives present the most difficulty in formulation, so it is important to examine them in some detail. Most authorities agree with

Mager's (1962) suggestion that there are three parts to any objective, namely a verb indicating the learner's observable behaviour, an indication of the conditions under which the achievement will be demonstrated and a standard or criterion by which the performance is evaluated. Let us take each of these and examine them in relation to nursing.

Learner's observable behaviour
Unless the learner's behaviour is observable it is impossible to assess whether or not an objective has been achieved. Take the objective which states: 'The learner will understand the structure of bone'. How will the nurse teacher know that the learner has achieved this objective? It is not possible to measure understanding as such, but it can be inferred from certain behaviours. For instance, if the learner can write a description of the structure of bone in their own words and without referring to notes or textbooks, then one might safely assume that they have comprehended or understood the material. Thus, it would be much more accurate to state the objective as follows: 'Describe in writing the structure of bone'. The word 'describe' is the action verb, which indicates the learner's observable behaviour. It is important to select verbs that are as unambiguous as possible and which do not rely on the interpretation of the individual who is reading them.

Conditions under which achievement will be demonstrated
Although not always strictly necessary, this can be an aid to clarity in an objective. Conditions are usually such things as time constraints, use of materials or special situations. For example, an objective may state that the condition under which achievement is demonstrated is 'on a patient in bed'. In the example quoted above, the condition is 'in own words, without notes or textbooks'.

Standard or criterion of performance
In the following objective the criterion of performance is 'without danger or discomfort to the patient': 'Remove a drain from the wound of a patient using aseptic technique and without danger or discomfort to him'. Note that the objective cannot be achieved simply by removing the drain; it must be done according to the criteria.

This objective contains all three components, the action verb 'remove', the condition 'using aseptic technique' and the criterion of 'without danger or discomfort to the patient'. Criteria and standards are useful whenever there is doubt as to the level of performance required in an objective.

The taxonomy of educational objectives
In order to perform their role adequately, nurses need a variety of behaviours. They must be able to remember and understand the theoretical aspects of nursing, such as pathophysiology, therapeutics and behavioural sciences. In addition, nurses must possess a wide variety of skills

that demand physical ability and co-ordination, such as assisting patients who have difficulty performing activities of living. But the behaviour that is most closely associated with the role of the nurse is the caring aspect, which involves feelings, emotions, attitudes and values, and which puts the nurse in a unique position with regard to helping patients. Of course, most aspects of nursing involve a combination of all three types of behaviour. In order to perform a blanket bath, the nurse must utilize certain theoretical behaviours such as remembering the patient's condition and relating it to the procedure to be adopted. An assessment of the patient will be needed before commencing. Is the patient in pain? Does he or she require specific help, etc.? Knowledge of the normal and abnormal responses is integrated with information gained from the assessment, to give an overall picture.

The nurse must perform many nursing skills, such as stripping the bed, removing the patient's clothing, altering their position and so on. There is an accepted way of washing and drying a patient that takes a little time to learn. In addition to these 'theoretical behaviours' and 'practical skills', there are the elements of caring, namely interpersonal skills, feelings of empathy, consideration and such. A simple blanket bath is far from simple when analysed, although it is often argued that anyone with common sense can perform it, as we each take care of our personal hygiene when in normal health. This procedure is often delegated to health care assistants because of this viewpoint, but I maintain that there is a world of difference between a blanket bath that merely leaves patients clean and one which leaves them clean, undistressed and with many of their queries or anxieties relieved.

If the role of the nurse requires this wide range of behaviours, then objectives will need to be stated for each of these categories of activity. In addition, it is important that they do not simply require factual recall of information, since nursing involves the ability to apply theoretical knowledge to a practical situation and also to analyse, synthesize and evaluate information.

In order to assist the teacher in formulating objectives at different levels and for different kinds of behaviours, Bloom (1956) developed a system of classification called the taxonomy of educational objectives. A taxonomy is a classification, and the best known one is that of Linnaeus, which classifies all living things according to general and then subsequently more detailed, similarities of structure and function. The taxonomy of educational objectives classifies objectives into three main spheres or domains and each of these is further categorized according to level of behaviour, progressing from the most simple to the highly complex. The levels are arranged in the form of a hierarchy, so that the behaviours at any given level will incorporate those of the levels below.

The three domains are cognitive, which is concerned with knowledge and intellectual abilities, affective, which is concerned with attitudes, values, interests and appreciations and psychomotor, concerned with motor skills. The taxonomy for the affective domain was published by Krathwohl et al. (1964) and taxonomies for the psychomotor domain have been developed by Simpson (1972) and Harrow (1972).

The cognitive domain

Table 6.2 gives the classification of the cognitive domain. There are six levels of objective, each of which is divided into subcategories.

Level		Category		Sub-category	
1.00	Knowledge	1.10	of specifics	1.11	of terminology
				1.12	of specific facts
		1.20	of ways and means of dealing with specifics	1.21	of conventions
				1.22	of trends and sequences
				1.23	of classifications and categories
				1.24	of criteria
				1.25	of methodology
		1.30	of the universals and abstractions in a field	1.31	of principles and generalizations
				1.32	of theories and structures
2.00	Comprehension	2.10	Translation		
		2.20	Interpretation		
		2.30	Extrapolation		
3.00	Application				
4.00	Analysis	4.10	of elements		
		4.20	of relationships		
		4.30	of organizational principles		
5.00	Synthesis	5.10	Production of a unique communication		
		5.20	Production of a plan, or proposed set of operations		
		5.30	Derivation of a set of abstract relations		
6.00	Evaluation	6.10	Judgements in terms of internal evidence		
		6.20	Judgement in terms of external criteria		

Table 6.2

Taxonomy of educational objectives: cognitive domain (Bloom, 1956)

Level 1.00 Knowledge. At this, the most basic level, all that is required is the bringing to mind of such things as specific facts or terminology, as stated in the subcategories. Typical verbs used to indicate this level are: defines, describes, identifies, labels, names, states, lists, etc. However, it is important to remember that it is the context of the verb rather than the verb itself that will decide the level, as some verbs can be used at more than one level.

```
Knowledge        = Knowledge
Comprehension    = Knowledge + Comprehension
Application      = Knowledge + Comprehension + Application
Analysis         = Knowledge + Comprehension + Application + Analysis
Synthesis        = Knowledge + Comprehension + Application + Analysis + Synthesis
Evaluation       = Knowledge + Comprehension + Application + Analysis + Synthesis + Evaluation
```

Table 6.3

The hierarchical nature of the cognitive domain

Level 2.00 Comprehension. This refers to understanding, which is usually demonstrated by the learner making limited use of the information. Such activities as paraphrasing a communication whilst maintaining the intent of the original would constitute translation. Interpretation can be observed by the learner summarizing or explaining information in their own words and extrapolation is involved when information is projected beyond the given data. Typical verbs used at this level are: paraphrase, translate, convert, explain, give examples, etc.

Level 3.00 Application. The learner is required to apply rules, principles, concepts, etc., to real situations. These should be sufficiently unfamiliar to avoid the mere recall of previous behaviours. Typical verbs used at this level are demonstrates, discovers, prepares, produces, relates, uses, solves, shows, etc.

Level 4.00 Analysis. This involves the ability to break down information into its component parts, which may be elements of information, relationships between elements, or organization and structure of information. Its purpose is to separate the important aspects of information from the less important, thus clarifying the meaning. Typical verbs are: differentiates, discriminates, distinguishes, etc.

Level 5.00 Synthesis. At this level the learner is required to combine various parts into a new kind of whole. Creativity is present because the learner produces something unique, such as a plan or design. Typical verbs used are: compiles, composes, creates, devises, plans, etc.

Level 6.00 Evaluation. This implies the ability to make judgements regarding the value of material and involves the use of criteria. Typical verbs are: compares, contrasts, criticizes, justifies, appraises, judges, etc.

Table 6.4 gives examples of nursing objectives for the cognitive domain.

Table 6.4

Examples of nursing objectives for the cognitive domain

Level 1.00 Knowledge
States the four stages of the nursing process
Defines the term psychoneurosis
Identifies the functions of the health education officer
Outlines the three stages of normal labour
Defines the term anaesthesia
Names the stages in child development as described by Piaget. It should be noted that all of these objectives are normally to be achieved without reference to notes or textbooks, so it is not necessary to include this in each statement

Level 2.00 Comprehension
Translates the term haematemesis into its English equivalent

Summarizes section 26 of the Mental Health Act 1959
Gives three examples of the facilities available for the elderly in the community
Explains in own words the methods available for contraception
Gives one example of a potential threat to patient safety in the operating department
Distinguishes between the clean and dirty dressing rooms in the Accident and Emergency Department

Level 3.00 Application

Given the characteristics of ageing, relates these to the needs of the elderly in hospital
Given the principles of care for a patient with pneumonia, relates these to the care of a particular patient with this condition
Given the guidelines for handling violence in hospital, applies these to the care of a patient with a psychopathic disorder
Using the rules for calculation of an infant feed, calculates correctly the feed requirements of an infant of given weight and age
Given a list of community facilities for the handicapped, formulates a plan for discharge of a handicapped child to the community
Given the principles of aseptic technique, applies these when preparing trolleys for surgical operations in the operating department

Level 4.00 Analysis

Given a list of twelve statements about the aetiology of diabetes mellitus, differentiates between those which are factual and those which are assumptions
From a videotape depicting the performance of a surgical dressing, points out two instances of unsafe technique
Given a series of 12 assertion-reason statements on psychiatric disorders, identifies at least four in which the reason is inaccurate
Given a simulated case history of a community patient, distinguishes two inappropriate interventions
Given a list of surgical instruments for laparotomy, identifies three omissions
Given a list of nursing interventions in the Accident and Emergency department, discriminates between those which are important and those which are unimportant, in relation to cardiac arrest

Level 5.00 Synthesis

Writes an original essay on 'The role of the nurse in care of the in-patient with multiple sclerosis'
Devises a nursing care plan which meets the needs of a patient who has undergone cholecystectomy
Produces an outline design for an Accident and Emergency department, which allows for the following:
  (1) one-way flow through the department
  (2) prevention of cross-infection
  (3) separate resuscitation area
Given a list of personnel, designs an off-duty rota for a labour ward, which gives adequate coverage on all shifts
Writes an original essay on 'The role of behaviourism in psychiatry'
Devises a plan to meet the needs of a newly discharged lower-limb amputee in the community

Level 6.00 Evaluation

Evaluates the arguments for and against the use of pertussis vaccine in infants
Given three methods of contraception, judges which one is best, stating how this decision was reached, and what criteria were used
Justifies the continued use of bottle feeding as opposed to breast feeding of infants
Compares and evaluates two approaches to the treatment of depression, stating the criteria used

The affective domain

This domain has particular significance for nursing because it deals with the realm of feelings and attitudes, which constitute the caring functions. It is perhaps useful at this point to clarify what is meant by the terms attitude and value. Both of these are constructs, that is terms invented by psychologists to explain things which cannot be observed directly, but which must be inferred from the person's own account or their behaviour. 'Values' refer to the person's concept of what he or she considers desirable, and so has a large emotional component. A person's values may include sincerity, compassion, respect, etc. 'Attitudes', on the other hand, are positive or negative feelings about certain things and consist of both cognitive and affective aspects. People who feel that smoking is antisocial and that it endangers health, are demonstrating a negative attitude towards smoking.

The affective domain consists of five levels, each of which is subdivided into categories, as shown in Table 6.5.

Table 6.5

Taxonomy of educational objectives: affective domain (Bloom, 1956)

Level		Category	
1.00	Receiving (Attending)	1.1	Awareness
		1.2	Willingness to receive
		1.3	Controlled or selected attention
2.00	Responding	2.1	Acquiescence in responding
		2.2	Willingness to respond
		2.3	Satisfaction in response
3.00	Valuing	3.1	Acceptance of a value
		3.2	Preference for a value
		3.3	Commitment
4.00	Organization	4.1	Conceptualization of a value
		4.2	Organization of a value system
5.00	Characterization by a value or value complex	5.1	Generalized set
		5.2	Characterization

When writing objectives for this domain, it is essential to include within the written statement both the attitude or value in question, and the behaviour that will indicate the particular value or attitude.

Level 1.00 Receiving (attending). At this level the learner is sensitive to the existence of something and progresses from awareness to controlled or selected attention. It is difficult to tell when a learner is receiving or attending to something, so the best indicator is verbal behaviour. Typical verbs are: asks, chooses, selects, replies, etc.

Level 2.00 Responding. This is concerned with active response by the learner, although commitment is not yet demonstrated. The range is from reacting to a suggestion through to experiencing a feeling of satisfaction in responding. Typical verbs are: answers, assists, complies, conforms, helps, etc.

Level 3.00 Valuing. Objectives at this level indicate acceptance and internalization of the values or attitudes in question. The learner acts out these in everyday life in a consistent way. Typical verbs are: initiates, invites, joins, justifies, etc.

Level 4.00 Organization. Having internalized the value, the learner will encounter situations in which more than one value is relevant. This level is concerned with the ability to organize values and to arrange them in appropriate order. Typical verbs are: alters, arranges, combines, modifies, etc.

Level 5.00 Characterization. This is the highest level, and having attained this level the learner has an internalized value system which has become their philosophy of life. These are the values that characterize an individual. Typical verbs are: acts, discriminates, listens, etc. Nurse students, unlike schoolchildren, will have acquired mature attitudes and values systems, because they enter nursing mature. However, this domain is still most applicable to nurse education, as the learner may have to acquire new attitudes and values, or modify existing ones. Table 6.6 shows a list of words that come under the heading of 'caring', and which might form the basis of affective objectives for nursing.

Appreciative	Empathic	Obliging
Attentive	Feeling	Patient
Charitable	Friendly	Respectful
Comforting	Gentle	Sincere
Compassionate	Helpful	Sympathetic
Condolent	Honest	Thoughtful
Considerate	Humane	Understanding
Consoling	Integrity	Valuing
Courteous	Kind	Warm

Table 6.6

Words associated with the affective process of caring

Table 6.7 gives examples of nursing objectives for the affective domain.

Level 1.00 Receiving (Attending)
Indicates an awareness of the value 'consideration for others' by contributing to a discussion on the subject

Level 2.00 Responding
Demonstrates interest in the value 'considerations for others' by reading the assigned literature for the topic

Level 3.00 Valuing
Shows a high degree of commitment to the value 'consideration for others' by actively encouraging colleagues to display consideration for others

Level 4.00 Organization
Demonstrates organization of the values 'consideration for others' and personal autonomy' by writing an essay which requires interaction of these two values

Level 5.00 Characterization
Indicates characterization of the value 'consideration for others' by consistently approaching others in a considerate way

Table 6.7

Examples of nursing objectives for the affective domain

The psychomotor domain

Taxonomies in this domain have been developed by Harrow (1972) and Simpson (1972), the latter having more application to the type of skilled performance involved in nursing.

Level 1 Perception. This basic level is concerned with the perception of sensory cues that guide actions and ranges from awareness of stimuli to translation into action. Typical verbs are: chooses, differentiates, distinguishes, identifies, detects, etc.

Level 2 Set. This is concerned with cognitive, affective and psychomotor readiness to act. Typical verbs are: begins, moves, reacts, shows, starts, etc.

Level 3 Guided response. These objectives refer to the early stages in skills acquisition where skills are performed following demonstration by the teacher. Typical verbs are: carries out, makes, performs, calculates, etc.

Level 4 Mechanism. At this level, the performance has become habitual, but the movements are not so complex as the next higher level. Typical verbs are similar to the previous level.

Level 5 Complex overt response. This level typifies the skilled performance, and involves economy of effort, smoothness of action, accuracy and efficiency, etc. Again, verbs are similar to Level 3.

Level 6 Adaptation. Here, the skills are internalized to such an extent that the nurse can adapt them to cater for special circumstances. Typical verbs are: adapts, alters, modifies, reorganizes, etc.

Level 7 Origination. This is the highest level, and concerns the origination of new movement patterns to suit particular circumstances. Typical verbs are: composes, creates, designs, originates, etc.

Table 6.8 gives examples of nursing objectives for the psychomotor domain.

Table 6.8 Examples of nursing objectives for the psychomotor domain	**Level 1. Perception** Detects the need for pharyngeal suction in a patient, by listening to the sound of his breathing **Level 2. Set** Demonstrates the correct bodily position for lifting a patient **Level 3. Guided response** Performs urine testing as demonstrated by the instructor **Level 4. Mechanism** Sets a tray for an intramuscular injection **Level 5. Complex overt response** Applies with skill a stump bandage to a lower-limb amputee **Level 6. Adaptation** Modifies surgical dressing technique to suit a particular patient's circumstances **Level 7. Origination** Devises an original way of securing a dressing which has tended to come loose soon after application

Gronlund (1978) has suggested an alternative approach to the detailed documentation of single objectives. A general instructional objective is first stated, such as:

Understands the structure and function of the human body.

Then a representative sample of the types of behaviour that constitute understanding of the subject in question are given. For example:

Identifies the organs of the body. Describes the structure of a given organ. Describes the function of a given organ.

This approach has the distinct advantage that the objectives can be used for more than one course. It is based on the premise that it is impossible to list all the behaviours that constitute understanding of something, so only a representative sample of behaviours is included. It also emphasizes that the main goal is understanding of the structure and function of the human body, the objectives are only means to this end, and not ends in themselves. Gronlund's system can be effectively applied to the formulation of objectives for the clinical field, where difficulties might be experienced with objectives for different wards. Rather than having exhaustive lists for each ward, general instructional objectives can be stated for the main areas, with a representative sample of behavioural objectives. For example, the following might apply to every ward in the hospital:

General instructional objective: 'carries out admission procedure for a waiting-list patient'. Specific behavioural objectives: 'prepares bed and bedside area; assembles charts and equipment; conducts patient to bedside, employing appropriate interpersonal skills to allay anxiety'.

A critique of the behavioural objectives model

Although remaining influential in the design of curricula, the behavioural objectives model has been the subject of considerable criticism in the literature. Table 6.9 summarizes the viewpoints of both proponents and opponents of the model.

Perhaps a real-life example may help to show how much of the richness of the learning experience is lost by adhering strictly to a behavioural objectives model. I sat in on a lecture entitled 'The Care of a Child with Leukaemia' and the teacher's stated objectives for the students were:

1. recall the normal leucocyte blood picture;
2. state how the blood picture is altered in leukaemia;
3. deduce some resulting signs and symptoms of leukaemia;
4. suggest appropriate nursing care for an eight-year-old child undergoing chemotherapy in hospital; and
5. demonstrate an interest in the bone-marrow transplant form of treatment.

These objectives seem perfectly acceptable outcomes for the lecture, but such was the skill of the teacher that by the end of the lecture I was feeling a range of emotions that I subsequently wrote down to try to capture their essence:

Table 6.9

Viewpoints of proponents and opponents of behavioural objectives model

Proponents
They provide the student with clear directions as to what must be learnt
Their use encourages the teacher to examine his or her goals more carefully
It is relatively easy to assess students' achievements, as behaviours are observable
They can aid self-instruction
They are accessible to public scrutiny
They offer a rational system for curriculum planning
Students on the whole tend to welcome the clarity that behavioural objectives bring to learning
They provide a basis for comparison between similar courses in different institutions
They offer a system for evaluating the performance of the teacher

Opponents
They act as a set of blinkers that narrow the learning field
They are difficult to formulate for higher-level outcomes and hence encourage trivialization of
    learning by focusing on lower-level outcomes
They are almost impossible to formulate in the affective domain
They ignore unanticipated outcomes of instruction
It is impossible to state objectives for every learning outcome, even if this was desirable
They are unsuitable for arts subjects such as music, poetry and drama
They are unsuitable for science subjects, as they emphasize the learning of factual information
    rather than scientific enquiry
Their use reflects a training approach rather than an educational one
They encourage conformity rather than diversity
It is wrong for one individual, i.e. the teacher, to dictate how another individual, i.e. the student,
    should behave
They are extremely time-consuming to formulate and require continuous updating

1. feelings of empathy and caring for those children with leukaemia;
2. admiration for medical science and its new technology, which can offer treatment for children who would have been considered incurable a few years ago;
3. real appreciation of the frightening nature of treatment for leukaemia, especially the necessary isolation of the child during treatment for bone-marrow transplant;
4. feelings of pride for the courage of my fellow man;
5. understanding of the principle of bone-marrow transplantation, and
6. motivation and a desire to help patients suffering from leukaemia and their relatives.

It does seem from the list that there were many outcomes that could not have been anticipated by the teacher, yet they were very important results for me. One might argue that in the longer term they are much more important than the behavioural list that the teacher gave to the students, since I am more likely to remember and understand the principles of the lecture because of these feelings.

Stenhouse's process model of curriculum

One of the major critics of the behavioural objectives model was the late Lawrence Stenhouse, who formulated an alternative approach known as the 'process' model. He saw the use of behavioural objectives acting as a filter that distorted knowledge in schools (Stenhouse, 1975, p. 86):

'The filtering of knowledge through an analysis of objectives gives the school an authority and power over its students by setting arbitrary limits to speculation and by defining arbitrary solutions to unresolved problems of knowledge. This translates the teacher from the role of the student of a complex field of knowledge to the role of the master of the school's agreed version of that field'.

Requirements for a curriculum

Stenhouse's (1975) minimum requirements for a curriculum are that a curriculum should offer:

1. *In planning*:
   (a) principles for the selection of content – what is to be learned and taught;
   (b) principles for the development of a teaching strategy – how it is to be learned and taught;
   (c) principles for the making of decisions about sequence;
   (d) principles on which to diagnose the strengths and weaknesses of individual students and differentiate the general principles (a), (b) and (c) above to meet individual cases;
2. *In empirical study*:
   (a) principles on which to study and evaluate the progress of students;
   (b) principles on which to study and evaluate the progress of teachers;
   (c) guidance as to the feasibility of implementing the curriculum in varying school contexts, pupil contexts, environments and peer-group situations;
   (d) information about the variability of effects in differing contexts and on different pupils and an understanding of the causes of the variation; and
3. *In relation to justification*:
   (a) a formulation of the intention or aim of the curriculum which is accessible to critical scrutiny.

Stenhouse's position on behavioural objectives

Stenhouse believed that it was possible to organize the curriculum without having to specify in advance the behavioural changes that should occur in students; indeed, he argued that the purpose of education was to make student outcomes unpredictable. Knowledge does not consist of 'known facts' to be remembered, rather, it provides a basis for speculation and conjecture about a discipline. The content of a curriculum can be selected on the basis that it is worthwhile in itself and not merely as the means to achievement of a behavioural objective. Hence, we could argue that the content in a nursing curriculum can be chosen for its worthwhileness in providing examples of the key concepts, procedures and criteria of nursing science. Similarly, teaching methods and learning experiences can be specified in terms of their worthwhileness as learning activities. Stenhouse refers to these statements of worthwhileness as 'principles of procedure' and it is important to note that the principles of procedure for teaching are couched in terms of what the teacher will do rather than what the students will be able to do. For example, 'to encourage students to reflect on their experiences'.

The role of assessment in a process curriculum is very different from that in a product model, being that of critic rather than marker. The teacher is cast in the role of critical appraiser of the student's work, with the emphasis on developing self-appraisal in the student. According to Stenhouse (1975, p.95):

> *'The worthwhile activity in which teacher and student are engaged has standards and criteria immanent in it and the task of appraisal is that of improving students' capacity to work to such criteria by critical reaction to work done. In this sense, assessment is about the teaching of self-assessment'.*

A critique of Stenhouse's process model

The most common reservation expressed in nurse education with regard to the process model centres on the issue of evaluation. If no terminal behaviours are prescribed, how can the teacher assess whether a student is competent or not? It seems that nurse teachers have forgotten that there was life before behavioural objectives! Indeed, it is only some twenty years since the movement towards the product model was endorsed by the General Nursing Council for England and Wales (1977). How did nurse teachers evaluate student progress prior to 1977? Interestingly enough, it was by reference of a specification of course content, namely, the 'syllabus for training'. This gave an outline of the main topic headings, e.g. 'The effects of the environment on health', but no fine detail was included, this being left to the individual teacher to decide. A 'schedule of practical skills' was also available to identify clinical skills required for nursing practice and such skills were assessed by both clinical nurses and nurse teachers. The criteria for these skills must have been internalized by each assessor, in the light of what was considered to be good nursing practice by the institution and the profession. It is also worth reminding ourselves that large sections of education never espoused the behavioural objectives model at all, although it is fair to say that most higher education institutions identify student learning outcomes for each course. Learning outcomes, however, tend to be couched more broadly than the strict observable behaviours that characterize the behavioural objectives model.

The greatest weakness of the process model is identified by Stenhouse as its dependence upon the quality of the teacher. In this model, the teacher's commitment to professional development is vital; teachers need to see themselves as learners rather than as experts, and to be continually striving to improve their performance and judgement.

Table 6.10 shows the main differences in approach between the two models, as a basis for comparison.

Product model	Process model
An output model, i.e. emphasis is on the achievement of behavioural objectives; the product of education	An input model, i.e. emphasis is on learning experiences; the process of education
Curriculum activities are seen as means to an end, i.e. achievement of terminal objectives	Curriculum activities are seen as being worthwhile in themselves
Learning is seen as a change in observable behaviour	Acknowledges that much learning is not observable
Teaching is geared to producing predictable outcomes	Teaching is geared to encourage unpredictable outcomes
Teacher specifies content in terms of the student's achievement of behavioural objectives	Teacher specifies content but cannot know in advance what the student will do with that content
Evaluation is done by assessing the student's achievement of behavioural objectives	Evaluation is done by critical appraisal of the student's work, using the criteria intrinsic to the discipline concerned; includes self-assessment by the student

Table 6.10

Comparison between key concepts of product and process models of curriculum

Lawton's cultural analysis model

Lawton's model was a reaction against what he saw as the dangers of the behavioural objectives model. As the name implies, this model proposes a curriculum planned on the technique of cultural analysis. Culture is defined as the whole way of life of a society and the purpose of education is 'to make available to the next generation what we regard as the most important aspects of culture' (Lawton, 1983). Cultural analysis is the process by which a selection is made from the culture and in terms of curriculum-planning, Lawton suggests cultural analysis will ask the following questions:

1. What kind of society already exists?
2. In what ways is it developing?
3. How do its members appear to want it to develop?
4. What kinds of values and principles will be involved in deciding on Question 3, and on the educational means of achieving it?

Stages in cultural analysis

Lawton (1983) offers a five-stage model for this analysis:

1. *Cultural in variants.* This stage examines all the aspects that human societies have in common, such as economic and moral aspects, beliefs and other systems.
2. *Cultural variables.* This stage involves analysing the differences between cultures in each of the systems.
3. *Selection from the culture.* This stage consists of comparing the

cultural analysis of the systems with the existing school curriculum.

4. *Psychological questions and theories.* This stage is not in direct continuity with the previous stages, but is seen as an important consideration for any curriculum development.

5. *Curriculum organization.* In this final stage the curriculum can now be planned on the basis of the cultural analysis carried out in the previous stages, bearing in mind the important psychological questions and theories that influence learning and instruction.

Critique of Lawton's cultural analysis model

Lawton's model of curriculum attempts to apply a rational system of analysis to the problem of curriculum content; it is designed for the school curriculum for children and approaches the task of curriculum planning in a broader way. As Lawton points out in his preface 'the problems of young people growing up in a complex urban, industrialized society have been seriously underestimated; schools have generally failed to take seriously the moral, social and political aspects of culture in relation to curriculum planning' (Lawton, 1983).

Beattie's fourfold model

Beattie's (1987) fourfold model of the curriculum draws upon his experience with nursing curricula. He suggests that there are four fundamental approaches to the task of planning a curriculum for nursing, each with its own particular strengths and weaknesses:

1. *The curriculum as a map of key subjects.* As the name implies, this approach consists of mapping out the key subjects in the nursing curriculum, preferably integrating them by means of themes such as 'the human lifespan' to avoid the danger of an isolated collection of topics.

2. *The curriculum as a schedule of basic skills.* This approach emphasizes the explicit specification of basic skills of nursing, these skills being culled from recent empirical research into nursing practice. A behavioural objectives approach can be appropriate here, provided that it is not used dogmatically for all aspects of teaching, particularly in relation to the knowledge base for clinical practice.

3. *The curriculum as a portfolio of meaningful personal experiences.* This approach puts the student at the centre of things by organizing the curriculum around their interests and experiences. This is done by using a variety of experiential techniques such as action-research, critical incidents, role-play and the like. There will always be a degree of tension between the unpredictability consequent upon student autonomy and the need to ensure sufficient opportunity to cover key areas.

4. *The curriculum as an agenda of important cultural issues.* This approach avoids giving detailed subject-matter, focusing instead

on controversial issues and political dilemmas in nursing and health care. These issues are chosen because they are open to debate and have no single correct answer, thereby stimulating discussion and enquiry, e.g. nurse power or patient power.

How can nurse teachers use these ideas in practical curriculum planning? Beattie suggests that there are three ways of combining the fourfold framework. The first one he calls the 'eclectic curriculum', in which the four approaches are mixed together in some sort of combination. The main problem with this is that the more traditional approaches tend to dominate, leaving only the marginal inclusion of student-centred ideas. Another way is to negotiate each of the key areas with the consumers, the 'negotiated curriculum'. The third way Beattie calls the 'dialectical curriculum', in which the curriculum designer 'goes out to do battle', as it were, to engage in a deliberate, principled and committed struggle to combat, challenge and contest the dominant codes of curriculum (Beattie, 1987, p.31). In his 'fourfold model of curriculum', Beattie argues that 'curriculum planners in nursing can and must move beyond simpleminded, "single-model" approaches and towards complex, multifaceted strategies' (Beattie, 1987, p .32).

Humphreys' 'new paradigm' curriculum model

The genesis of this model lies in the NHS reorganization in the early 1990s which led to the NHS internal market, and more specifically in the Government White Paper *Working for Patients: Education and Training Working Paper 10* (HMSO, 1989). The latter had given employers a major say in the process of educational contracting, and Humphreys and Quinn (1994) claim this triggered a revolution in healthcare education. Humphreys (1994) expresses the essence of the new paradigm:

> 'the political and ideological climate of health care delivery is not just an important component of, or context for, educational change – it is the origin and driving force of it. In this situation, educators are beginning to act in different ways, consider new values and work from new ideologies – in short, to operate within what can loosely be described as a new paradigm' (Humphreys, 1994, p. 142).

Humphreys identifies a new dominating ideological stance, 'corporate instrumentalism', which reflects the important influence that NHS employers have on curricula. He maintains that this must be 'the ideological basis for effective models of curriculum development' (Humphreys, 1994, p. 150).

Curriculum as product

Humphreys utilizes modern concepts of marketing as a basis for his curriculum model. He defines the purpose of marketing as 'to enable or facilitate voluntary and mutually advantageous exchange relationships', and this includes the importance of purchaser satisfaction, and the fact that educational institutions should provide services that the service providers want to buy. This emphasis on the mutual satisfaction of both purchaser and provider is the cornerstone of a marketing approach. Humphreys sees curriculum as a product, but qualifies this:

> *'In marketing terms the concept of the "product" refers to more than simply the basic nature of what is being sold. To the purchaser, the "product" represents a combination of perceived benefits that will meet her/his needs. In designing a product, care is taken to ensure that the full range of the product's attributes are collectively sufficient to interest the purchaser. In educational terms, these attributes include the availability of the course (time, location, frequency etc) and the price' (Humphreys, 1994, p.153).*

A new model for curriculum development

Humphreys' model consists of three stages:

1. *Planning.* This stage involves the identification of an unsatisfied client need, and is followed by a survey of market information to make sure the development is worthwhile. This stage also includes an analysis of the educational institution's strengths in relation to the client need.
2. *Development.* This stage consists of three interrelated elements:
   (a) Resourcing: the total available resources and costs need to be calculated.
   (b) Regulations: the requirements of appropriate academic and statutory bodies must be taken into account.
   (c) Design: this must identify the coverage specification in relation to client need, decide which aspects of applied human sciences should be included, and systems innovations such as flexibility, APL and APEL.
3. *Validation and operation.* Validation includes not only the formal academic validation, but also checking that the curriculum still matches client need. Once the curriculum is operational, monitoring and evaluation processes ensure the continuing match between the curriculum and client need.

The shortcomings of curriculum models in nurse education

The classic models outlined above were, with the exception of the Beattie and Humphreys models, developed with the education of children in mind. The various educational ideologies underpinning the models are beliefs about childhood education, as evidenced by references to 'transmission of the cultural heritage of the nation', 'creation of a common democratic culture', 'meeting the needs, aspirations and personal growth of the individual' and 'education relevant to the social and economic needs of society'. The classic models are usually adapted in some way to meet the needs of curriculum developers in nursing and midwifery, but these tend to be relatively superficial adaptations which leave the essential principles of the model unchanged. The only model that actively considers the educational needs of service providers is that of Humphreys, which was developed to specifically address the short-comings of the child-centred curriculum models in the NHS internal market.

MODELS OF TEACHING

Teaching is a deliberate and purposeful activity directed towards the promotion of learning. It normally comprises two basic elements: the teacher, i.e. the individual doing the promoting of learning, and the student/learner/recipient, i.e. the one whose learning is thus promoted. However, these elements are commonly combined from time to time, as when individuals teach themselves. Teaching can be, and is, carried out by any member of society, e.g. parents, trainers, etc., but there is also a profession called teaching that includes teachers of children and adults. The element called 'teacher' need not refer exclusively to a human being; there are many non-human teaching resources available, such as computers, video, etc.

A number of models exist that attempt to represent the nature of teaching, and a selection is outlined below.

The transmission model of teaching

This model conceptualizes teaching as a process in which the teacher transmits knowledge, skills and attitudes to the students, who are subsequently considered to have learned these capabilities. This model has been the basis of teaching for centuries, and is still very much evident in the lecture method used in higher education. However, the model is not without its critics, who question the relatively passive role of the student in the process. Their reservations are neatly expressed in the aphorism 'the lecturer's notes are transmitted to the students' notes without passing through the brains of either'. Indeed, the model is often termed the 'empty vessel' model, implying that the students are empty vessels waiting for the teacher to fill them up with learning. One eminent proponent of the transmission model of teaching is David Ausubel (see Chapter 4, p. 91), who argues that the model is the most efficient means of transmitting the culture of a society from one generation to another.

The facilitation model of teaching

In this model, the teacher is seen as a facilitator of learning rather than a transmitter of information, and one of the key originators is Carl Rogers (see Chapter 3, p. 53). The facilitation of learning requires the setting up of an environment conducive to learning, including interaction between teacher and students in a challenging but non-threatening environment. Proponents of this model emphasize its appropriateness for individual learning, and its relevance to life-skills. Opponents cite the time-consuming nature of such activities, and the consequent inability to adequately cover the syllabus.

Teaching styles

There is no such things as an ideal teaching style, since individual teachers differ widely in personality and approach to teaching. Nevertheless, research has shown that it is possible to categorize teaching styles to some degree; the following classic examples relate to the teaching of children.

Getzels and Thelen's teaching styles

Getzels and Thelen (1960) describe three teaching styles: nomothetic, idiographic and transactional. The nomothetic leader is one who places emphasis on the requirements of the institution rather than on the individual. Education is perceived as the handing down of information. The idiographic style is the opposite to this, in that the individual is stressed rather than the institution and education is seen as assisting him to learn what he is motivated to learn. There is an intermediate style called transactional, which implies an appreciation of the limitations of the individual and the institution, and attempts to make a sensible compromise between the two.

Bennett's teaching styles

Neville Bennett (1976) analysed nearly 500 junior school teachers by both observation of classroom activities and interviews about educational issues and teaching methods. He categorized these teachers into three types (formal, mixed and informal) based upon their approach to the following aspects:

1. integration or separation of subjects;
2. pupils given choice of work and/or seating;
3. use of testing and grading;
4. teacher's class control and discipline; and
5. use of class or small-group teaching.

Having classified the teaching styles of teachers, Bennett then classified primary school children into groupings according to personality testing and proceeded to correlate the pupils' progress, pupil type and teacher style. Bennett concluded that the teaching style was more influential than the effects of personality type, but the study has been the subject of extensive criticism on the grounds of methodological and statistical problems.

ORACLE and teaching styles

The 'observation research and classroom evaluation' project (ORACLE) was carried out at the University of Leicester (Galton and Simon, 1975). In total, 58 classrooms were observed, from inner-city, urban, village and housing estate areas. The project used systematic observation plus interviews with teachers, and four teacher styles and four pupil styles were identified. The four teaching styles were as follows.

1. *Individual monitors (22% of the sample)*. Teachers showed a high level of one-to-one interaction with pupils.
2. *Class enquirers (15% of the sample)*. Teachers showed a high proportion of class teaching.
3. *Group instructors (12% of the sample)*. Teachers interacted with groups of pupils rather than individuals.
4. *Style changers (50% of the sample)*. Teachers were able to change their teaching style in a number of ways.

The ORACLE project found that teaching style was the most important variable in pupil progress and the results showed the characteristics of successful teaching to be:

1. a high level of teacher–pupil interaction;
2. a high level of task statements and questions by the teacher;
3. regular feedback to pupils;
4. encouragement for pupils to work by themselves;
5. use of higher-order and open-ended questions; and
6. avoidance of the overuse of instructions.

NURSING MODELS

Nursing models are used to plan, implement, and evaluate nursing care in a wide range of practice settings, and will therefore feature significantly in curriculum documentation for nursing programmes. Indeed, a nursing model may well function as the over-arching model for an entire curriculum, and it is here where the boundary between curriculum models and other models becomes blurred. The majority of models originated in North America, with the notable Scottish exception of the Roper, Logan and Tierney Model of Activities of Living. The most commonly-used American models are the Orem Self-Care model; Roy's Adaptation model; Neuman's Health Care Systems model, and Johnson's Behavioural Systems model. Fraser (1996) advocates the use of a multiple-model approach to practice, as no single model is capable of covering all the problems experienced by clinical nurses.

CURRICULUM DEVELOPMENT

The basic principles of curriculum development apply to both pre-registration and post-registration provision, although there are some differences in approach between these. Pre-registration courses or programmes in nursing and midwifery tend to be offered in both full-time and part-time modes, whereas post-registration continuing education programmes are largely part-time.

Since pre-registration programmes form the entry gate to the nursing or midwifery professions they must meet the criteria laid down by the UKCC and the appropriate National Board for Nursing, Midwifery and Health Visiting. Post-registration programmes and courses are, on the whole, less constrained by such requirements and provide scope for curriculum designers to be much more flexible and imaginative.

Curriculum development needs to be distinguished from curriculum design at this point:

1. *Curriculum development* is a broad concept that encompasses all the processes involved in the production and implementation of a curriculum, from the initial idea through to monitoring and review of its operation.
2. *Curriculum design* is a focused activity concerned with questions of structure, content and process, e.g. curriculum philosophy and model, content-mapping, organization and sequencing of content, etc. It is a sub-component of curriculum development.

Although nursing curricula within the UK will differ one from another, there will be certain things in common. For example, the English National Board describes a documentary analysis of nursing degree curricula undertaken by University College, Suffolk (ENB, 1999a) which describes the similarities and differences between nursing degree curriculum documents from 32 institutions. The ways in which the documents were comparable included:

1. the graduate nurse was conceptualized as an innovative leader, flexible, and able to manage change;
2. level descriptors were comparable, but there was difficulty in articulating higher levels of practice;
3. preparation of practice assessors was similar;
4. students were required to undertake a substantial piece of independent work over a period of time;
5. for post-registration programmes, a common emphasis on flexible delivery.

The documents differed in a number of ways including:

1. considerable variation in whether or not practical skills were assessed by direct observation, particularly in post-registration degrees;
2. fundamental differences in course structure;
3. lack of comparability of distribution of the 360 credits throughout degree programme components;
4. no sense of common currency of credits in either learning time or student achievement;
5. variation in whether or not students were required to undertake research within their dissertation.

Before proceeding to discuss curriculum development in detail, it may be helpful to highlight the context in which higher education curricula operate, including the important concept of accreditation of prior learning (APL).

Higher education credit schemes in relation to curriculum development

Many higher education institutions use the concept of credit schemes to structure their academic awards. Programmes within a credit scheme are composed of large numbers of discrete, self-contained courses of learning that are designated either core or option. Core courses are compulsory, whereas option courses offer the student a degree of choice. Each course is described in the form of a course specification, and the typical components are shown in Table 6.11.

Course title	Should concisely indicate the nature of the course
Department	
Credit points and learning time	Proportion of a full-time year
Level	CATS level 1, 2, 3 or M
Code	For computer records
Co-ordinator	Individual responsible for delivery
Pre-requisite and co-requisite	Courses that must be taken before of concurrently with the course
Rationale	Justifies the inclusion of the course in the programme
Aims	Identify the overall purpose of the course
Learning outcomes	State what the student can do as a result of learning, e.g. 'Analyse the factors which influence the effectiveness of nurse-patient interaction'
Process of learning and teaching	Range of activities to achieve learning
Assessment	Means of testing achievement of learning
Indicative content	List of key topics
Indicative reading	List of representative texts

Table 6.11

Typical components of a course specification

The complete set of core and option courses will differ from student to student, according to the option courses they choose. The basic criterion for the inclusion of an option course within a student's programme of study is that she must be able to demonstrate its coherence and relevance to her overall programme.

Take the example of a nurse working within the field of sexually transmitted diseases who is undertaking a post-registration degree in nursing studies. This particular nurse may choose to study an option course from a social science degree programme on human sexuality, since this would be relevant to his or her particular professional needs and interests. Similarly, an option course on personnel management from a diploma in management studies may be undertaken so as to improve both knowledge and skills as a departmental manager.

In credit schemes, a specified number of credit points is awarded to the student on successful completion of appropriate learning, and this can be gained in three ways:

1. through formal study on a programme;
2. from existing qualifications;
3. from professional or life experience.

The system of credit points takes as its standard a three-year full-time undergraduate degree with honours, which is credit rated at 360 credit points, 120 for each of the three years of the course. Each year represents a specific level of learning:

First year = level 1

Second year = level 2
Third year = level 3

There is also a Level M for postgraduate study at master's degree level. Credit points gained from appropriate learning can accumulate towards a higher education award such as a diploma or degree, and the amount and level of credit normally required for these in England, Wales and Northern Ireland is shown below.

- Certificate of higher education: 120 credit points at level 1;
- Diploma of higher education: 240 credit points, 120 at each of levels 1 and 2;
- Unclassified degree: 360 credit points, of which a minimum of 60 must be at level 3;
- Degree with honours: 360 credit points, of which a minimum of 120 must be at level 3;
- Postgraduate diploma: 70 credit points, of which a minimum of 50 must be at master's level;
- Master's degree: 120 credit points, of which a minimum of 80 must be at master's level and the remainder at level 3.

The system in Scotland differs from that in the three countries above, in that there are four levels: SD1, SD2, SD3 and SD4. The first three levels equate with the certificate, diploma and unclassified degree as shown above, but the degree with honours requires 480 credit points, 120 at each of the four levels.

The Dearing Report (1997) proposed a framework for higher education qualifications consisting of eight levels as shown in Table 6.12, which were subsequently endorsed by the Government in its response to Dearing.

Table 6.12

The Dearing framework for higher education qualifications

H1	Certificate
H2	Diploma
H3	Bachelor's degree
H4	Honours degree
H5	Higher honours/Postgraduate Conversion Diploma
H6	Master's degree
H7	M.Phil
H8	Doctorate

The proposed framework includes both academic and vocational qualifications, and provides for progression through the whole range of achievement. It also embraces credit accumulation and credit transfer between institutions, and each level in the framework must have recognized standards.

Accreditation of prior learning

One of the fundamental principles of credit schemes is that students who have been awarded credit points from one institution can transfer them to studies in another institution.

APL

The contribution of existing credits, gained outside the awarding institution, towards a higher education award is termed APL (accreditation of prior learning). In order for credit to count towards an award it must be relevant to that award, and be at an appropriate level. The length of time since the course was completed also affects its current relevance, so APL is normally confined to courses completed within the previous five years. There is a maximum percentage of APL that can be counted towards an award and this is normally between 50% and 75% of the total credit required for that award. In credit schemes a distinction is made between general credit and specific credit, and the following vignette illustrates this.

> *Tara was halfway through the second year of a degree in Nursing when her husband's company decided to transfer him to the north of England office. She contacted the university nearest to her new address who explained that there was currently no degree in nursing available, but that a degree in health studies was well established. Tara had earned a total of 240 credit points from her previous nursing degree studies, 120 at each of Levels 1 and 2. However, because the focus was nursing rather than generic health studies Tara was allowed to count only 80 of her Level 2 credit points towards the health studies degree.*

Credit awarded to a student for specified learning in one institution is termed *general credit* and can be transferred to studies in other HE institutions. The receiving institution, however, may decide that only a proportion of this general credit is actually relevant to their course, and this proportion of the general credit is termed specific credit. If any specific credit matches the learning outcomes of a unit on the course to which the student is transferring, then he or she can be given exemption from that unit.

Deciding the amount of credit

Course leaders in institutions are often faced with the task of deciding how much credit should be allowed for previous qualifications, and this is doubly difficult in the case of courses that do not carry a national credit rating. There are two aspects to be considered when examining sources of evidence about courses:

1. *Quantity of learning.* This is based upon a full-time higher education academic year, with adjustment for variations in length of NHS-related courses.
2. *Quality of learning* In order to appraise the quality of learning it is necessary to scrutinize:
   (a) level of learning as defined in the scheme definitions, for example, the University of Greenwich Level 3 definition for health schemes is: 'Practitioners are specialists within their chosen areas, who have developed new professional skills,

knowledge and understanding; who have utilized existing research; whose practice is enquiry based and who promote innovative practice';

(b) apropriateness of the aims and outcomes of the course and the relationship between these and the definitions of learning;

(c) appropriateness of the learning and teaching processes; and

(d) reliability and validity of course assessment in relation to (a), (b) and (c) above.

Accreditation of prior experiential learning

Earlier, the concept of APL was discussed. This was concerned with learning gained from previous qualifications, but prior learning can also be gained from the day-to-day experience of professional practice or of life generally, as in rearing a child or writing a book. It is important to note that experience alone is insufficient; the student must demonstrate how he or she has learned from the experience. A useful theoretical basis for APEL is given by Kolb (1984) in his experiential learning cycle. This is discussed in Chapter 3 (p. 62).

Credit points can be given for such experiential learning provided that it is relevant to the award which the student is seeking to achieve, and that a portfolio of evidence for such learning has been presented for accreditation to the awarding institution.

Butterworth (1992) describes two models of practice used to accredit prior experiential learning: the credit exchange model, and the developmental model. The widest application of the former is in the NVQ (National Vocational Qualifications) field, where the emphasis is very much on the production of satisfactory evidence of previous performance by the claimant.

In the developmental model, evidence of past achievements must also be produced by the claimant, but in addition he or she must produce an analysis of that evidence, including its significance to their professional development. This analysis must be supported by relevant theoretical perspectives. Butterworth argues that the developmental model is more appropriate for the accreditation of learning derived from professional practice.

Making an APEL claim

There are seven steps in making a claim for Accreditation of Prior Experiential Learning (Butterworth, 1993).

1. Focus on the area of learning and summarize it in a learning claim. The first step in putting together an APEL claim is for students to decide upon which part of their past experience they wish to base their claim, and this can be one large experience or more than one, provided that it is reasonably substantial. It is not possible to use many small experiences to build up a claim, as this would lack the necessary coherence.

2. Clearly identify and list the learning outcomes derived from the

experience. Learning outcomes need to be stated in a precise form rather than vague, general statements, and must encompass all the knowledge and skills that were learned.

3. Check that the learning is relevant and at the right level for the award which is being sought. The claim must be current, i.e. the experience should have been within the last five years, sufficient, and relevant to the award being sought.

4. Collect sufficient documentary evidence to support the claim, together with at least one suitable testimonial authenticating it. Direct evidence constitutes the student's own work, such as reports, plans, materials that have been designed, etc., that will demonstrate achievement of the learning outcomes. Indirect evidence refers to testimonials and other evidence from external sources.

5. Produce a reflective commentary which describes the experience(s) and analyses them to show how they produced the learning that is being claimed. This is a very important stage, as it demonstrates the student's ability to reflect upon and conceptualize the experiences.

6. Present an outline of APEL portfolio at a formative assessment tutorial. This involves discussion with the APEL counsellor about the appropriateness and sufficiency of the claim, and the quality of the reflective commentary.

7. Collate all this material and organize it in the form of a portfolio that can be presented to an assessor. The portfolio is not assessed by the APEL counsellor, but by a 'gatekeeper' who has not been involved with the student's preparation. The portfolio should contain a contents page and each chapter should be clearly labelled.

Stages of curriculum development

There are four stages in the curriculum development process: exploratory, design, implementation, and monitoring and review.

Exploratory stage

It is important that education providers liaise closely with service providers to identify gaps in the provision of nursing and midwifery education so that new courses or programmes can be developed to meet those needs. Ideas for new provision need to be carefully explored before either adopting or rejecting them, and a core team should be set up to this effect. Market research is vitally important to ascertain the views of employers and other interested parties such as statutory bodies. The availability of resources and expertise within the university needs to be explored, and the estimated costs of development will have to calculated for eventual inclusion in any contract. It is useful to undertake an initial critical path analysis for the development so that a realistic idea of the timescale is gained.

Design stage

If a decision is made to go ahead with the development, a curriculum planning team should be set up to prepare the course or programme for validation and subsequent implementation. The actual process of design and validation is discussed in the next section of this chapter.

Implementation stage

In this stage students have been recruited, all systems are in place, and the curriculum is fully operational. In the early days of implementation a few teething troubles can be expected until the systems have been fine tuned. For example, the offering of a choice of option courses to students may result in some courses being under-subscribed and others oversubscribed. During the implementation stage, curriculum evaluation is ongoing by means of course evaluation. This does not refer to the assessment of students' achievement of course outcomes, but to the systematic collection of opinions about the quality and usefulness of the courses.

Monitoring and review stage

Although the evaluation of programme courses is an ongoing process, the monitoring and review stage can be usefully seen as a distinct phase in the curriculum. In HE, programme leaders – in consultation with programme committees – are required to produce an annual programme monitoring report. This report is retrospective for the previous academic year, and requires the programme director to reflect upon the quality of the programme using data gathered from a variety of sources such as students' evaluations of courses, external examiners' reports, and the views of employers. This report is scrutinized at a series of meetings before being discussed at a Faculty Board or Academic Board. Annual programme monitoring is therefore an important mechanism for ensuring quality on the programme. Programme monitoring is further discussed in Chapter 12 (p. 318).

When a programme receives approval following validation, a timescale for programme review will be proposed. The length of approval ranges from as little as one year through to indefinite approval, but regardless of length, continuation of the programme is dependent upon a satisfactory programme review. A review is very similar to a validation event, but the programme team are required to produce a detailed review of the operation of the programme over the prescribed timescale. Proposals for changes must be accompanied by a well-argued rationale and supporting evidence.

CURRICULUM DESIGN

This constitutes the second stage of the curriculum planning process as outlined above. The core team, formed during the exploratory stage to consider the feasibility of the development, now needs to be augmented by a small number of other individuals possessing the required knowledge and experience with reference to the curriculum in question. In curriculum development groups for nursing and midwifery, particularly for pre-registration programmes, the range of representation commonly includes teaching staff, students, and hospital and community service managers. The latter represent the various specialisms of nursing, such as learning difficulties, community nursing, and children's nursing, and are usually chosen to reflect representation from each health district or trust to which the university relates. The curriculum development group should have a chairperson, and it is sufficient to have notes of the decisions made at meetings rather than formal minutes.

Critical path analysis

One of the first issues to be addressed by the group should be a critical path analysis which identifies deadlines for each aspect of the development. It is useful to work backwards from the proposed date of the validation event, allowing several weeks before the event for the documentation to be available to validation panel members. Other deadlines that need to be included are the first draft of the validation document, the internal validation event, and the printing of the document. A specimen critical path analysis for curriculum development is shown in Figure 6.2.

Figure 6.2

Specimen critical path analysis for curriculum development

Oct	Nov	Dec	Jan	Feb	Mar	Apr	May	Jun	Jul	Aug	Sep

Formation of planning team

Curriculum development

Unit writing

Document writing

Internal validation

Document to panel

Validation event

Response to validation conditions

Start intake

Incorporating statutory body guidelines into the curriculum

Another issue that needs to be addressed early in the development is the question of curriculum 'givens', i.e. the university's regulations on programme development and validation, and the requirements and guidelines of the UKCC and of the relevant National Board for Nursing, Midwifery and Health Visiting. For example, the UKCC has produced Guidelines for Mental Health and Learning Disabilities Nursing (UKCC, 1998) that address a range of relevant issues such as inter-disciplinary working, evidence-based practice, advocacy, autonomy and confidentiality.

Approval in principle, and statement of intent

Institutions of higher education and statutory bodies both have mechanisms for granting approval in principle, which is normally required before the team can proceed with curriculum development. In the higher education sector, approval in principle normally requires the completion of a planning proposal form which outlines the academic rationale and the resource implications of the proposed programme. The proposal is then considered by the appropriate body at Faculty level.

The English National Board for Nursing, Midwifery and Health Visiting requires institutions to forward a statement of intent for the proposed programme to the designated education officer at the outset of the development. The statement of intent specifies the following (ENB, 1997):

1. a summary of the aims, processes and outcomes of the proposed programme;
2. intended programme participants;
3. staff and physical resource allocation for the development and implementation;
4. evidence of education purchaser demand;
5. overall timescale for development and process of approval;
6. name and contact number of designated lead person and individuals with lead responsibilities for specific aspects.

The Board then communicates its decision as to whether or not the development is approved; if approval is granted, then an appropriate timescale for the approval process is agreed with the education officer.

Writing the validation submission document

Another key component of curriculum development is the validation submission document, and the writing of this should be the responsibility of one person, although informed by the team. The document should be written in parallel with the development so that key aspects are captured as they happen. HE institutions differ in their requirements for validation documents, but there is a general structure common to all. The format for programme documentation used in the University of Greenwich is shown in Table 6.14

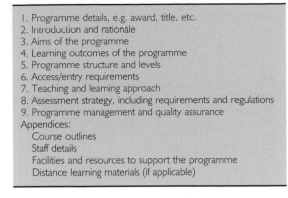

1. Programme details, e.g. award, title, etc.
2. Introduction and rationale
3. Aims of the programme
4. Learning outcomes of the programme
5. Programme structure and levels
6. Access/entry requirements
7. Teaching and learning approach
8. Assessment strategy, including requirements and regulations
9. Programme management and quality assurance
Appendices:
    Course outlines
    Staff details
    Facilities and resources to support the programme
    Distance learning materials (if applicable)

Table 6.13

Format for validation submission document (University of Greenwich, 1996)

For conjoint validation with the ENB, the validation submission document must address the ENB standards and criteria for programme approval.

Curriculum rationale and model

One of the key sections of the validation document is Section 2, the rationale of the programme. The purpose of the rationale is to outline the philosophy and model upon which the curriculum is based, and all other components of the programme must be congruent with this rationale. For example, the rationale for a nursing curriculum may define the student as an autonomous, reflective individual who is responsible for his or her own learning. Hence, the timetable should provide adequate time for private study and reflection, but if the day is fully programmed with lectures and teaching contact, then there is clearly a mismatch between the rationale and the teaching and learning process. Such incongruence would be seriously questioned at a validation event. The development team may decide to use any one of the curriculum models outlined earlier in this chapter, in their curriculum. On the other hand, they may wish to adapt an existing model to fit their ideas, or devise an entirely new one. Curriculum development teams may be tempted to include a model in their validation document simply because it is expected, but unless the model helps to conceptualize the curriculum it will quickly be detected as irrelevant by the panel.

Devising a curriculum model is not difficult, and an example is shown in Figure 6.3.

The example I have devised is a generic model of curriculum for nursing and midwifery, consisting of three main components, inputs, process, and outputs.

1. *Curriculum inputs*. These are the elements influencing the curriculum design, and consist of educational perspectives, employer requirements, national and local culture, and professional culture including requirements of statutory bodies.
2. *Curriculum process*. This is the curriculum as experienced by the student, and consists of learning outcomes, content, teaching and learning strategies, and assessment/evaluation.

Figure 6.3

Example of a model of curriculum
for nursing and midwifery

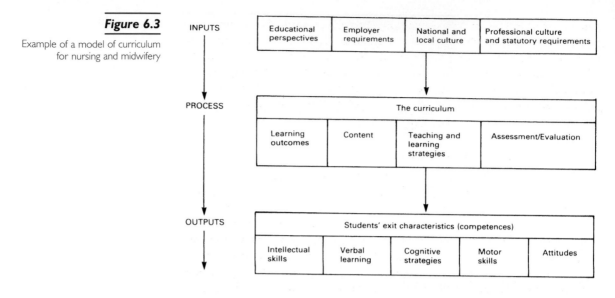

3. *Curriculum outputs.* These can be subsumed under the general
   heading of professional competence, but in the model I have used
   Gagne's five learning capabilities which together constitute the
   students' characteristics on exit from the curriculum.

This model can therefore be used to conceptualize curricula for nursing
and midwifery, and being a generic model could apply to a wide range
of curricula at different levels. For example, it could be equally appropriate for a pre-registration midwifery course or a post-registration
course in intensive-care nursing. The nature of the curriculum inputs,
process and outcomes would differ markedly between these two
examples, but the basic structure of the model would remain the same.

Organizing and sequencing of curriculum content

The curriculum rationale guides the selection of content, but not the
sequence and organization of that content into some form of logical
order. The latter is important if students are to be able to make sense of
the programme of study and is achieved by means of a conceptual
framework or model. Bernstein (1971) identifies two approaches to
content organization in curricula: collection and integration. In a
'collection' curriculum, subjects are taught as separate, isolated entities
with clear-cut boundaries, the emphasis being on depth of treatment. In
contrast, 'integrated' curricula focus on common themes that unite
various subjects and the emphasis is on breadth of coverage. Collection
curricula are typified by timetables containing 'slots' with separate
subjects such as 'anatomy' and 'physiology' and 'psychology'. Integrated
curricula, on the other hand, consist of broad themes such as 'the individual in pain'. Simmons and Bahl (1992) describe an integrated approach
to curriculum development at post-registration level. In nurse education,
they see integration having two main meanings. Integration of content

can be achieved by linking academic disciplines, and also theory and practice. Integration also applies to student groups, where students from different branches of nursing, or from other professions, learn together. They describe their PEP curriculum model for post-registration education as developing individual practitioners in three areas: professional development, educational development, and personal development.

Academic validation of curricula

Academic validation is the programme or course approval process used in HE. It consists of a carefully selected panel of academics that engages the programme team in discussion about the programme curriculum, and decides whether or not the programme is approved to run. Validation needs to be distinguished from an allied concept, accreditation. Many programmes and courses in HE involve professional education and training, and as such are subject not only to university regulations, but also to the requirements for professional recognition by the appropriate professional body. These requirements are safeguarded by the process of professional accreditation, which may consist of scrutiny of the programme documentation alone, or by an accreditation event. The latter is usually combined with a validation event, so that both academic validation and professional accreditation are undertaken at the same time.

In nursing and midwifery, however, there is an additional category called conjoint validation, in which HE and a National Board for Nursing, Midwifery and Health Visiting are equal partners in the validation process. Once the curriculum development work has been completed the programme can be advertised provided that it states 'subject to validation'.

The validation event is seen as the culmination of the work of the curriculum development team, and if carried out in the right spirit can be a stimulating academic debate between peers. There are three types of validation: internal, mock and full validation.

1. *Internal validation* is a formal component of the quality assurance mechanism of the institution, and consists of a meeting between the curriculum development team and selected members of the institution. The curriculum submission is scrutinized in a similar way to a final validation, using a small panel of internal members of the institution who have no direct involvement with the curriculum in question. Feedback from internal validation is incorporated into the draft validation document, after which it is sent for printing.
2. *Mock validation* is the name given to a practice validation event which is conducted exactly like a real event, the aim of which is to test the team's cohesiveness and ability to defend their curriculum design.
3. *Full validation* is a major academic event in which a panel of

academic staff is assembled to engage and challenge the programme team on their curriculum design.

Membership of validation panels

The HE sector has strict guidelines for the choice of panel members, and typical membership is as follows:

- chair: a senior member of staff drawn from the committee responsible for academic standards in the university, who is not from the faculty submitting the programme;
- one academic from the host school, who was not involved in the development;
- one academic from outside the host school;
- an external practitioner who is a practising professional in an appropriate field, or a potential employer of graduates from the programme.

The validation event

Programme development teams usually experience some anxiety when approaching a validation event, since it is important for them to achieve a successful outcome. However, a validation event is one of the few opportunities that educators have to engage in real academic debate about philosophical and practical educational issues. The programme development team will have received in advance the key agenda issues that the panel wish to cover, but should be prepared also for other issues to be raised during the event.

The most important aspect of a programme is the quality of the staff who will be teaching on it, so the programme team must project a confident, informed and cohesive impression. This means that contributions should be distributed amongst the entire team, and not dominated by any one individual. Having said this, it is equally important that the programme director designate should maintain a high profile during the event, and this can be done by taking the lead in some areas of questioning, and by inviting other members of the team to answer particular questions. It is useful to have decided in advance of the event which team member will answer questions on a particular area, such as assessment or admissions. This ensures that no team member should be caught out by not having a satisfactory answer ready. Self-confidence and conviction are the keys to successful validation; the panel are fellow educationalists and peers, so the programme team need not feel intimidated by them. The chair of the event has an important role in keeping the dialogue constructive rather than confrontational, although it is important to encourage an atmosphere of rigorous challenge and debate.

There are a number of possible outcomes of a validation event:

1. approval for an indefinite length of time, with review at a given time, e.g. every five years;
2. approval for a fixed length of time, e.g. five years, after which the programme is then subject to review;

3. approval that is conditional upon fulfilment of certain requirements within a specified time scale; and
4. approval withheld.

Conditional approval is a very common outcome of validation events,
and conditions can be imposed for any aspect of the curriculum. For
example, the assessment strategy may need to be amended, certain regulations modified, an evaluation carried out by the end of the first year,
or a students' handbook produced. Conditional approval will always
carry a date by which the conditions must be met, and this can vary
from a few weeks to a whole year. The programme development team
must make a satisfactory response to the conditions, and this is sent to
all panel members. Once the panel has agreed that the conditions have
been met, the amendments are incorporated into the validation
document, and this then becomes the definitive programme document.
This is housed in the library for general access by students and anyone
else who is interested in the programme.

Curriculum monitoring and evaluation

This is dealt with in Chapter 12, Quality Assurance and Evaluation.

Staff development for practice supervisors

Whilst the curriculum group is developing its work, there needs to be a
parallel development with the in-service training department to plan for
the anticipated training needs of qualified staff who will be involved in
the new curriculum. Opportunities must be made available for such staff
to spend time in workshops and study days that relate to specific aspects
of the new curriculum.

EQUAL OPPORTUNITIES:THE INCLUSIVE CURRICULUM

Equality of opportunity is a central tenet of modern education, and
relates to all aspects of higher education curricula as well as to wider
aspects of institutional management. The term 'equal opportunities' can
be interpreted in a number of ways, and the difficulty of pinning down a
definition is highlighted by Farish *et al.* (1995):

> '*One of the problems with examining the effectiveness or otherwise
> of equal opportunities policy-making is that the term "equal
> opportunities" itself is so elusive. It can be applied to a wide variety
> of contexts within educational institutions: for instance, to staff
> issues, curriculum, pedagogy, assessment, access and recruitment,
> priorities in funding, staff-student relationships, the general work
> environment and so on'.*

Powney *et al.* (1997) suggest that higher education institutions should
have an equal opportunities policy that covers the following aspects:

1. the recruitment, induction, support and career development of
students;

2. the content and methods for learning and teaching;
3. the recruitment, employment, support, and staff development of academic staff and support staff;
4. the management and governance of the institution.

Equal opportunity practice in higher education is supported by legislation in three main areas: race, sex and disability, and the relevant acts are the Sex Discrimination Act 19975, the Race Relations Act 1976, and the Disability Discrimination Act 1995. Higher education institutions are required to ensure that no unlawful discrimination on the grounds of race or sex occurs in the institution.

Curriculum provision for students with disabilities

It is important that nurse teachers have an understanding of approaches to disabled students if the latter are not to be disadvantaged. Lloyd (1998) points out the difference between the traditional view of disability as a deficit, and the new approach that is emerging:

> 'In educational terms, the provision of access, or the integration of disabled students, has been concerned with normalization i.e. assisting and supporting the student to fit into existing structures with the minimum of modification. Provision has, in the old model, involved a focus on remediation, extra support, withdrawal groups, and extra technological aids. It compensates for disability, and tries to eliminate differences. Currently a different model is being proposed, whereby genuine access to learning for disabled students is planned within an inclusive framework. This provision will recognize difference and diversity as enriching and will begin to offer access for all to the full curriculum. All our learning and teaching approaches should support this aim. The result will be a celebration of difference'.

Candidates for nursing or midwifery education are required to possess the physical and mental ability to carry out the demands of the role of nurse or midwife, so this precludes the selection of candidates with severe disabilities. However, candidates may have a degree of disability that does not prevent them from carrying out the role, e.g. visual impairment, hearing impairment, a physical disability, or dyslexia. Nurse teachers need to take the needs of such students into account during their teaching. For example, she may need to provide paper copies of overhead transparencies for students with visual impairment, and ensure that when talking to students with a hearing impairment, she faces the student and speaks clearly.

Nurse teachers may encounter students with dyslexia, both diagnosed and undiagnosed; in the latter case the following indicators may suggest dyslexia (University of Greenwich, 1998):

1. discrepancy between academic achievement and practical performance;

2. excessive spelling errors in written work, such as confusion of letter order;
3. difficulty in writing lecture notes;
4. difficulty with working memory, e.g. problems taking down a phone number;
5. forgetting a sequence of instructions, and/or getting them in the wrong order.

Universities will have a member of staff who has expertise in dealing with dyslexia, and students should be referred to this individual in the first instance. The student may then be referred for in-house assessment, or psychometric testing by an educational psychologist. Dyslexic students need special help with writing their assignments, and nurse teachers need to provide careful feedback on how to construct an essay. It may be necessary to arrange for extra time during examinations, or even to make arrangements for students to be examined by a viva rather than a written examination. Most dyslexic students benefit from using a computer, and software packages are available to augment standard word-processing software in terms of spelling and syntax.

The multicultural curriculum

The term *culture* refers to the civilization and customs of particular people or groups, their whole way of life, in fact. Great Britain is very much a multicultural society by virtue of its rich mix of individuals and groups with ethnic differences. This does not refer solely to differences in skin colour, since cultures can vary considerably within a relatively small area. There are marked differences in customs between the North, the Midlands and the South of England and such cultural differences form part of the richness of society.

Immigration has brought a much wider range of cultures to British society, each with its own particular values, beliefs and customs, and a true multicultural society will give equal status to every culture. In practice, however, it appears that ethnic minorities, particularly black people, are exposed to racial discrimination and racism in their daily lives in Britain. Racial discrimination means that an individual or group receives less favourable treatment in comparison to another by virtue of their racial origins. Discrimination is not always obvious, as in the case of regulations regarding nurses' uniforms, which forbid certain forms of dress in violation of cultural requirements. Racism is a broad term that implies the use of power to support racist beliefs, such as the superiority of white people.

Nurse educators need to be aware of the implications of multicultural education in nursing and these can be thought of in terms of two specific aspects, the students' own cultural requirements and their need to understand aspects of the culture of patients with whom they will come into contact. It is common to find that curricula in nursing deal with aspects of diet in relation to other cultures and also the specific beliefs and procedures to be followed when a patient dies. Awareness of cultural values as a topic needs to be seen as crucial if nurses are to practise their profession effectively in a multicultural society.

Nursing draws its recruits from a variety of cultural backgrounds and they will practise very much in a multicultural setting in both hospitals and community. The ENB commissioned a study on the recruitment of minority ethnic groups into nursing, midwifery and health visiting (ENB, 1998) in which the recruitment and selection practices of eight education centres in England were investigated through case studies. The main findings in relation to applications are as follows:

- Substantial proportions of applicants were resident outside Great Britain.
- Amongst female applicants resident in Great Britain at the time of their application, each of the Black Groups was over-represented relative to the population as a whole; there was a very strong degree of over-representation for the Black African group.
- Amongst male applicants there was no single pattern for Black Groups, but Black African males were more strongly over-represented than female applicants from the same group.
- Both females and males in Asian Groups are consistently under-represented amongst applicants for nursing and midwifery.
- In relation to ethnic minority applicants, higher proportions of applications were rejected before interview, at the shortlisting stage, in comparison to whites.
- There was little targeting of recruitment on minority ethnic communities, and only a patchy understanding of rationales for a more focused approach to recruitment of minority ethnic groups.

Curricula in nursing and midwifery education should acknowledge the multicultural nature of an NHS Trust by including study of the cultures represented in that particular community. This should not be represented as a minority interest, but as part of a balanced approach to the study of society in general.

Another way in which multicultural aspects can be brought into nurse education is during actual classroom teaching; when presenting materials and information, the teacher should present ideas and examples from a variety of cultures rather than solely from Western European culture. It is important that visual media and books contain members of ethnic minorities as well as the indigenous white population and that case studies and simulations should include names and characters from ethnic minorities. The Further Education Curriculum Unit offers a comprehensive checklist on the multicultural curriculum (FEU, 1988), and a selection from this is shown in Table 6.14.

The multi-professional curriculum

The increasing need for practitioners to work as part of a multi-disciplinary team has fuelled interest in the concept of multi-professional education. The English National Board for Nursing, Midwifery and Health Visiting commissioned a study of the role of collaborative/shared

A. Curriculum development, evaluation and review
1. Has the content of the curriculum been examined in terms of ethnocentrism or eurocentrism?
2. Does the content reflect the multicultural nature of British, European and world contexts?
3. Is feedback sought from students on their reaction to content, materials and resources?

B. Books and resource materials
1. Are people from different ethnic groups shown in a variety of roles?
2. Are there strong role models with whom students from different ethnic groups can identify?
3. Are illustrations free from stereotyping?

C. Teaching and classroom interaction
1. Is the teacher aware of the different racial/ethnic/religious/linguistic backgrounds of students without making stereotyped assumptions about these?
2. Are students' names remembered and pronounced correctly?
3. Does the teacher have a clear understanding of, and commitment to, race equality?

Table 6.14

Checklist for a multicultural curriculum

learning in pre- and post-registration education in nursing, midwifery and health visiting (ENB, 1999b). The project focused on three key questions:

1. What qualities and skills are needed by practitioners to work effectively in a multi-professional context?
2. What is the extent and interpretation of shared learning provision in higher education?
3. What is the fit between the knowledge and skills needed in multi-professional practice, and the teaching and learning which takes place in educational preparation?

The data was collected using case studies of six multi-professional teams, surveys and telephone interviews with higher education institutions, interviews with Trust managers, and information from professional bodies. The findings included the following:

- very little of the current provision of multi-professional education in universities addressed inter-professional issues;
- content was chosen because it was defined as common across different professions;
- the most frequent shared provision was biological and behavioural sciences;
- in initial education, commonality was associated with large group, didactic teaching;
- geographical separation of disciplines and organizational incompatibilities presented problems in shared learning;
- timetabling was also problematic, i.e. the need to find common learning needs that two or more professional groups could do jointly at the same point in time;
- disparity between educational entry requirements;
- differences in the period of time required for professional education, e.g. medicine is five years, nursing three;
- numerical dominance by one professional group could mean courses tailored to majority needs;
- there was a need for greater role flexibility;

- multi-skilling initiatives were progressing primarily with nurses;
- vested professional interests may lead to disputes about new interpretations of roles.

REFERENCES

Beattie, A. (1987) Making a curriculum work, in *The Curriculum in Nursing Education*, P. Allan and M. Jolley (eds), Croom Helm, London.

Bell, R. (1973) *Thinking About the Curriculum*, Open University Press, Milton Keynes.

Bennett, N. (1976) *Teaching Styles and Pupil Progress*, Open Books, London.

Bernstein, B. (1971) On the classification and framing of educational knowledge, in *Knowledge and Control: New Directions for the Sociology of Education*, M. Young (ed.), Collier Macmillan, London.

Bloom, B. (1956) *Taxonomy of Educational Objectives: The Classification of Educational Goals, Handbook One: Cognitive Domain*, McKay, New York.

Butterworth, C. (1992) More than one bite at the APEL: contrasting models of accrediting prior learning., *Journal of Further and Higher Education*, **16**(3).

Butterworth, C. (1993) *Introduction and Self-assessment Guide to Claiming APEL by Distance Learning*, University of Greenwich, London.

Davies, I. (1969) Education and social science, *New Society*, May 8th.

Dearing, R. (1997) *Higher Education in the Learning Society*, The Report of the National Committee of Inquiry into Higher Education, HMSO, Norwich.

English National Board for Nursing, Midwifery and Health Visiting (1997) *Standards for Approval of Higher Education Institutions and Courses*, ENB, London.

English National Board for Nursing, Midwifery and Health Visiting (1998) *Evaluation of Equal Opportunties Policy: The Recruitment of Minority Ethnic Groups into Nursing, Midwifery and Health Visiting*, ENB, London.

English National Board for Nursing, Midwifery and Health Visiting (1999a) *A Documentary Analysis of Nursing Degree Curricula*, Research Highlights 38, ENB, London.

English National Board for Nursing, Midwifery and Health Visiting (1999b) *The Role of Collaborative/Shared Learning in Pre-and Post-Registration Education in Nursing, Midwifery and Health Visiting*, Research Highlights 39, ENB, London.

Further Education Unit (1988) *Staff Development for a Multicultural Society*, FEU, London.

Farish, M., McPake, J., Powney, J. and Weiner, G. (1995) *Equal Opportunities in Colleges and Universities: Towards Better Practices*, SRHE/OUP, Milton Keynes.

Fraser, M. (1996) *Conceptual Nursing in Practice: A Research-Based Approach*, Chapman and Hall, London.

Galton, M. and Simon, B. (1975) *Observation Research and Classroom Behaviour*, University of Leicester, Leicester.

General Nursing Council for England and Wales (1977) *A Statement of Educational Policy*, Circular 77/19, GNCEW, London.

Getzels, J. and Thelen, H. (1960) A conceptual framework for the study of the classroom as a social system, in *The Social Psychology of Teaching*, Penguin, Harmondsworth.

Gronlund, N. (1978) *Stating Behavioural Objectives for Classroom Instruction*, Macmillan, New York.

Harrow, A. (1972) *A Taxonomy of the Psychomotor Domain*, McKay, New York.

HMSO (1989) *Working for Patients, Education and Training, Working Paper 10*, HMSO, London.

Humphreys, J. and Quinn, F.M. (1994) *Healthcare Education: The Challenge of the Market*, Chapman and Hall, London.

Humphreys, J. (1994) New models in a corporate paradigm, in *Healthcare Education: The Challenge of the Market*, J. Humphreys and F.M. Quinn (eds), Chapman and Hall, London.

Kerr, J. (1968) Changing the curriculum, in *The Curriculum: Design, Context and Development*, R. Hooper (ed.), Oliver and Boyd, Edinburgh.

Kolb, D. (1984) *Experiential Learning*, Prentice Hall, London.

Krathwohl, D., Bloom, B. and Masia, B. (1964) *A Taxonomy of Educational Objectives: the Classification of Education Goals, Handbook 2: Affective Domain*, McKay, New York.

Lawton, D. (1983) *Curriculum Studies and Educational Planning*, Hodder and Stoughton, London.

Lewis, A. and Miel, A. (1972) *Supervision for Improved Instruction: New Challenges, New Responses*, Wadsworth, Belmont.

Lloyd, C.M. (1998) *Access to Learning for Students With Disabilities: The FOSL Project*, University of Greenwich, London.

Mager, R. (1962) *Preparing Instructional Objectives*, Fearon, California.

Powney, J., Hamilton, S. and Weiner, G. (1997) *Higher Education and Equality: A Guide*, Commission for Racial Equality/Equal Opportunities Commission/CVCP.

Quinn, F.M. (1988) *The Principles and Practice of Nurse Education*, 2nd edn, Chapman and Hall, London.

Quinn, F.M. (1994) The Demise of Curriculum, in *Healthcare Education: The Challenge of the Market*, J. Humphreys and F.M. Quinn (eds), Chapman and Hall, London.

Saylor, J., Alexander, W. and Lewis, A. (1981) *Curriculum Planning for Better Teaching and Learning*, 4th edn, Holt, Rinehart and Winston, New York.

Scrimshaw, P. (1983) *Educational Ideologies. Unit 2 of Educational Studies*, Open University, Milton Keynes.

Simmons, S. and Bahl, D. (1992) An integrated approach to curriculum development, *Nurse Education Today*, **12**, 310–15.

Simpson, E. (1972) The classification of educational objectives in the psychomotor domain, in *The Psychomotor Domain*, Vol. 3, Gryphon House, Washington, DC.

Skilbeck, M. (1984) *School Based Curriculum Development*, Harper and Row, London.

Stenhouse, L. (1975) *An Introduction to Curriculum Research and Development*, Heinemann, London.

Tanner, D. and Tanner, L. (1980) *Curriculum Development: Theory into Practice*, 2nd edn, Macmillan, New York.

Tyler, R. (1949) *Basic Principles of Curriculum and Instruction*, University Of Chicago Press, Chicago.

University Of Greenwich (1996) *Quality Assurance Handbook*, University of Greenwich, London.

University of Greenwich (1998) *Access to Learning for Students With Disabilities: The FOSL Project*, University of Greenwich, London.

7 Planning for Teaching

Professional teaching in nursing, midwifery and health visiting is an intentional enterprise that aims to facilitate learning. It is characterized by an acceptance of responsibility for facilitating other people's learning by means of planned and purposeful educational interventions. This is not to say that teaching ignores the possibility of unplanned learning; indeed, there are powerful arguments to support the view that teaching must provide an atmosphere for students in which unpredictable or creative outcomes can emerge. However, even this example shows evidence of broad teaching intentions, namely, the provision of a climate in which unpredictable outcomes are encouraged.

Within nursing, midwifery and health visiting there is a wide range of teaching contexts, ranging from the delivery of lectures in a university through to one-to-one teaching sessions with individual students, practitioners, patients and clients. It must also be acknowledged that many teaching encounters in clinical and community settings are opportunistic, arising spontaneously during the day-to-day delivery of care. It is therefore difficult to be specific about what should be included when planning for such a diverse range of teaching, but there are a number of generic factors that might be taken into account, as shown in Table 7.1. However, the relevance of each of these will vary according to the nature of the teaching encounter.

Defining the Purpose of a Teaching Session

In Chapter 6 (p. 137), aims and learning outcomes were discussed in some detail, so only a brief overview is given below. The practice of stating aims and learning outcomes is now almost universal within the higher education sector; these are normally of two kinds, general aims and learning outcomes for the programme as a whole, and those for specific modules or units of learning. It is important to state aims and learning outcomes even if the teaching session is not related to an academic programme, since they help the learner to understand the purpose of the session.

Educational aims are broad, strategic statements of intent, which include reference to the value of achieving the aim. For example, 'To assist the students to develop the appropriate knowledge and skills that will enable them to deliver high- quality care to patients suffering from cancer'. Note that no details of the 'knowledge and skills' are given in the aim; fine detail such as this are contained within the learning outcomes. Note also that there is a value included in the aim, i.e. 'enable them to deliver high-quality care'.

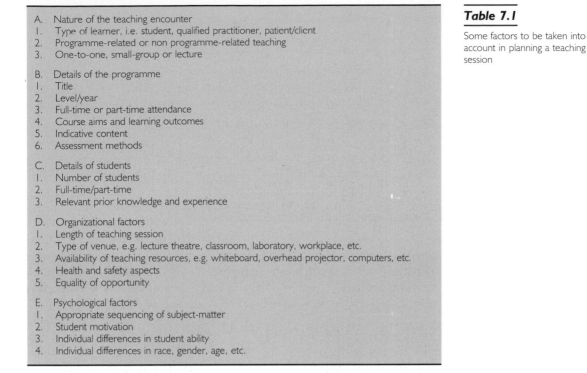

A. Nature of the teaching encounter
1. Type of learner, i.e. student, qualified practitioner, patient/client
2. Programme-related or non programme-related teaching
3. One-to-one, small-group or lecture

B. Details of the programme
1. Title
2. Level/year
3. Full-time or part-time attendance
4. Course aims and learning outcomes
5. Indicative content
6. Assessment methods

C. Details of students
1. Number of students
2. Full-time/part-time
3. Relevant prior knowledge and experience

D. Organizational factors
1. Length of teaching session
2. Type of venue, e.g. lecture theatre, classroom, laboratory, workplace, etc.
3. Availability of teaching resources, e.g. whiteboard, overhead projector, computers, etc.
4. Health and safety aspects
5. Equality of opportunity

E. Psychological factors
1. Appropriate sequencing of subject-matter
2. Student motivation
3. Individual differences in student ability
4. Individual differences in race, gender, age, etc.

Table 7.1

Some factors to be taken into account in planning a teaching session

Learning outcomes are specific statements about what the student should have achieved by the end of a module or unit, and are often stated in terms of student behaviours. For example, 'Defines the terms transient, acute and chronic pain, with reference to the relevant literature'. The behavioural verb here is 'defines', which indicates very clearly what the student is expected to achieve. This would normally be either in written form or by oral explanation. The outcome also contains a criterion for performance, i.e. 'with reference to the relevant literature'.

It would not be sufficient for the student to simply be able to 'define the terms'; she must also meet the criterion for performance of the outcome.

Academic level of learning outcomes

Learning outcomes are formulated at the appropriate level for the unit or module in question. Academic levels and definitions may vary between higher education institutions; Table 7.2. gives the levels and definitions in use at the University of Greenwich. Levels 1, 2, and 3 correspond to years 1, 2, and 3 of an undergraduate honours degree programme.

Learning outcomes and assessment

Learning outcomes and assessment of learning are inextricably linked, in that assessment normally requires the student to demonstrate achievement of the learning outcomes. One advantage of learning outcomes is

Table 7.2

Definitions of academic levels
(University of Greenwich, 1999)

Level 0	Meeting required levels of literacy and numeracy and acquiring understanding in core areas allowing access to defined programmes of study in post school education
Level 1	Acquisition of basic knowledge, skills and competence
Level 2	Builds on level 1 and involves an extension and reinforcement of those experiences
Level 3	Reflects the synthesis of basic knowledge, skills and competence and equips students with tools of analysis and evaluation
Level M	Provides opportunities to: (i) reflect on the significance and inter-relationships of knowledge acquired from a variety of sources (ii) to use such sources, with critical insight, to evaluate findings of a small-scale enquiry or other activity (iii) to provide explanations within identified frameworks and/or general theory (iv) formulate innovative proposals (v) achieve all outcomes with a large degree of autonomy

that they provide learners with clear goals for their studies, but they can shift the focus of study too heavily towards assessment, to the detriment of wider reading.

SELECTING THE SUBJECT MATTER (CONTENT) OF A TEACHING SESSION

It must be acknowledged from the outset that subject-matter is not necessarily synonymous with content. The term *subject-matter* is normally attached to the various fields of knowledge that comprise the science and art of nursing, midwifery and health visiting and in this sense it equates with the term content. However, some teaching sessions in nursing and health have as their content a variety of group processes and interactions which are not subject-matter *per se*, but which still require careful planning. This aspect is dealt with in Chapter 14 (p. 353) on small-group teaching and experiential learning.

It goes without saying that a teacher should possess a thorough understanding of the subject matter to be taught; in higher education the minimum benchmark for a lecturer is normally the possession of a first degree or equivalent. This level of knowledge does, in itself, present problems in the selection of subject matter for teaching. The more expert a teacher is, the more difficult it is to decide what must go in, and more importantly what has to be left out, of a teaching session.

This may result in the inexperienced teacher cramming far too much information into sessions. The secret of successful teaching is to place severe limits on the amount of content in a given session by the judicious selection of the most important aspects of the topic, and the ruthless pruning of other, less crucial material.

Concept mapping

In Chapter 4 (p. 76), the nature of concepts was discussed. When planning teaching sessions, one of the most difficult decisions confronting the teacher is deciding what *must* go in, what *should* go in, and what *could* go in; concept sorting and mapping can be a helpful tool in this regard. Lawless *et al.* (1998) offer the following definition:

> '*Concept sorting is a simple, yet powerful, way in which to generate, sort, arrange and rearrange any set of elements, i.e. ideas, concepts, events, statements or procedures, in a visually explicit manner, namely a concept map*' (Lawless et al., p. 219).

Hence, the terms have largely the same meaning, but the writers point out that the term 'concept-sorting' is used in business and public administration, whereas 'concept mapping' is the preferred term in education because the emphasis is on the relationships between concepts.

Concept mapping provides a way of prioritizing concepts in a concrete, visual way. The simplest way of making a concept map is to write each concept on a small square of paper and then place the squares on a flat surface. The squares are then arranged in order of their relationship to each other, with the most closely-related concepts being place next to each other. This pattern is then transferred to a diagram, and the relationships between concepts are shown by connecting lines, usually annotated.

Figure 7.1 shows an example of a concept map for the topic 'coronary heart disease', and a range of first-order, second-order and third-order concepts are included. When making a decision about which concepts to include and which to omit, the teacher will need to judge the appropriate level of information for the learners in question, and also the amount of time available for the session.

When sorting the concepts, lecturers draw upon the relevant literature and their specialist knowledge and experience of the topic, and the end result should be a prioritizing of concepts into key concepts (must be included), second-order concepts (should be included) and third-order concepts (could be included). At the level of the key concepts, selection is usually fairly straightforward; it is at the level of the second- and third-order concepts that the danger of over-inclusion of information is most likely to occur. There are all kinds of fascinating facts and anecdotes attached to the key concepts of nursing and health, and as such these can be important elements in the maintenance of students' interest and motivation.

Problems may arise when the teacher perceives that there are so many key concepts to include, leaving no time for these interesting, but non-essential aspects of the topic. This dilemma can be lessened if the aim of the session is taken into account. Provided sufficient book and periodical resources are available in the college, there should seldom be the need for the teacher to attempt to cover all aspects of a topic in detail. By the judicious use of references and further reading, the teacher can limit the number of concepts within the session, and in so doing will free up time for inclusion of anecdotes and other interesting facets of the topic.

Although the foregoing information has focused on the planning of a single teaching session, concept mapping is equally appropriate for

181

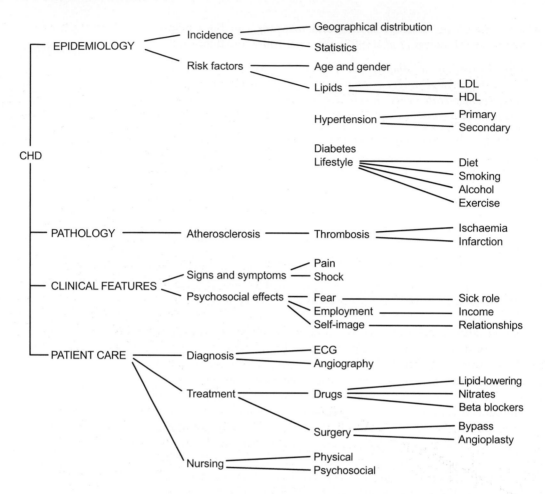

Figure 7.1

Concept map for coronary heart
disease

planning a scheme of work for a series of sessions on a broad topic area. It can actually be easier to make a selection from a concept map if more than one session is available, as the time constraints may be less evident.

SELECTING APPROPRIATE TEACHING STRATEGIES

There is a wide range of strategies available to the teacher and these are discussed in detail in the relevant chapters of this book. Hence, for this section I will simply provide an overview of the basis on which teaching strategies might be selected. The starting point for selection of teaching and learning strategies is the broad purpose of the session(s). The strategies must be compatible with the aims of the session; lecturing is very commonly used as a vehicle for conveying subject matter to students, but there may well be more effective ways involving individualized instruction. If the intention of a session is to encourage discussion or debate about issues, student-centred activities should predominate; for skills teaching, demonstration followed by student practice is an appropriate strategy.

Encouraging a deep approach to learning

Evidence suggests that there is an over-reliance on those teaching methods involving the transmission of information, often combined with assessment methods that encourage the superficial reproduction of facts.

The Improving Student Learning Project (CNAA, 1992) identified ways in which teachers can encourage students to adopt a deep approach to learning as opposed to the superficial approach referred to above. A deep approach to learning involves a search for understanding, and there are four elements of courses which foster this:

1. *Motivational context*. Students experience a need to know, and are intrinsically motivated;
2. *Active learning*. Active involvement in learning is encouraged;
3. *Interaction with others*. Opportunities exist for exploratory discussion; and
4. *A well-structured knowledge base*. Content is taught in integrated wholes and related to other knowledge.

The CNAA project identified several strategies which contain one or more of these elements, and these are shown in Table 7.3.

The CNAA project makes the point that existing curricula need not necessarily be abandoned, but can be modified to include the above strategies.

Independent learning	This involves the use of learning contracts that give the student a greater measure of control of the learning process.
Personal development	Student motivation and the involvement of feelings as well as intellect are key elements in this strategy,
Reflection	This includes use of reflective diaries and journals, video and observers for skills learning.
Independent group work	The emphasis here is on interactive group methods such as peer tutoring and group projects.
Learning by doing	This is experiential learning and includes role play, gaming and work experience.
Learning skills	These are not merely study skills per se, but a sense of purpose and awareness of task demands and flexibility.
Projects	These involve activity and application of knowledge, and require a high level of student motivation.

Table 7.3

Strategies encouraging a deep approach to learning (CNAA, 1992)

Deductive and inductive teaching of concepts

There are two main ways of teaching concepts, deductively and inductively. When teaching a concept *deductively*, the teacher begins by giving a definition of the concept and then follows this up with a number of examples. Thus, when teaching the concept of 'cell' a definition would be given, followed by a number of examples of various cells such as nerve cells, epithelial cells and so on. Examples would also be

Table 7.4

Sequence for teaching a concept by deductive method

1.	Define the concept to the student
2.	Show an example of the concept, or a representation of it
3.	Give two different examples of the concept along with two non-examples and check the student's discrimination
4.	Help the student to identify the critical attributes of the concept
5.	Give novel examples to check concept attainment

given of non-cells to aid discrimination of the concept. Table 7.4 summarizes the sequence for teaching a concept by the deductive method.

When teaching a concept *inductively*, the teacher first gives a number of instances (examples) of the concept and then draws out from the students a definition of the concept. The teacher might begin with illustrations or descriptions of a number of patients, some grossly over-weight, some extremely thin, others with specific physical or nervous disorders such as scurvey and bulimia. The students then try to ascertain any factors that are common to all the instances, eventually coming up with a definition of the concept 'malnutrition'.

The following is a useful mnemonic for remembering the difference between inductive and deductive teaching:

*De*ductive teaching begins with a *de*finition and then gives instances (examples);

*In*ductive teaching begins with *in*stances (examples) and then arrives at a definition.

PLANNING AN EXPLANATION

Explanations form the greater part of the teaching of subject-matter, yet the study of explanations is still in its infancy (Bligh, 1998). When an explanation is given to students, the teacher links what the students already know to the new information that is being given. This principle is nicely captured by Ausubel *et al.* (1978):

> *'If I had to reduce all educational psychology to just one principle it would be this: The most important single factor influencing learning is what the student already knows. Ascertain this and teach him accordingly' (Ausubel* et al. *1978, p. 163).*

Classification of explanations

Within the literature there are a number of ways in which explanations are classified; for example, Bligh (1998) identifies eleven kinds of explanation, but for everyday practice a much more useful classification is that of Brown and Atkins (1988):

1. interpretive, i.e. answers the question 'What?'
2. descriptive, i.e. answers the question 'How?'
3. reason-giving, i.e. answers the question 'Why?'

Brown and Atkins describe explaining as a three-stage process consisting of:

1. *A problem to be explained (problem identification).* The term 'problem' relates to concepts in the subject-matter to be taught to students.
2. *A series of statements (transmission).* These are linked statements made by the lecturer containing the examples, principles and other material relevant to understanding of the problem, and must be stated at an appropriate level for the students in question. They must be conveyed with clarity, and should arouse students' interest in the explanation.
3. *An understanding of the problem (outcome).* If the explanation is successful, students will understand the problem. If not, the lecturer will have to deliver a new series of statements that offer a different perspective on the problem.

When planning an explanation, Brown and Armstrong (1984) suggest that initially, the lecturer should analyse the topic into its main parts or 'keys' and then establish any links between these, including any rules that might be involved. The particular type of explanation required is identified and incorporated into the teaching plan. Brown and Armstrong found that better explanations had more keys and a greater variety of cognitive levels of keys, so that the lecturers in the study placed more varied demands on the pupils, particularly higher levels of cognitive demand. Better explanations also involved the use of examples, visual aids and rhetorical questions and were more appropriately structured and stimulating.

Sequence for planning an explanation

George Brown (1978) is one of the few writers to have offered a sequence for planning an explanation:

1. Decide precisely what is to be explained, in the form of a question, for example what, why, how?
2. Identify any hidden variables. These might be prerequisite concepts which, although not immediately obvious in the problem, will influence understanding of the explanation. For example, a hidden variable in the question 'How does oxygen from the air reach the tissues?' would be the concept of diffusion of a gas.
3. State the key points.
4. Design the 'keys'. This involves taking each of the key points and writing each one as a simple statement. Each statement should have one or two examples to illustrate it and also elaborations or qualifications, as appropriate. It is useful to include a restatement or extension of the main point, using different words.
5. Write a summary of the key points, to be used at the end of the explanation.

6. Write the introduction to the explanation. Brown suggests that this is done last so that a motivating and interesting introduction can be devised, which is appropriate to the sequence. It is useful to use such devices as a provocative question or an interesting anecdote to capture attention.

Table 7.5 shows a planning sequence for an explanation, with the problem stated in the form of a question in Step 1. Step 2 shows the attempt to identify hidden variables by stating the relationship between the parts of the question. It can be seen that the explanation needs more than the four points made here, because there is a hidden variable namely the fact that gallstones do not always cause jaundice. Step 3 is a list of the key points of the explanation, and these are expressed in Step 4 as statements or keys. Each of these keys would need to have some examples to illustrate the point and also elaboration or qualifications. For instance, the teacher might give examples of the kind of people who are likely to suffer from gallstones, possibly including the aphorism 'fair, fat, forty, fertile and flatulent'. Having designed the explanation, all that remains is for the teacher to incorporate it into the teaching plan, taking care to provide a motivating introduction.

Table 7.5

Planning sequence for explaining 'How gallstones cause jaundice'

Step 1	How do gallstones cause jaundice?
Step 2	Common bile duct conveys bile from liver to intestine via gall bladder Obstruction to bile flow causes jaundice Gallstones block the common bile duct Gallstones cause jaundice
	Hidden variable = gallstones do not always cause jaundice. Thus, the explanation must make clear in what circumstances gallstones cause jaundice.
Step 3	Secretion of bile; storage and passage of bile; formation of gallstones; migration and impaction of gallstone; results of obstruction to flow of bile.
Step 4	(a) Bile is secreted by hepatocyes and conveyed to the gall bladder via the hepatic duct and cystic duct. (b) Bile is stored and concentrated in the gall bladder, from whence it is ejected by muscular contraction, and conveyed by peristalsis into small intestine via cystic duct and common bile duct. (c) In some people, gallstones form from precipitation of bile constituents, for example cholesterol, in gall bladder. (d) Small gallstones may be ejected during contraction of the gall bladder, passing by peristalsis into the common bile duct, where they may impact in the lumen. (e) This implication may cause obstruction to the flow of bile, with a resultant rise in back-pressure to the liver. (f) This back-pressure will eventually cause reversal of flow of bile into the bloodstream, raising the serum bilirubin and discolouring the skin and mucous membranes, i.e. jaundice.

Explaining complex medical jargon

The term *jargon* is often used in a derogatory way to indicate incomprehensible technical language, but a more appropriate definition is the specialist vocabulary of professions such as law and medicine. Indeed, the professions of nursing, midwifery and health visiting draw extensively upon the vocabulary of medicine, and this 'language of the priest-

'hood' must be mastered by students before they can understand the concepts upon which their practice is based. To the student, this is like being confronted with a totally unintelligible form of communication out of reach of the vocabulary of ordinary people in society.

It is possible for a student to know the word for something without understanding the concept it represents, the so-called 'empty verbalism'. The role of the teacher is to make this unfamiliar language meaningful to the student so that it can be remembered and recalled when required. The best way to help students remember jargon is to link it to what they already know, but the problem with medical jargon is that there may be no existing knowledge with which to link the new terminology.

One way to overcome this problem is to use the literal meanings of the Graeco-Roman terms as a link to their everyday lives. The word 'acetabulum' has no meaning to a student in its existing form, but its literal translation is 'vinegar cup' and this is a nice description of the cup-shaped hollow in the pelvis where the femoral head sits. The word is easily remembered if it is associated with words that the student is already familiar with, i.e. acetic acid (vinegar). Similarly, the term 'nausea' literally means 'seasick' although its meaning has now generalized to all feelings of sickness, and it can be remembered by linking it to the word 'nautical'.

Table 7.6 gives a list of examples of medical jargon together with

Graeco-Roman word	Literal meaning
Physiotherapy	Healing by nature
Physiology	Science of nature
Epithelium	Upon the nipple
Pupil	Little doll
Nausea	Seasickness
Atheroma	Porridge-like tumour
Syndrome	Running together
Scaphoid	Boat-shaped
Lumen	Light
Acetabulum	Vinegar cup
Epididymis	Upon the twins
Eosinophil	Dawn, to love
Ectopic	Out of place
Sagittal	Arrow
Coronal	Crown
Trochanter	To run
Ischaemia	To check
Sesamoid	Sesame seed
Coccyx	Cuckoo-beak
Reticulum	Little net
Hemiplegia	Blow to half
Collagen	Glue
Decubitus	Lie on the elbow
Pathology	Science of suffering
Malaria	Bad air
Hypochondriac	Below the cartilages
Hysteria	Womb
Fontanelle	Little fountain
Hypercapnia	High level of smoke (CO_2)

Table 7.6

The original literal meanings of some examples of medical jargon

their original Greaco-Roman meanings, which might give students a more meaningful way of remembering the terms. It may also give a glimpse of the richness of language in the dim-and-distant past, alas now largely forgotten.

DESIGNING EFFECTIVE QUESTIONS

Questioning forms part of the canon of teaching, and it is useful to distinguish between two major types of questions: educational and management questions. Educational questions are those directly concerned with the educational outcomes of the student, such as subject-matter, feelings and opinions, whereas management questions are used to organize or control the classroom environment. Examples of the latter might be questions that are really commands, such as 'Would you please stop talking during my lecture?', or 'Would someone like to open a window?' This section focuses on educational questions.

Purposes of educational questioning

The purposes of educational questioning can be grouped under four main headings.

1. *Social purposes*:
   - to promote active involvement of the students during a lesson;
   - to encourage closer relationships between teachers and students;
   - to elicit any special interests or experience from the students.
2. *Motivational purposes*:
   - to develop the student's interest and motivation, e.g. 'How do you think that this problem might be overcome?';
   - to focus attention upon an aspect of the session;
   - to provide a change of stimulus.
3. *Cognitive purposes*:
   - to encourage the students to think at varying levels of complexity, and in a logical, analytical way.
4. *Assessment purposes*:
   - to assess the previous knowledge or skill of a student; to assess the student's ability to use the higher levels of cognitive functioning such as analysis, synthesis and evaluation;
   - to provide the teacher with feedback on the learning taking place during the course of a lecture.

These four categories emphasize the wide-ranging uses of questioning, but in practice, it seems that most teachers use mainly factual and closed questions (Delamont, 1983).

Classification of questions

There are many different ways of classifying questions, none of which is entirely satisfactory because questions depend very much on the context in which they are asked. Although none of the following examples are particularly recent, they are probably the most useful ones in the literature.

Bloom's taxonomy classification

In Chapter 6 (p. 139) the work of Benjamin Bloom (1956) is discussed in connection with educational objectives. The taxonomy of educational objectives can be used to formulate questions at different intellectual levels. Bloom classified intellectual or cognitive functions into a hierarchy of levels of increasing complexity, from simple recall of facts to evaluation and judgement of ideas.

The most basic level is called 'knowledge' and questions aimed at this level will ask the student to recall a definition or term, state a fact, or identify certain things.

The next level is 'comprehension', and the teacher can test this level by asking questions that require the student to restate meanings in his or her own words or to predict consequences or effects.

The third level is 'application', which requires the student to apply rules, methods and principles to specific situations. In a first aid lecture, for example, the teacher may have already given the rule for casualties, which states that they should be given nothing by mouth. Later in the lecture the teacher may give a specific example of a casualty with a fractured femur and ask the question, 'How would you deal with the casualty's request for a drink?'

'Analysis', the fourth level, requires questions to be phrased in such a way as to make the student break down concepts or situations into their component parts, whereas the fifth level, 'synthesis', asks the student to do the opposite, i.e. to build up a whole from a series of constituent parts. For example, a question such as 'From what we have done so far, can you tell us what the main areas of your nursing-care plan would be?' is an example of a synthesis-level question. The highest level of intellectual functioning, according to Bloom, is that of 'evaluation' and consists of questions that ascertain from the students their judgements about the best or most effective arguments or courses of action.

Brown and Edmondson' types of questions

Brown and Edmondson (1984) classify questions into two broad categories: 'cognitive' and 'speculative, affective and management'. Cognitive level questions are arranged in a way similar to Bloom's above, with five subcategories:

1. *data recall* includes recall of knowledge, tasks, naming, and classifying;
2. *simple deductions* from data, such as comparing, describing, and interpreting;
3. *providing reasons*, i.e. causes or motives that have not been taught in the lecture;
4. *problem-solving*;
5. *evaluating*.

Speculative, affective and management questions comprise such aspects as speculation, intuitive guesses, expression of emotions, class control, attention and checking understanding.

Kerry's classification

Kerry (1980) has devised a ten-item classification of questions:

1. *data-recall* questions, i.e. facts are recalled but not used;
2. *naming* questions, i.e. things are named;
3. *observation* questions, i.e. what the student observes;
4. *control* questions, which is part of classroom management;
5. *pseudo-questions*, where the teacher seems to give the impression that a range of answers will be acceptable, but in reality his or her mind is made up;
6. *speculative or hypothesis-generating* questions, which invite the student to speculate about a hypothetical situation;
7. *reasoning* questions, which ask for reasons as to why things occur;
8. *personal response* questions, which ask how the student feels about an issue;
9. *discriminatory* questions, which look for the points for and against an issue; and
10. *problem-solving* questions, which are geared to finding out about things.

The various classification systems outlined above are not exhaustive and there are other types of questions that have been identified. Probing questions encourage the student to develop his or her first answer, and prompting questions give students hints about the direction they might take. Convergent questions are those that narrow down to a specific answer, whereas divergent questions open out a number of possibilities.

Making questioning more effective

Questioning is often a rather haphazard affair, with questions being thrown out without too much thought as to their purpose. There are a number of criteria that apply to the formulation of good questions. The question should be short so that it can be remembered by the students whilst they are working out their answers, and it should be stated in language that can easily be understood. The question must also be appropriate to the level of the student, as it is unfair to expect an answer to questions that are at too high a level for his or her particular stage of education. On the other hand, the teacher must try to include questions that require more than simple recall of factual material, by posing questions containing problems that need a thought-out solution.

Needless to say, a question should never be ambiguous, and should contain only a single question. For example, it is confusing for a student to be asked a question like 'What are the main points in the pre-operative care of this patient, and why are they important?' Another example of a poor question is 'Are models of nursing useful in planning patient/client care?' The student need simply say 'Yes' or 'No' to answer the question and the teacher will then need to probe further to elicit the actual 'answer' required.

'Pose, pause and pounce' technique

A useful tip for improving questioning technique is to write out the questions beforehand, and include them on the lesson plan. This ensures that the questions have received some careful thought before being included and so the teacher is less likely to ask poor questions. It is good teaching technique to explain to the students that, whenever a question is posed during a lesson, each of them is to think about the answer and that then one of them will be selected by name to answer it. This is sometimes referred to as the 'pose, pause, pounce' technique, and is useful in that it ensures that each student thinks about the question, just in case it is he or she who is selected. This method is superior to the overhead type of question technique, where the question is posed and students volunteer the answer, because any given student may well decide not to answer the question, leaving the bright members of the audience to vie for the privilege.

The teacher's response to the answers given by students is very important, as the act of questioning is highly threatening from the student's point of view. Teachers often seem unaware of the power they possess in a lecture; their responses can have a devastating effect on the individual student.

Individuals can be made to feel humiliated by a thoughtless response from the teacher, so sensitivity is needed when dealing with this aspect. Correct answers must be reinforced adequately and this should also include the correct parts of a partially correct answer. An incorrect answer should not be left, but should be followed by a rephrased version at a lower level. A partially correct answer can usefully be referred to another student for further elaboration.

One problem that requires careful handling is that of the students who do not answer at all. It is tempting to try to relieve their discomfort by moving on to another person, but it is well worth rephrasing the question at a lower level of difficulty so that the reluctant student gains a little success if he or she answers. If the rephrased question still evokes no response, then the best strategy may well be to leave such students for the moment and then to see them privately after the lecture in order to attempt to find a solution to their difficulty.

The most common failing of questioning is that the response called for is at a low level of intellectual functioning, such as simple factual recall of information. It is therefore necessary for the teacher to plan for the inclusion of questions that test the higher intellectual functions.

DRAFTING A TEACHING PLAN

It is interesting to watch how teachers and other public speakers use notes; these are often written on very small cards secreted in the palm of the hand, to which furtive glances are directed from time to time when a prompt is required.

From this behaviour we might conclude that generally, people feel they should be able to speak without notes, their use being somewhat akin to cheating! However, it is the needs of the audience, not his own prestige, that should be at the forefront of the teacher's mind, and a teaching plan can help to minimize the chances of omitting some vital part of the session and ensure that all the necessary factors have been considered.

Teaching plans need to be distinguished from a closely related concept, that of the teacher's subject-matter notes. Subject-matter notes are used to provide a reminder to the teacher of the actual details of the subject matter during a session and eliminate the possibility of forgetting some crucial aspect. It is quite possible for a teacher to present a teaching session without having teacher's notes, depending on the type of subject-matter and the degree of expertise of the teacher. Indeed, many teachers do not use subject-matter notes per se, but put the key headings on overhead-projector transparencies, using these as prompts to their memory of the subject-matter. It is tempting for a newly qualified teacher to write down every word of what he or she plans to say, but this may well result in their notes being read aloud rather than delivered, and it is also easier for the teacher to lose their place! If anxious not to omit any detail, it is still possible to include all the major headings and subheadings, with suitable indicators of examples, etc., without writing the whole plan in prose form.

Proforma for a teaching plan

Figure 7.2 shows a proforma for a teaching plan which will suit any type of teaching situation. It fits on two sides of A4 sheet and contains spaces for all the essential details on one side, with room for the actual structure and sequence of delivery on the reverse.

The side headed 'Sequence and process' is for the main headings only, as finer detail should be contained in the teacher's notes, as should the questions that one is planning to ask. (I always use bright colours for the main headings, and write the notes in a much larger script than the normal writing style so that they are easily visible from a waist-height table or desk top when standing up.)

The 'Activity' column is a useful indicator of the amount of interaction and activity during a lesson and should also include any use of learning resources as well as teacher talk. Although a 'Timing' column is included, the timing is meant to be an approximate guide only and the plan must be sufficiently flexible to allow for unplanned events.

Space is allowed also for the teacher's immediate reactions at the end of the session, so that key aspects are recorded whilst fresh in his or her mind, which can then form the basis for later reflection.

Sequencing of subject-matter content

There are many different approaches to the sequencing of subject-

---

TEACHING PLAN (Side one)

Title of session: Date:

Time and duration: Venue:

DETAILS OF LEARNER(S)

Type of learners (students/qualified staff/patients etc):

Programme and level (where appropriate):

Number of learners:

AIMS AND LEARNING OUTCOMES

Aims:

Learning outcomes:

TEACHING RESOURCES REQUIRED

LAYOUT OF VENUE

---

matter in a teaching plan, but the Herbartian principles are useful as a general approach when considering the sequencing of the session. Johann Herbart was a nineteenth century German philosopher and educator who formulated a number of principles for teaching, and it is interesting to compare these with Ausubel's assimilation theory of meaningful learning outlined in Chapter 4 (p. 91). The Herbartian prin-

Figure 7.2a

Proforma for a teaching plan

TEACHING PLAN (Side two)			
SEQUENCE AND PROCESS			
TIMING	CONTENT	TEACHER ACTIVITY	LEARNER ACTIVITY

TEACHER'S INITIAL SELF-EVALUATION

Figure 7.2b

ciples are as follows:

1. *Teaching should proceed from the simple to the complex.* The sequence should start with the easiest concepts first, so that students acquire the basic building-blocks before tackling complex concepts.

2. *Teaching should proceed from the known to the unknown.* The starting point for the sequence should be what the student already knows about the subject. New material is then introduced to build upon their existing knowledge.

3. *Teaching should proceed from the concrete to the abstract.* Concrete concepts are normally easier to understand than abstract ones, and they are often pre-requisites for abstract concepts. It is therefore useful to teach the concrete concepts first before moving on to the more abstract ones.

Reece and Walker (1997) list 23 ways in which teaching sessions

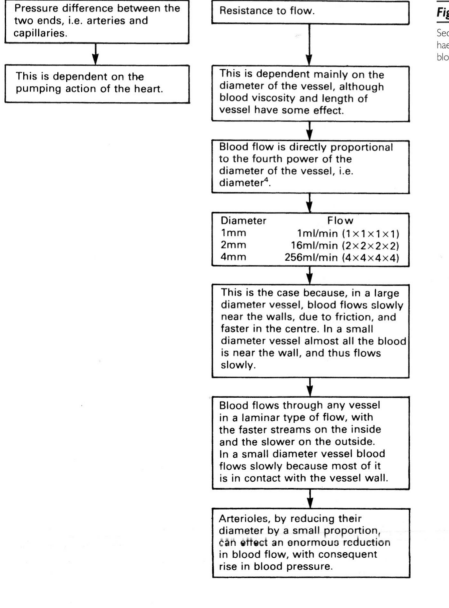

Figure 7.3

Sequence for a teaching session on haemodynamic determinants of blood flow through any vessel

might be sequenced, including sequencing by themes, by historical and chronological order, by theory/practice, by order of a textbook, etc. Figure 7.3 shows the sequencing for a teaching session on haemodynamics, which is based upon a logical step-by-step explanation of each concept.

DRAFTING A SCHEME OF WORK

Within nursing and midwifery education, teachers are normally responsible for the delivery of a specific area of the curriculum, such as a module or unit of study, being of a defined size and duration, and consisting of a series of sessions centred around a common theme or topic area. It may be difficult to maintain the overall continuity and coherence of a module if the teacher plans each session individually, so it is preferable to use a scheme of work that encompasses the entire module.

A scheme of work is a document that gives an overview of the key components of each teaching session within the module, and this would normally include the title, goals or learning outcomes, sequence of content, teaching and learning activities, assessment, and media resources. Table 7.7 shows an example of a scheme of work for a course entitled 'Teaching research and enquiry skills for staff development of community practitioners'. By considering each of these components for a given session in relation to the others within the scheme, the teacher

Table 7.7

Example of a scheme of work

Session	Outcomes	Content	Teaching methods	Assessment
Introduction to research	Understand nature of knowledge	Mutual knowledge, formal knowledge, informed consent, confidentiality	Lecture Issue-centred groups Resource material	Multiple-choice test
Types of research	Understand principles of experimental research Describe the nature of experimental research	Experimental research non-experimental research	Lecture/discussion Carousel exercise	Nil
Action research	Understand nature of action research Discuss potential projects in own field	Principles: exploratory, practical, problem-centred	Problem-centred groups Case-study material	Quality of feedback from group work
Basic statistics	Awareness of uses and limitations Understanding of basic statistics	Uses and abuses, basic concepts, centrality, variability, correlation, probability, sampling	Activity workshop Handout material	Monitoring of activities
Research critique	Understanding of principles of a critique Undertake an elementary critique	Guidelines, academic fraud	Lecture/discussion Practical exercise	Assessment of critiques
Writing a research proposal	Identify sources of funding Write a draft proposal	Sources of funding DOH, NHS, HEA, etc. Guidelines	Lecture/discussion Workshop on writing a proposal	Assessment of draft proposal Essay assignment on course outcomes

can ensure integration and coherence of the whole module. The scheme of work is a useful tool for checking on other important aspects of the module, such as whether or not there is sufficient variety of teaching and learning activities across the module, and the amount of assessment within the module as a whole.

ORGANIZING THE TEACHING ENVIRONMENT

As the poet Robert Burns said: 'the best-laid schemes o' mice an' men gang aft agley', and this is particularly appropriate in the context of organizing the teaching environment. All a teacher's careful planning can be undone if he or she neglects the environment within which the session takes place. The amount of organizing that can be done will depend upon whether the teaching session is in a formal classroom or in the clinical or community areas. It is much easier to organize a classroom than it is to set up a treatment room or consulting room for teaching, and in the latter case all the teacher may be able to do in advance is to bring some chairs into the room.

When teaching in formal classrooms it is always good practice, wherever possible, to prepare the room in advance of the students' arrival, but this assumes that the previous teacher vacates on time. In reality sessions often overrun, but even so the incoming teacher should take a few minutes to check the teaching materials and set up any media resources before commencing the actual teaching. The problem may be compounded if the seating arrangements need to be changed, as this can be a time-consuming exercise. However, it can be accomplished more quickly if the students are asked to move their own desks and chairs.

It is useful to switch on the classroom lights, even if the daylight is adequate, since this can have the effect of focusing students' attention; the overhead projector is designed to operate in normal lighting and is therefore not affected.

Sunlight, however, can bleach out the image on the screen if shining directly onto it, so window blinds or blackout curtains need to be closed if this occurs.

Institutions vary in the quality of their resources so teachers should be aware that their carefully prepared teaching plans may be ruined if vital media fail to arrive. Overhead projectors may not be available in every classroom; they may have to be projected onto an adjacent wall if a screen is not available; video replay facilities may not arrive when ordered, and do not always work when they do arrive.

Finally, one of the most frustrating situations a teacher can face is that, having prepared the classroom in advance, it transpires that another class has booked the room. Tense negotiations with the other teacher usually follow, taking up valuable time from the lesson and often resulting in a mass move to another room. In these situations, the interpersonal skills of the teachers are severely put to the test, but such events are all part and parcel of the work of teaching.

PLANNING FOR OPPORTUNISTIC ONE-TO-ONE TEACHING

By opportunistic teaching, I mean the kind of spontaneous teaching that occurs as part of everyday professional practice, with either students, qualified staff, or patients and clients. Planning for this may seem to be a contradiction in terms, but it is possible to state some general principles that teachers can draw upon whenever opportunities for spontaneous teaching arise.

1. *Initiating spontaneous one-to-one teaching.* Whilst accepting that opportunities for teaching during professional practice will arise spontaneously, it is normally possible to predict the broad areas within which such teaching will fall. For example, if the teacher is working on an acute surgical unit, she will know the patients' conditions and the nature of their care requirements. Similarly, if the context is a community nursing visit to a client's home, the teaching opportunities will again be broadly predictable. This allows the teacher to do some advance preparation in anticipation of possible teaching opportunities within the specific practice context.

   Teaching opportunities can arise in a number of ways; for example, students may ask the teacher to go through some aspect or procedure with them, or simply ask questions about the care of specific patients. On the other hand, the teacher may herself initiate teaching by asking questions or by explaining aspects or procedures. Teaching can also be initiated by the teacher if she perceives that a student or qualified member of staff is experiencing difficulty with procedures or understanding.

2. *Using appropriate questioning.* This has been dealt with in a general way earlier in this chapter, but it is useful to consider questioning with specific reference to spontaneous teaching. It is good practice for the teacher to review the types and levels of questions in advance (e.g. Kerry's classification described above), so that she can select appropriate types and levels for the individuals who are likely to be involved in spontaneous teaching opportunities.

3. *Planning explanations of difficult concepts or procedures.* In clinical and community practice contexts there are inevitably concepts and procedures that most people find difficult to grasp, for example, biochemistry or pharmacology concepts that are important for the understanding of particular treatments. It is likely that the teacher will encounter again and again requests for an explanation of these concepts, so it is useful to prepare an explanation in advance that can be 'wheeled out' as required. The guidelines on planning an explanation given earlier in this chapter will be helpful in this regard.

4. *Planning ways to assess learning.* Assessment is not usually thought of in the context of spontaneous teaching, but there are some situations where feedback on what has been learned is

important. This is particularly the case when teaching patients and clients about aspects of continuing care such as long-term drug compliance following discharge, but it is also important for students and qualified staff in some circumstances.

Ausubel, D., Novak, J. and Hanesian, H. (1978) *Educational Psychology: A Cognitive View*, 2nd edn, Holt, Rinehart and Winston, New York.

Bligh, D. (1998) *What's the Use of Lectures?*, 5th edn, Intellect, Exeter.

Bloom, B. (1956) *Taxonomy of Educational Objectives: The Classification of Educational Goals, Handbook One: Cognitive Domain*, McKay, New York.

Brown, G. (1978) *Lecturing and Explaining*, Methuen, London.

Brown, G. and Armstrong, S. (1984) Explaining and explanation, in *Classroom Teaching Skills*, E. Wragg (ed.), Croom Helm, London.

Brown, G. and Edmondson, R. (1984) Asking questions, in *Classroom Teaching Skills*, E. Wragg (ed.), Croom Helm, London.

Brown, G. and Atkins, M. (1988) *Effective Teaching in Higher Education*, London, Methuen.

CNAA (1992) *Improving Student Learning Project*, Oxford Centre for Staff Development, Oxford.

Delamont, S. (1983) *Interaction in the Classroom*, Methuen, London.

Kerry, T. (1980) *Effective Questioning*, Nottingham University School of Education, Nottingham.

Lawless. C., Smee, P. and O'Shea, T. (1998) Using concept sorting and concept mapping in business and public administration, and in education: an overview, *Educational Research*, **40**(2), 219–31.

Reece, I. and Walker, S. (1997) *Teaching, Training and Learning*, 3rd edn, Business Education, Sunderland.

University of Greenwich (1999) *Academic Regulations for Taught Awards: August 1999*, University of Greenwich, London.

8 ASSESSMENT OF LEARNING

The setting, marking and moderation of students' written assessment work constitutes a very significant part of the lecturers' role in higher education, but in nurse education there is the added dimension of workplace assessment to be considered. Given that both success and failure have important consequences for their future development, students often perceive assessment as the most important aspect of their course or programme, and the one that causes them most anxiety. It is almost inevitable, therefore, that students will see the assessment tasks as the main priority of their studies, to the possible detriment of their wider reading and exploration of topics.

This point is nicely made by Brown *et al.* (1997):

> *'Assessment defines what students regard as important, how they spend their time and how they come to see themselves as students and then as graduates. Students take their cues from what is assessed rather than from what lecturers assert is important'.*

However, if the assessment has been carefully planned, it will form an integral part of the teaching and learning experience for the student rather than something that distracts from the main business of studying. Brown *et al.* cite examples of studies showing that the type of assessment can influence whether students adopt a reproductive style or deeper strategies of understanding.

PURPOSES AND AIMS OF ASSESSMENT

> *'Assessment is the exercise of judgement on the quality of students' work, as a way of supporting student learning and of appraising its outcomes' (HEQC, 1996).*

However, whilst this is the main purpose of assessment there are a number of others that are considered important in higher education. For example, assessment can provide valuable feedback to students about their progress, and point out ways in which they could develop further. Also, the successful achievement of a publicly-recognized award can enhance an individual's status, and may lead to employment opportunities or confer eligibility to undertake further academic study.

There is no doubt that assessment can act as a powerful motivator of study; students expect to be assessed, and plan their studies accordingly. Assessment also provides feedback to the higher education funding bodies about the effectiveness of an institution, and in that sense is a performance indicator of quality.

Regardless of the type, there are three basic aims of assessment:

1. It should assess student performance in relation to the aims of the particular programme in question.
2. It should be regarded as an integral component of the teaching and learning process, and not simply a means of measuring attainment.
3. It should encourage the students to undertake self-assessment and reflection on their learning.

These aims are set in a context of equality of opportunity and anti-racism, and it is a fundamental tenet of higher education that no student is assessed on the basis of their race, religion, politics, gender or sexual orientation.

THE TERMINOLOGY AND DIMENSIONS OF ASSESSMENT

One of the most confusing aspects of assessment is the number of different terms used for what is essentially the same thing. Table 8.1 gives the main distinctions between the most commonly used terms.

Measurement	A quantitative process involving the assigning of a number to an individual's characteristics
Assessment	A term used instead of measurement when a numerical value is not involved, e.g. checklists of behaviours
Evaluation	The process of judging the value or worth of an individual's characteristics obtained by measurement or assessment
Test	An instrument or tool for obtaining measurements or assessments, e.g. an essay
Examination	A formal situation in which students undertake one or more tests under specific rules

Table 8.1

Terminology of assessment

In addition to this basic terminology, it is useful to look at the dimensions of the concept of assessment, as shown in Table 8.2.

Formal	Informal
Quantitative	Qualitative
Episodic	Continuous
Formative	Summative
Teacher-centred	Student-centred
Norm-referenced	Criterion-referenced
Achievement	Aptitude/personality
Paper and pencil	Practical/oral

Table 8.2

Dimensions of assessment

Formal assessment involves the use of tests to obtain data that is then made available to the institution; the data is often subjected to statistical analysis and comparisons drawn between other students. Examples of formal assessment in nurse education are modular or unit assessments, unseen written components, and clinical practice assessments.

Informal assessment, in contrast, does not involve comparisons with other students, but is essentially private and subjective to the teacher concerned. Such informal assessment is gleaned from the day-to-day observation of students' behaviour, examination of students' notes, and from informal contact and interviews. Informal assessment, then, is for the private use of a particular teacher and forms an essential part of the total assessment process.

Quantitative assessment refers to the use of numerical data in the assessment of students, whereas *qualitative assessment* is concerned with the properties or qualities that an individual possesses. Scores obtained on a written test constitute quantitative data; a student's views on what constitutes effective relationships with a patient would be qualitative data. There are two dimensions that are concerned with the timing of assessment, the first being 'episodic' versus 'continuous' assessment.

Episodic assessment involves testing the student at specific times or occasions during an educational programme, such as an end of year assessment or a number of specific clinical assessments in particular aspects of nursing. One of the major drawbacks of this system is its reliance on a student's 'one-off' performance on the day of the test and this performance may not reflect the student's typical performance over a longer period. In other words, episodic assessment generates data that is based on a very small and possibly unrepresentative sample of a student's behaviour. A further criticism, which relates particularly to the clinical setting, is that of artificiality, in that episodic clinical assessments are often seen as 'set pieces' which the student may rehearse until 'word perfect' and which bear little resemblance to the student's normal working practices.

Continuous assessment attempts to overcome these weaknesses by sampling all of a student's outputs in a course on a continuous basis. In the college setting, this might involve assessing all of a student's coursework, including tests, projects and seminar presentations. In the clinical setting, continuous assessment samples a student's nursing practice on a continuous basis, so that no particular nursing skill can be said to have been 'passed' on a 'once-and-for-all' basis.

The second time-related dimension is that of 'formative' versus 'summative' evaluation and these terms are used in two distinct ways. First, they can be applied to the assessment of a particular student's achievement and second, to the evaluation of a particular aspect of curriculum design, such as teaching media.

Formative assessment provides feedback about the progress a student is making whilst the course or unit is being followed, so that modifications can be made to the teaching if necessary.

Summative assessment, on the other hand, is done at the end of a course or unit to see if the student has achieved the objectives of the programme and is usually done as a formal test covering the content of the course. Many teachers feel that formative assessment should not be graded for assessment purposes, but used only as feedback or diagnosis of student needs. With regard to the use of these terms for curriculum evaluation, formative evaluation means that instructional material intended for eventual use with students is tested during its formation and modified in the light of these pilot studies. Summative evaluation is the evaluation of such material after it has been used with students in its intended setting.

Another useful dimension to consider is that of 'teacher-centred assessment' versus 'student-centred assessment'. Traditionally, the teacher has been the key figure with regard to the assessment of students in nursing, but with the growth of interest in student-centred learning, there is a move towards much greater involvement of the student in his or her own assessment. Indeed, self-assessment seems to be one of the hallmarks of a professional practitioner in any field, so this is a practice that should be encouraged from the outset.

The next dimension to be considered is that relating to the interpretation of the results of assessment; there are two main ways that these results can be referenced: norm-referencing and criterion-referencing.

Norm-referenced assessment means that an individual student's score on a test is compared with scores of other students in a given group, and a rank order assigned. Cut-off points for pass and fail are built into the assessment. In norm-referenced assessment, a student could be in the top 10% of scores in one year, but the same score in the following year may not achieve the top 10% if the general scores of the group are higher than the previous year.

Criterion-referenced assessment implies that the score is compared with some criterion or learning task such as achievement of behavioural objectives and is also termed 'content referenced' or 'domain-referenced' assessment. The main difference between these two forms of referencing is that norm-referenced assessment means that the score obtained by the student is influenced by the performance of the group to which he or she is compared. Criterion-referencing, on the other hand, does not depend on any form of comparison with others, only with achievement in relation to a specific criterion or standard.

Assessment is not only concerned with the measurement of student achievement, but includes such aspects of an individual as attitudes, aptitudes, personality and intelligence. Achievement refers to how well a student has performed in the past; aptitude refers to how well he or she will perform in the future. Assessment of personality and intelligence is usually done using published standardized tests.

A useful distinction can be made between the kinds of tests employed in the assessment of nurses. On the one hand we have the so-called 'paper-and-pencil' tests, which include essays, objective tests and a host of other kinds of written instruments. At the other end of the scale, there are the practical, clinical forms of assessment and oral examinations. Practical assessment usually involves observation combined with some form of checklist or rating scale to guide the observer. Oral, or viva voce, tests rely on the spontaneous answering of questions by the student and allow for follow-up and further elaboration on answers given.

Cardinal criteria for assessment

Regardless of the type of assessment employed or the purpose for which it is used, every effective assessment must meet the four cardinal criteria described below.

Validity

This is the most important aspect of a test and is the extent to which the test measures what it is designed to measure. In other words, validity is the relevance of a test to its objectives.

Content validity

Assessments should sample adequately the content of the syllabus and if this is the case, then the examination is said to have content validity.

Predictive validity

If a test is designed to predict the future performance of a student and it fulfils this function, then it is said to have predictive validity.

Concurrent validity

Concurrent validity is the extent to which the results of a test correlate with those of other tests administered at the same time.

Construct validity

The fourth kind of validity is construct validity. A construct is a quality that is devised by psychologists to explain aspects of human behaviour that cannot be directly observed. For example, such things as attitudes, values and intelligence are constructs. Construct validity is the extent to which the results of a test are related to the data gained from observations of individuals' behaviour with regard to the construct in question.

Reliability

Reliability is the term used to indicate the consistency with which a test measures what it is designed to measure. In other words, it should yield similar results when used on two separate occasions, provided that the other variables remain similar. The main way in which reliability is assured is by using more than one type of assessment to measure student achievement.

Test–retest reliability

If a test is administered to a group of students and then re-administered, either immediately or after an interval of time, and the scores are similar on both occasions, then the test is said to have high test-retest reliability.

Parallel-form reliability

If the group is given a different test in the retest phase, but one that measures the same thing, then a positive correlation indicates parallel-form reliability.

Split-half reliability

A third type of reliability is termed split-half reliability, in which the test items are divided into two halves and the correlation calculated between the two sets of scores.

The importance of validity and reliability is self-evident, but it might be helpful to give an example to show the inter-relationship between them. One of the most common measuring instruments to be found in the home is the bathroom scales. Just like any other assessment tool, the measurement of human weight by the scales must be valid and reliable. To check the validity (accuracy) of the measurement of an individual's weight, it is necessary to record the weight as registered by the scales, and then to check the weight again using a different scales, such as can be found in most chemist shops. If the two weights are identical, then the measure is valid, i.e. it is demonstrating accuracy and fitness for purpose.

If the measurement of an individual's weight by the bathroom scales is reliable (consistent) then the scales should register the same weight when the individual weighs themselves again and again (provided, of course, that their weight has remained constant since the last measurement).

It is possible, however, for an assessment test to be valid but not reliable, or reliable but not valid. Referring again to the bathroom scales example, the scales may register the same weight each time (reliability), but that weight may be several pounds above the actual weight of the individual (i.e. not valid). Alternatively, the scales may register the correct weight of the individual on some occasions (validity), but the incorrect weight on others (i.e. not reliable).

Discrimination

The purpose of any test is to discriminate between those who answer correctly and those who don't. The term discriminate is used in the sense of 'distinguish between', and not in the equal opportunities sense. If a test makes no discrimination between students, then it has no purpose. The discrimination index will be examined later in this chapter.

Practicality or utility

It is important that a test is practical for its purpose. This implies such factors as the time taken to conduct the test, the cost of using it and the practicality for everyday use.

PLANNING ASSESSMENTS

Given that assessments have significant implications for students, it is essential that considerable time and care is given to their formulation and implementation.

Students' assessment workload

One of the aspects of higher education programmes most commonly highlighted at validation events is the assessment workload of students. Whilst assessment is clearly an important aspect of teaching and learning, over-assessment has a number of undesirable consequences; Brown and Knight (1994) point out that excessive assessment may result in superficial coverage of content rather than understanding in depth. Over-assessment becomes a treadmill for both students and markers, demanding a considerable time-commitment from both parties. There is a danger that students and tutors become subject to assessment fatigue, thereby reducing the quality of the former's assessment work, and the latter's marking.

Brown *et al.* (1997) suggest seven questions to ask oneself when designing written assessments:

1. What are the outcomes to be assessed?
2. What are the capabilities/skills implicit in the outcomes?
3. Is the method of assessment chosen consonant with the outcomes and skills?
4. Is the method relatively efficient in terms of student time and staff time?
5. What alternatives are there? What are their advantages and disadvantages?
6. Does the specific assessment task match the outcomes and skills?
7. Are the marking schemes or criteria appropriate?

Learning outcomes and assessment

The statement of learning outcomes for programmes and modules is now an almost universal practice in higher education, and these form the basis for planning assessments. It is important that each of the learning outcomes is assessed, although this need not be by formal written assessment for every outcome. The assessment must be appropriate for the level of learning outcome and also for the domain of learning covered by the learning outcome. It is also necessary to bear in mind the general aims of higher education, and to ensure that these are incorporated into assessment strategies. Table 8.3 shows the general aims of higher education.

Table 8.3

General aims of higher education (University of Greenwich, 1999)

1. Development of students' intellectual powers, understanding and judgement
2. Development of students' ability to see relationships within what they have learned
3. To stimulate an enquiring, analytical and creative approach
4. To encourage independent judgement, critical self-awareness, and problem-solving skills

Levels of learning outcomes

Learning outcomes are stated at one of a number of academic levels, and these levels and definitions may vary between higher education institutions. It is important that the assessment takes account of the level of the learning outcome, as the level may not be apparent within the statement itself. In order to ensure that students achieve the outcome at the appropriate level, the assessment must utilize the level-definition of the institution. Table 8.4 gives the levels and definitions in use at the University of Greenwich.

Level 0	Meeting required levels of literacy and numeracy and acquiring understanding in core areas allowing access to defined programmes of study in post school education
Level 1	Acquisition of basic knowledge, skills and competence
Level 2	Builds on level 1 and involves an extension and reinforcement of those experiences
Level 3	Reflects the synthesis of basic knowledge, skills and competence and equips students with tools of analysis and evaluation
Level M	Provides opportunities to: (i) reflects on the significance and inter-relationships of knowledge acquired from a variety of sources (ii) To use such sources, with critical insight, to evaluate findings of a small-scale enquiry or other activity (iii) to provide explanations within identified frameworks and/or general theory (iv) formulate innovative proposals (v) achieve all outcomes with a large degree of autonomy

Table 8.4

Definitions of academic levels (University of Greenwich, 1999)

Learning outcomes are discussed in more detail in Chapter 6 (p. 138).

Domains of learning

Some higher education institutions use Bloom's (1956) taxonomy as a basis for their definitions of the level of learning outcomes. The taxonomy is discussed in detail in Chapter 6 in relation to educational objectives.

ASSESSING KNOWLEDGE AND UNDERSTANDING USING ESSAYS

Essay assessments require the learner to supply an answer that is organized in his own words and presented in his own style and hand-writing, with few restrictions imposed, and no single correct answer. The term 'essay-format' covers a number of forms of written assessment; for example, it is used to describe negotiated course-work as well as formal written examinations.

The use of essay tests

Because of the factors indicated above, essays are inefficient for testing recall of knowledge, but are useful for assessing higher levels of cognitive functioning, such as application, analysis, synthesis and evaluation.

There are a number of weaknesses in this form of assessment that may limit its usefulness.

Weaknesses of essay tests

Low content-validity
In essay tests, only a small number of questions are answered, hence only a small proportion of the total syllabus is sampled by this method.

Low marker-reliability
Essay tests are notoriously unreliable from the point of view of marking. Every learner knows that some teachers are easy markers and others hard, and the final mark depends to a large extent on the marker. There is often wide variation between markers, and between the same marker at different times.

Often ambiguous or unclear
Essay questions are often difficult for the learner to understand because they do not spell out clearly enough exactly what is required.

Marking is difficult
The marking of essay tests is time-consuming and often tedious, which may adversely affect the marker's judgement about the quality of the essay.

Student fatigue
This aspect is rarely mentioned in connection with essay tests, but in my opinion it is a very serious disadvantage. Examinations are commonly time-tabled in three-hour slots, so students are required to write for three hours without a break. If a student has a three-hour examination in both the morning and afternoon of the same day, the test may be more a measure of stamina than of academic prowess.

Marks are affected by students' writing ability
The learner's ability to write good prose can influence the mark that is awarded. It is often difficult to separate the content of an essay from the literary style, with the result that a learner may bluff the marker into giving a higher grade than she deserves. On the other hand, a learner may be penalized for poor grammar or expression, even though she knows the content adequately. Of course, the essay must be legible, but I feel that marks should not be taken off for the grammar or spelling. The teacher may draw attention to this aspect by adding a comment in the margin, without this affecting the mark awarded.

Choice is often included
In any essay examination a choice of questions is invariably included, but this practice is open to question on a number of counts. First, it is difficult to construct questions which have the same degree of difficulty,

so that in effect a different test is being offered to each learner. This obviously makes comparison difficult between the achievements of students. Secondly, the more able students may well be attracted to the difficult questions and suffer penalties if they fail to do well.

Using a specification grid (blueprint) for designing essay tests

Planning a written examination paper requires careful formulation to ensure that it has high content validity for the course or unit in question. One way to do this is by use of a specification grid or blueprint, based upon the Bloom taxonomy of educational objectives (see Chapter 6, p. 139). The best time to formulate the blueprint is during the planning phase for the particular unit, when the learning outcomes have been formulated. Table 8.5 shows a blueprint for planning an examination paper for a module on 'Nursing the burned patient'.

| Subject matter | Cognitive domain categories | | | | | | Total % |
	1	2	3	4	5	6	
Admission of patient	2	4	8	1	1	4	20
Structure of skin	0.5	1	2	0.25	0.25	1	5
Pathophysiology of burns	1	2	4	0.5	0.5	2	10
Observations	1.5	3	6	0.75	0.75	3	15
Infection control	0.5	1	2	0.25	0.25	1	5
Pre- and post-operative care	2	4	8	1	1	4	20
Fluids/drugs	1.5	3	6	0.75	0.75	3	15
Rehabilitation	1	2	4	0.5	0.5	2	10
Total %	10	20	40	5	5	20	100

Table 8.5

Test specification grid or blueprint: 'Nursing the burned patient'

The blueprint is a two-way matrix, with content areas derived from the objectives down one side and the categories of Bloom's cognitive domain across the top. The right-hand side shows the amount of weight given to each aspect of content in terms of a percentage of the total content of the unit. For example, the item 'admission of a burned patient' is weighted at 20%, whereas structure of the skin is only given 5%. At the foot of each of the cognitive-domain categories, there is another total percentage that applies to the percentage weighting given to each category of intellectual functioning. For example, this unit emphasizes the application of knowledge, rather than the mere recall of specific facts, so category 3 (application) receives a weighting of 40%. The two columns of percentages should both add up to 100 and the percentage of test items for each aspect of the unit can now be calculated.

For example, taking the component called 'admission of the patient'' we see that it has a total weighting of 20% of the unit; this figure is now multiplied by each of the figures at the foot of the cognitive-domain categories to give the percentage for each cell in the matrix. Thus, under the category of knowledge, admission of a burned patient receives 20% of 10%, i.e. 2%. This means that 2% of the total test must comprise questions about terminology relating to the admission of a burned patient. If we wish to know the percentage of the test that should be devoted to pre-operative/post-operative care of a burned patient, at the level of application (category 3), we calculate 20% of 40%, i.e. 8%.

The use of a test blueprint ensures that the test reflects the weighting given to both the subject matter and the level of objectives during the particular unit.

EXAMPLES OF TYPES OF ESSAYS

Interpretive essay

Example: *'The accompanying table relates accidents at work to the type of industry, i.e. manufacturing, construction, railways, coal mining and agriculture. Comment on the relative risk of accidents for the types of industry represented in the table'.*

When answering this type of question, the student has to interpret the table in order to come up with the relative risk for each industry, and this requires high-level cognitive functioning.

Hypothesis-formation essay

Example: *'Imagine that you are the chair of a committee charged with making recommendations for the siting of a new home for brain-injury patients in a quiet suburban area of town. Speculate on the likely planning objections to your proposal'.*

In this case, the student has to consider all the relevant facts and come up with a hypothesis about the likely planning objections. This essay cannot be written by a simple reliance on memorized facts, but requires higher order synthesis.

Questioning assumptions' essay

Example: *'Read this article from the* Journal of Advanced Nursing *and comment on the author's underlying assumptions'.*

This assessment requires the student to explore the article thoroughly and to search for the writer's assumptions. These assumptions may not be obvious, and the student may have to analyse the text deeply before they become apparent.

Inquiry-based assessments

As the name suggests, this type of assessment requires the student to undertake some form of enquiry, the results of which must be written up in the form of a report.

Example: *'Carry out an investigation into the provision for disabled people in terms of access to public buildings within the Newhampton district. Write up your findings in the form of a report to go to the Newhampton District Council'.*

Assessments requiring synthesis

This kind of assessment requires the student to synthesize information gained by both experiential learning and study in order to identify any gaps between them, and requires high-level cognitive functioning on the part of the student.

Example: *'Select a patient or client within either a hospital or community setting in consultation with your mentor. Participate in the care for this patient/client over a period of one week, maintaining a diary of your interactions and interventions. Write a commentary on the care given, within the context of relevant theory from both nursing and social and biological science. Make particular reference to any incongruities between your experiences and your theoretical analyses'.*

MARKING AND GRADING OF ESSAY TESTS

In relation to marking and grading of assessments, the University of Greenwich makes the following helpful points:

1. Assessment is a matter of judgement, not simply computation.
2. Marks and grades are not absolute values, but symbols used by examiners to communicate their judgement of a student's work.
3. Marks and grades provide data for decisions about students' fulfilment of learning outcomes.

Marking and grading criteria

Higher education institutions normally use an institution-wide grading scale for undergraduate programmes, whereas postgraduate programmes tend to be graded on a pass/fail basis or a pass/fail/distinction basis. Grading scales tend to incorporate both percentage grading and literal grading; the latter meaning letters such as A, B, C, etc. The grading scale used in the University of Greenwich is shown in Table 8.6.

Mark on a 0–100 scale	Comments
70+	Work of exceptional quality
60–69	Work of very good quality
50–59	Work of good quality
40–49	Work of satisfactory standard
30–39	Compensatable fail
0–29	Failure

Table 8.6

Grading scale for undergraduate assessment (University of Greenwich, 1999)

Undergraduate grading scales are likely to be very similar in other higher education institutions. It is interesting to compare this scale with the percentage equivalents for the class of honours degree, as shown in Table 8.7.

Marks or grades are assigned to students' essays to indicate the degree of achievement they have attained and there are two systems for assigning grades.

Table 8.7

Percentage equivalents for class of honours degree (University of Greenwich, 1999)

0–34%	= Fail
35–39%	= Pass Degree
40–49%	= Third Class Honours
50–59%	= Lower Second Class Honours
60–69%	= Upper Second Class Honours
70% or more	= First Class Honours

Absolute grading gives the student marks for her essay answer, depending on how well the essay has met the assessment criteria, and is usually expressed as a percentage or letter, e.g. 60% or B.

Relative grading tells the student how his essay answer rated in relation to other students doing the same test, by indicating whether or not he was average, above average or below average. Relative grading usually uses a literal scale such as A, B, C, D and F. Some teachers would argue that two grades are the best way of marking, so that students are given either a pass or fail grade.

This gets over the problem of deciding what constitutes an A or a C grade but does reduce the information conveyed by a particular grade, since no discrimination is made between students who pass with a very high level of achievement and those who barely pass at all.

Analytical method of marking (marking scheme)

When using absolute grading to specific criteria, it is useful to use the analytic method of marking. In this method, a marking scheme is prepared in advance and marks are allocated to the specific points of content in the marking specification. However, it is often difficult to decide how many marks should be given to a particular aspect, but the relative importance of each should be reflected in the allocation.

This method has the advantage that it can be more reliable provided the marker is conscientious, and it will bring to light any errors in the writing of the question before the test is administered. Table 8.8 gives an example of an analytical marking scheme for a nursing essay.

Global method of marking (structured impressionistic marking)

The global method is also termed structured impressionistic marking, and is best used with relative grading. This method still requires a marking specification, but in this case it serves only as a standard of comparison. The grades used are not usually percentages, but scales, such as 'Excellent/Good/Average/Below average/Unsatisfactory'. Scales can be devised according to preference, but it is important to select examples of answers that serve as standards for each of the points on the scale. The teacher then reads each answer through very quickly and puts it in the appropriate pile, depending whether it gives the impression of excellent, good, etc. The process is then repeated and it is much more effective if a colleague is asked to do the second reading. This method is much faster than the analytical one and can be quite effective for large numbers of questions.

When marking essay answers it is important to eliminate the 'halo'

Pressure sores constitute one of the biggest challenges for nursing care. Critically discuss the role of the nurse in risk assessment and prevention of pressure sores (3000 words).

ANALYTICAL MARKING SCHEME

Element		Marks Allocated (out of a hundred)
ELEMENT 1.0: INTRODUCTION (10%)		
1.1	Definitions and prevalence	2
1.2	National context e.g. DH targets and strategy	3
1.3	Nursing context	5
ELEMENT 2.0: RISK ASSESSMENT (30%)		
2.1	Factors implicated in pressure sore development e.g. poor nutrition; immobility; incontinence, etc.	10
2.2	Nursing rationale for use of tools for risk assessment e.g. Norton Scale, Waterlow Scale, etc.	10
2.3	Critique of tools, including criteria used for critique	10
ELEMENT 3.0: PREVENTION (30%)		
3.1	Nurse's role in reducing risk factors at home and in hospital	10
3.2	Methods available to nurses e.g. turning, alternating-pressure mattress etc.	10
3.3	Critique of preventive measures, including criteria used for critique.	10
ELEMENT 4.0: PRESENTATION AND SCHOLARSHIP SKILLS (30%)		
4.1	Spelling, Grammar and Syntax	3
4.2	Citing and Listing References	7
4.3	Coherence of arguments and discussion	10
4.4	Reference to appropriate theoretical perspectives	10

Table 8.8

Example of an analytical marking scheme for a CAT level 3 module assessment

effect, which is the term used to describe the influence that the preceding answer has on the marker. If all the answers from one learner were marked together, then the chances are that this would create an impression, favourable or otherwise, that would influence the marking of the remainder of the answers for that learner. It is thus important to mark all the answers for one question before proceeding to the next. It has been suggested that answers should be shuffled randomly after each question has been marked, so that the position of any paper will not consistently be affected by the quality of the preceding ones.

Anonymous marking helps to eliminate bias, by avoiding the use of students' names, substituting a number instead.

Assessing students' written presentation and scholarship skills

Marking an essay assignment involves more than simply checking the content for accuracy; it also requires the marker to make a judgement about the quality of the students' scholarship skills.

Spelling, grammar and syntax

Assessment work in higher education requires students to be able to express themselves adequately in written English. It is therefore important that errors of spelling, grammar, syntax or punctuation are pointed out to the student by markers. Poor use of grammar, syntax and punctuation can interfere with the student's communication of the content of the assessment, preventing it from being fully understood unless an extra effort is made by the marking lecturer. This can adversely affect the final grading of the assessment, since communication is an essential core academic skill.

Citing and listing references

It is standard procedure in higher education that students must adhere to a given format for citing and listing references in their assessment work. Such consistency facilitates the marking and moderation of assessment work.

Scholarship skills

The content of students' assessments in higher education must be appropriate and relevant to the assessment specification. The arguments and discussion must be presented coherently and logically, and in the context of relevant theory.

Giving feedback to students about their presentation and scholarship skills

It is important that, from the outset of their studies, students' attention is drawn to any problems of presentation and scholarship skills. If lecturers ignore such problems this may be perceived by the students as tacit acceptance, reinforcing the likelihood of errors in future assessments. However, it would not be feasible for marking lecturers to point out all the grammatical errors in a student's assessment work, given the length of assessments and the numbers of scripts requiring to be marked. However, it is good practice for markers to correct such errors on the first two or three pages of an assessment, and then to note at the end that there are problems in this area. If lecturers identify students with problems in the area of presentation and scholarship skills, they should ensure that such students are made aware of the sources of help available to them within the institution.

Giving formative feedback to students

Formative feedback is that which is given to students during the process of preparing their work for assessment, i.e. prior to their handing in the final draft. It is important that a clear policy exists with regard to the provision of formative feedback to students about their assessments. It is appropriate that students should be able to seek advice about their assessments, but the danger exists that the teacher may influence the subsequent draft to such an extent that the assessment is no longer the students' own work, but a collaborative effort of both student and teacher. Teachers should not accept written drafts of entire assignments from students for formative comments; it is, however, appropriate to comment on outline assignment drafts, or one section of an assignment.

Writing summative feedback comments on students' assessments

Formal summative examinations are designed solely to assess students' achievement, so feedback comments are not offered and the papers are not returned to the students. However, in assessment by coursework it is common practice to provide written as well as verbal feedback. The question of how much feedback to give is a difficult one, since for some answers the teacher would have to write out the entire essay again to indicate the improvements required. In addition, feedback is time-consuming, whereas it is fairly easy simply to assign a mark without comments. However, feedback is very important for students' learning, provided they review such feedback rather than just filing their essay away. It is often better to return marked essays to the student during a tutorial so that the main feedback points can be discussed.

Brown *et al.* (1996) offer a number of suggestions for giving student feedback, including:

1. the need to target feedback on those aspects that could be improved;
2. the importance of making feedback positive rather than overly critical;
3. the need to provide feedback promptly so that the student has less chance of forgetting what she has written in her answer.

VARIANTS OF ESSAYS

The 'seen-paper'

Some essay examinations allow the candidate to see the paper some weeks prior to the examination and may even allow them to bring notes into the examination up to 100 words. The test is used to evaluate the candidate's ability to select sources and to organize the information in a meaningful way.

The 'open-book' examination

The candidate is allowed to look up information in a book during the examination. It removes over-reliance on memorizing facts and is closer to the reality of professional behaviour, where information has to be looked up most of the time. Gray (1993) suggests that there are several benefits of open-book examinations, such as deeper study of course notes, development of important professional skills, easier marking of exam scripts, and a reduction in students' exam anxiety.

USING OBJECTIVE TESTS

The limitations of the essay test led to the development of the objective test, the word 'objective' referring to the marking of the test, which is not influenced by the subjective opinion of the marker. However, the actual writing of the test may be as subjective as an essay, depending on the expertise of the writer. In current terminology, an objective-test question is termed an item and this seems quite logical, since many items are written in the form of statements.

In comparison with essay tests, objective tests have perfect marker reliability, because the answer is predetermined. Content validity is also very high in this form of test, as the large number of items ensure that the syllabus is adequately sampled. Furthermore, the marking can be done very quickly by using hardware such as optical scanners, and items can be kept in a bank and used time after time. The question of student fatigue does not arise, as objective tests take much less time to answer. However, they are very time consuming to write, and tests of the higher levels of intellectual functioning are difficult to formulate. Objective tests are commonly classified into those that require the answer to be selected from amongst alternatives and those that require the answer to be supplied by the learner.

Multiple-choice item

This consists of three parts; the 'stem' containing the problem or statement, the 'key', which is the correct response, and 'distracters', or incorrect responses. There should be at least three options given, to reduce the chances of guessing. Example:

(Stem)	The type of epithelium that lines the colon is called:
(Distracters)	a squamous
	b cuboidal
	c transitional
(key)	d columnar

The multiple-choice item is a very versatile test that can measure a variety of levels of functioning. It is less susceptible to guessing, as there is only a one in four chance of getting it correct.

Matching item

This consists of two lists in columns, and the learner is required to match items from column A with responses in B. For example:

A		B	
1	Yellow discoloration of skin	a	Bile salts
2	Severe itching of skin	b	Unconjugated bilirubin
3	Clay-coloured stools	c	Bilirubinaemia
4	Dark urine with yellow foam	d	Jaundice
		e	Haemolysis
		f	Obstruction

Matching items are useful for testing both knowledge of terminology and specific relationships between facts.

True–false item

True–false items are statements which the learner has to decide are true or false. There is a large risk of guessing in this type of item and it is often difficult to select items that are categorically true or false. For example:

The commonest form of mental illness in Great Britain is schizophrenia. True/False

Assertion–reason item

This test presents two statements, an assertion and a reason. The learner is required to decide whether (a) each statement is true and (b) whether the reason is a correct explanation of the assertion. For example:

Assertion	**Reason**
Pressure in the glomerular capillaries is 70 mm Hg	The efferent arteriole has a smaller calibre than the afferent.

Short-answer (missing-word) items

In this item, there is a statement or question that has a missing word that the learner must supply. For example:

The part of the brain which contains the visual cortex is called the................ lobe.

This type is used to test knowledge of terms, but is not very useful for higher levels of functioning. There is often more than one answer which will fit the blank and this item may encourage rote learning.

Multiple completion items

This involves the selection of more than one correct response, from a choice of combinations. The learner is looking for the incorrect option, so this item is often termed reverse multiple-choice. For example:

Which of the following would indicate occurrence of cardiac arrest?

a   Apnoea
b   Dilated pupils
c   Chest pain
d   Absence of pulse

GUIDELINES FOR WRITING OBJECTIVE TESTS

Writing multiple-choice items

The stem should include:

1. the clearly stated problem;
2. only material which is essential for clarity;
3. Novel material to test higher levels.

The options should:

1. be three or more, to limit guessing;
2. be in logical or quantitative order;

3. be as short as possible, but clear;
4. avoid repetition;
5. be homogeneous;
6. make limited use of negative forms; and
7. avoid 'all of these' and 'none of these'.

The distractors should be plausible.

The key should be:

1. the single best or most likely answer; and
2. free of specific determiners.

Specific determiners are clues contained in the item, but not linked to knowledge of content. There are several types to be aware of:

1. constant position of key in options;
2. length of key in relation to distractors;
3. opposite options;
4. grammatical inconsistency; and
5. use of words like 'never' and 'always'.

Students will often see the key as being one of the opposites, as item writers commonly choose statements which are opposite to the one they have selected. It can be remedied by including another pair of opposites.

Worked examples and comments on their construction

Example	Comments

Example 1
Vitamin B12:
  a. contains iron
  b. is absorbed by mouth
  c. is stored in liver
  d. is given for haemolytic anaemia
	Stem does not contain the problem.

Example 2 Vitamin B12, one of the water-soluble B group of vitamins, is necessary for: a. prevention of haemolytic anaemia b. formation of haemoglobin c. formation of thrombocytes d. maturation of red corpuscles	Stem contains non-essential material, namely 'one of the water-soluble group of vitamins'.
Example 3 A female patient aged 60 is admitted with history of fatigue, dyspnoea on exertion, and fainting attacks. Her Vitamin B12 is low and tests reveal	Stem contains a novel problem which requires application and synthesis of knowledge

achlorhydria. The likely diagnosis is:
a. iron deficiency anaemia
b. haemolytic anaemia
c. pernicious anaemia
d. folic acid deficiency anaemia

Example 4

The normal range of haemoglobin level for men (g/l) is:
a. 320-380
b. 30- 80
c. 230-280
d. 130-180

Options should be in rank order.

Example 5

A patient's blood pressure when lying down is charted using:
a. 2 black dots joined by an interrupted horizontal line
b   2 black dots joined by a continuous vertical line
c. 2 black dots joined by a continuous horizontal line
d. 2 black dots joined by an interrupted vertical line

Options are repetitious.

Example 6

The inferior boundary of the thoracic cavity is:
a. sternum
b. thoracic vertebrae
c. diaphragm
d. peritoneum

Options not homogeneous, i.e. peritoneum not part of thoracic cavity.

Example 7

Which of the following are not found in normal urine:
a. urea
b. albumin
c. phosphate
d. chloride

Negative should be clearly indicated by capitals or underlining.

Example 8

Which of the following is found in dehydration:
a. inelastic skin
b. oliguria
c. constipation
d. all of these

Poor use of 'all of these', i.e. option (d) can be discarded if student recognizes one wrong option, or two correct ones.

Example 9
The secretion of the sebaceous glands is called:

a. cerumen
b. sebum
c. semen
d. sweat

Option c. is implausible.

Example 10
A patient in the ward develops diarrhoea. The nurse's first priority is:

a   increase his fluids
b. isolate him
c. send stool to laboratory
d. commence fluid balance recordings

None of the options are clearly right or best.

Example 11
Hypertension is a state of:
a. high blood sugar
b. high blood pressure
c. low blood sugar
d. low blood pressure

Two pairs of opposites are included, to reduce chance of guessing.

Example 12
Diaphragmatic breathing is usually seen when a patient is:

a. running
b. standing
c. sleeping
d. in pain

Option d. is grammatically inconsistent.

Writing matching items

When writing matching items, there are two specific points to watch out for. The number of choices should always exceed the number of statements, so that guessing is reduced. Also, the longer statements should be used as the premises, so that the student has the shorter responses to scan when searching for the answers.

Writing true–false items

The specific points when writing these are to:

1. have an equal number of true and false statements;
2. ensure that items are clearly true or false; and
3. avoid trick questions.

Writing short-answer (missing-word) items

The specific points when writing these are:

1. Leave only important words blank.

2. Avoid excessive blanks in a statement.

3. Ensure that it is factually correct.

ANALYSIS OF OBJECTIVE-TEST ITEMS

One of the more useful characteristics of objective-test items is that they can be stored and used again, but this can only be the case if the item has been validated. Validation is performed after the test has been marked, and there are two aspects that are considered, facility and discrimination. The facility index is the percentage of students who answer the item correctly, and the discrimination index indicates the extent to which an item discriminated between the more knowledgeable and the less knowledgeable students.

Facility index

This is calculated by the following formula:

$$\frac{\text{Number of students who answered correctly}}{\text{Total number of students tested}} \times 100$$

For example, if 40 students take the test, and 20 get the item correct, then the facility index is

$20/40 \times 100 = 50\%$.

Discrimination index

This is normally calculated by arranging the test papers in order from the highest to lowest mark, and then putting them into high and low groups. The top 27 per cent from the high group and the bottom 27 per cent of the low group are used to calculate the index, as follows:

[(No. of students who answered item correctly in top 27 per cent) minus (No. of students who answered item correctly in bottom 27 per cent)] divided by (27 per cent of total number of students tested).

The figure of 27 per cent is not rigidly fixed, and if the number of students is less than about 40 it is better to use the top and bottom halves of the group. The index range is from + 1.00 to –1.00.

Example: if a batch of 200 test papers is used and the number of correct answers for the top 27 per cent is 40, and for the bottom 27 per cent 20, then the calculation will be as follows:

$$\frac{40 - 20}{54} = 0.37$$

Interpretation of indexes

The facility index is generally considered ideal when it is 50 per cent, but the acceptable range is from about 25 to 75 per cent. It is often desirable to include some easy items at the beginning of the test and then make it progressively more difficult.

The index of discrimination ranges from + 1.00 to – 1.00 and zero indicates no discrimination. Positive discrimination is accepted at 0.3 and above. If the index shows a negative figure, this implies that the less knowledgeable students are getting more correct answers for an item than the more knowledgeable ones and may indicate that the item is ambiguous or the wrong key has been chosen.

The writing of objective-test items is made easier if regular 'shredding' sessions are conducted, consisting of three of four lecturers who look at new test items to decide whether or not they are suitable for inclusion in pre-testing.

ASSESSMENT OF GROUP PROJECTS

Group projects can take many forms depending upon the subject being studied, but the fundamental principle is that a small number of students work collaboratively on a common problem or task, e.g. the design and production of artefacts such as a computer program, with each student in the group receiving the same overall grade. Group projects can help students to experience teamwork at first hand, and also to develop interpersonal communication skills and management skills. There are also advantages to the teacher, in that the number of assessments to be marked is considerably reduced. There are, however, some disadvantages associated with assessment of groups (PCFC, 1992):

1. In the end, it is students not groups who gain academic awards, so marks have to be awarded to individuals.
2. By giving all students in the group the same grade, there is a danger that some students will opt out of the work.
3. Outstanding students can be dragged down by poor or lazy group members.

One way to overcome the problem of non-contributing group members is for each individual's contribution to the project to be taken into account. The advantage of the latter is that lazy students do not get the same reward as those students who have worked diligently. Brown *et al.* (1997) suggest a way of dealing with this issue using a soccer analogy. Students who contribute little to the group project in the early stages are shown a yellow card, and their potential group mark reduced by ten per cent. If their commitment does not improve by the end of the project, they are shown a red card and marked at zero!

When attempting to assess projects it is important that a clear set of criteria is used. The nature of the criteria will depend upon the subject specialism; for example, assessment of a project report might use the following criteria:

1. identification and context of the issue or problem;
2. use of appropriate literature to inform project design
3. design of the project methodology;
4. collection and analysis of data/information;
5. discussion of findings and implications.

STUDENT SELF-ASSESSMENT

Self-assessment is an important strategy for students to acquire, as it forms the basis of life-skills and lifelong learning. It could be argued that students already engage in self-assessment when, for example, they write successive drafts of assignments until they are satisfied with the quality.

Student marking of their own essays can be a very useful way of encouraging self-evaluation. In this method, the student is given the opportunity to mark his own essay according to the criteria that the teacher has devised and then they both discuss their respective marking with each other. Interviews are another useful way of getting students to undertake self-assessment; the teacher can facilitate this by careful use of probing questions that focus attention upon aspects of the student's performance.

Questionnaires provide an alternative method for this and are less time-consuming, but both methods are open to distorted reporting by the student. It is best not to grade these self-assessments to ensure honest and unbiased reporting, although the teacher may wish to negotiate with the student about the final grade of work, taking into account these self-assessments. Another method is to keep a self-assessment diary or commentary about progress on a course and this involves writing down the reflections of the student about his experiences and feelings.

PEER-ASSESSMENT

Peer-assessment is the assessment of a student by her peer group, and is already familiar to students in the form of quiz assessment, where students exchange answer papers with each other and then mark them correct or incorrect. Essays can be exchanged between students and then marked by them prior to returning to the writer, but peer assessment need not be confined to this contentious area. It can be used in a range of other, less sensitive areas of assessment; for example, it is commonly used to facilitate students' report-writing ability, where peers are invited to constructively comment on draft reports. A similar use is that of peer-assessment of students' presentations to an audience; in this case, peer feedback may be more acceptable to the presenters than that provided by the tutor.

Peer-assessment is also useful for assessing practical skills; groups of three or four students are briefed on how to assess their peers' practical skills, and then each student performs the skill whilst the other group members observe. Feedback is given after each performance, and the whole cycle may be repeated so that students can remedy any mistakes or deficits.

One of the problems with any kind of peer-assessment is the potential for collusion amongst the students to raise the level of marks. Students might soon realize that if each of them gives a high mark to

1. What past work and training experiences do I have?
2. What have I learned from these experiences?
3. Which of this learning is relevant to this course?
4. Which of the course outcomes can I claim to have already achieved?
5. How can I prove that I have achieved them? What evidence do I have?

AP(E)L portfolios are assessed and moderated according to the same standards as other programme assessments.

Management structures for the operation of APL/APEL

Responsibility for awarding APL or APEL credit resides with the relevant programme board of examiners, but the business of assessing and moderating claims is normally delegated to an accreditation sub-committee. The sub-committee is responsible for monitoring the pathway leader's recommendations for the award of credit for APL and APEL, and is also responsible for accrediting courses from external providers. There are two roles that are essential in any APEL system, the APEL counsellor and the APEL assessor. The APEL counsellor's main role is to assist the claimant to formulate his or her learning claim in accordance with the procedures of the institution. Because of this close involvement in the process, the actual assessment of the claim is undertaken by the APEL assessor or gatekeeper, a different person who has had no previous involvement with the claimant in relation to the learning claim.

Reliability and validity of AP(E)L assessment

Higher education institutions approach the assessment of prior learning in a variety of ways, and nurse education has been at the forefront of developments in this area. One major study of AP(E)L in relation to nursing, midwifery and health visiting (ENB, 1997) identified a number of key points:

1. AP(E)L assessment appears to be as valid and reliable as other forms of assessment in higher education.
2. Portfolios are the main method of assessment for AP(E)L.
3. APEL is not normally graded, nor does it count towards the degree classification.
4. Reflection is an important aspect of portfolio construction.
5. The AP(E)L co-ordinator role is a crucial one in ensuring the quality of the system.
6. The costs of operating an AP(E)L system are not adequately reflected in the charges made.

ASSESSMENT IN THE NURSING, MIDWIFERY AND HEALTH VISITING WORKPLACE

Within the UK, practice-placements constitute 50 per cent of the total hours of study on programmes for pre-registration nurse education, so work-based assessment is a major component of the overall assessment strategy.

The ENB Standard 12, criterion bvi, states that: 'The assessment strategy for each educational programme demonstrates that practice has equal value with theory in terms of academic credit awarded to ensure parity within the total assessment strategy' (ENB, 1997). However, work-based assessment presents a challenge to nurse educators in terms of the validity and reliability of the assessment methods used to determine students' competence. Unlike classroom assessment, work-based assessment is not controlled entirely by academic staff from the institution; employers, supervisors and workers may all be involved to some extent in the context of the assessment. There are also clients, patients and relatives forming part of this context, and this presents a very different assessment scenario from that of essay assessments in the higher education institution.

Competence

The term *competence* has a range of meanings according to the context within which it is discussed. The Further Education Curriculum Unit defines it as follows: 'Competence is the possession and development of sufficient skills, knowledge, appropriate attitudes and experience for successful performance in life roles' (FEU, 1984). Benett (1989) suggests that the term has several dimensions such as task competence, job competence, functional competence, occupational competence, and vocational competence.

Eraut (1998) suggests that common usage of the term applies to two kinds of situation. In situation 1, an implicit binary scale operates, i.e. an individual is either competent or not competent. This is the meaning of competence as used in competence-based assessment systems such as the National Vocational Qualifications (NVQ) framework. In situation 2, competence means 'adequate but not excellent', and this view is reflected in the expression 'mere competence' which indicates mediocrity.

Assessment by observation

By far the most common, and valid, method of assessment for work-based learning is observation by the assessor. However, the mere presence of an observer is often sufficient to raise students' anxiety levels so that the quality of their performance is adversely affected. On the other hand, the presence of an observer can, in some circumstances, enhance performance. One of the weaknesses of assessment by observation is the subjectivity of the observer, so it is of paramount importance to have specific assessment criteria in the form of a check list or rating scale that serves as a guide for the assessor, and allows a second observer, when present, to assess the same aspects as the first.

Checklists

A checklist is simply a list of student behaviours associated with a

Fearon, M. (1998) Assessment and measurement of competence in practice, *Nursing Standard*, **12**(22), 43–7.

Flanagan, J. (1954) The critical incident technique, *Psychological Bulletin*, **51**, 327–58.

Further Education Curriculum Unit (1984) *Towards A Competency-Based System*, FEU, London.

Gray, T. (1993) Open book examination, *The New Academic*, **3**(1), 6-9.

Higher Education Quality Council (1996) *Guidelines on Quality Assurance*, HEQC, London.

Latane, B. and Darley, J. (1968) Group inhibition of bystander intervention in emergencies, *Journal of Personality and Social Psychology*, **10**, 215–21.

Murrell, K., Harris, L. and Tomsett, G. (1998) Using a portfolio to assess clinical practice, *Professional Nurse*, **13**(4), 220–3.

Polytechnics and Colleges Funding Council (1992) *The Teaching More Students Project*, Oxford Centre for Staff Development, Oxford.

Redfern, E. (1998) The power of the professional profile, in *Continuing Professional Development in Nursing: A Guide for Practitioners and Educators*, F.M. Quinn (ed.), Stanley Thornes, Cheltenham.

Stenhouse, L. (1975) *An Introduction to Curriculum Research and Development*, Heinemann, London.

University of Greenwich (1999) *Academic Regulations for Taught Awards, August 1999*, University of Greenwich, London.

Information and Communication Technology 9

Information and communication technology (ICT) is a term encompassing the full range of teaching and learning resources encountered by students in higher education and nursing. It has replaced former terms such as *educational technology* and *media resources*, however, it is important to remember that the new term embraces not only computers, but more modest media also. The field of computing is replete with terminology, and there are two other terms that nurses will encounter in the literature, i.e. *health informatics* and *nursing informatics*. Severs and Pearson (1999) define the former as follows:

> *'Health informatics (HI) is the term used to describe the science of information management in health care and its application to support clinical research, decision-making and practice'.*

Nursing informatics is a sub-category of health informatics, and can be seen as a combination of computer science and nursing science.

The context of ICT

This section highlights ICT in the context of three key documents relating to the following areas of education: the NHS, higher education, and further education. These documents may help the reader to understand the wider background of this important development.

'Learning to Manage Health Information' (Severs and Pearson, 1999)

This document is published by the NHS Executive, and is the result of discussions held over two years between the Education and Training Programme in Information Management and a number of organizations including the United Kingdom Central Council for Nursing, Midwifery and Health Visiting (UKCC); the English National Board for Nursing, Midwifery and Health Visiting (ENB), the Royal College of Nursing; the Royal College of Midwives, and the Community Practitioners and Health Visitors Association (CPHVA).

The aims of the paper are as follows:

1. to propose health informatics as a theme for career-long learning for health care professionals;
2. to suggest some key components towards an education framework for health informatics in career-long clinical education;
3. to elicit discussion about the practicalities of achieving a continuum for the health informatics component of clinical education.

The report points out that clinical education and health informatics are inextricably linked in terms of curriculum content, process and infra-structure, and makes suggestions for core content for health informatics in clinical education. The approach taken by the paper is to identify eight areas of health informatics, and to identify 'key points for good practice' and 'expectations for learning' for each area. The 'expectations for learning' are what higher education would term learning outcomes. The eight areas are:

1. communication;
2. knowledge management;
3. data quality and management;
4. confidentiality and security;
5. secondary uses of clinical data and information;
6. clinical and service audit;
7. working clinical systems;
8. telemedicine and telecare.

The paper offers a number of key assumptions and issues for education providers, including a pre-requisite requirement that participants possess basic computer skills; advice about teaching informatics in a more creative way than beginning with basic concepts; the availability of resources; and the encouragement of multi and inter-professional programmes.

'Communication and Information Technologies for Teaching and Learning in Higher Education' (CTI, 1998)

This document is published by the Computers in Teaching Initiative (CTI), an organization funded by the higher education funding councils for England (HEFCE), Scotland (SHEFC), Wales (HEFCW) and the Department of Education for Northern Ireland (DENI). The CTI consists of 24 subject-based centres which act as advice centres for academics wishing to incorporate information and communications technology into their curricula, and the services include publications, databases, workshops, and consultancy.

The CTI world wide web (WWW) home page address is http://www.cti.ac.uk/ and one of the 24 centres is the CTI Nursing and Midwifery. The centre offers text, video and internet services, and also offers workshops, visits to departments, and open days for visitors to network on matters relating to NHS information management. The centre web site address is http://www.shef.ac.uk/uni/projects/ctinm/index.html and the site has the backing of the University of Sheffield School of Nursing and Midwifery.

'The Use of Technology to Support Learning in Colleges' (FEFC, 1998)

This document is the report of a national survey undertaken by the Further Education Funding Council (FEFC) on a representative sample of 44 colleges across nine FEFC regions. The aim of the survey was: 'to investigate the use and effectiveness of technologies to support teaching and learning in colleges and the factors influencing developments'. The findings of the survey include the following:

1. *Management issues*. The report shows a correlation between the staff understanding of possible applications of technology, and the range of vision for use of technology found in the colleges. Effective use of technology is best achieved when there is strong corporate support and a senior manager with overall responsibility for planning and implementation. However, monitoring and review of policy implementation does not always occur.
2. *Teaching issues*. 'Intranets' for accessing databases and materials are beginning to develop within colleges and their remote bases, but there is as yet little application of technology to independent learning. The use of technology to enhance learning in the classroom was not a routine feature of teaching, and the main use of technology by students was for presentation of assessments.
3. *Staff development issues*. Staff development events to disseminate good practice did not always result in the college taking action, and the lack of time for curriculum development in this area was highlighted.

GENERAL ISSUES IN THE USE OF ICT

Before moving on to discuss the main applications of ICT in nurse education, it is necessary to make some general points.

Anti-racist and anti-sexist resources

Over the last decade there has been a growing awareness amongst educators of the need to ensure that ICT resources do not perpetuate stereotypes and prejudice. Whilst few teachers would design or select media that were deliberately racist or sexist, they may quite innocently use such materials because they have never thought about their potential to promote stereotyping. When considering resources for teaching, it is useful to check the following aspects:

1. Do pictures of social groups actually represent the multicultural nature of society e.g. are all the people white?
2. Are ethnic minorities portrayed in positions of power, or only white people?
3. Does the language use reflect all strata of society, or simply middle-class?
4. Are there stereotypes portrayed, e.g. a male doctor and a female nurse?

The teacher should be familiar with the university's policy in relation to equal opportunities, racism and sexism, which can be a useful source to help teachers to avoid inadvertent stereotyping.

Manufacturer's instructions for use of ICT

It is of the utmost importance from a health and safety point of view that teachers ensure they have read the manufacturer's instructions for the use of ICT equipment, and preferably, have received some instruction in their use. It is also important from the point of view of damage to expensive equipment if used incorrectly.

University facilities for ICT production

Universities have sophisticated facilities for the production of ICT, including professional recording studios and graphics departments staffed by skilled technicians. Teachers may simply have to put in a request to these in order to have them produced by experts in these departments. However, it may not always be convenient or possible to utilize such facilities, so the following sections explain how teachers should set about producing their own media.

The chapter takes a Herbartian approach to sequencing, in that it starts with the most basic types of ICT, moving on to progressively more technically-sophisticated media, and culminating in the latest computer technology for teaching and learning.

Using a whiteboard in teaching

The whiteboard or inkboard is now the most common type of board in use in higher education teaching rooms. When using a whiteboard for teaching, it is important to have the correct type of marker pen. Most boards utilize dry marker pens that can be wiped off with a dry cloth; if ordinary marker pens are used they will not wipe off without the use of some form of spirit.

The purpose of the whiteboard is to record, in semi-permanent form, the key points and explanations during a teaching session. This enables the student to see as well as hear the points and to copy them down as a source of reference for the future.

Positioning and illumination

Before the teaching session begins, the board should be checked for glare by walking around the room and looking from various angles. If glare spots are identified, then, in the case of a fixed board, the seats should be re-positioned in that section until glare is eliminated. If the board is portable, then it can be re-positioned as required. Illumination serves as a spotlight, focusing the attention of the audience on the message, so the room lights should be switched on whenever one is teaching.

Lettering

The art of writing on a whiteboard is to forget your normal style of handwriting, concentrating instead on making lines and loops from the shoulder. This involves considerable practice, but will pay dividends in clarity and legibility. The size of lettering is often quoted as between one and a half to three inches high, but this will depend mainly on the size of the room in which one is teaching. It is useful to write a specimen heading on the board before the class begins and then to check from the rear of the room for visibility. Lettering is classified into two main types in whiteboard work, upper and lower case. The former are capital letters, and the latter small and the terms are derived from the printing trade, where the cases of letters were placed one above the other, with the capitals in the upper case.

Upper-case letters should be used for main headings and also to emphasize key words. All other writing should employ lower case, since the shape of the word is easier to read in this format. When writing on the board the teacher should stop talking, as the voice will not project when the teacher has his back to the audience.

Teachers may feel uncomfortable with silences, so tend to write as quickly as possible, with a resulting loss of legibility. The period spent writing on the board can be used as a mini-break for the students, so that their arousal will increase when the teacher faces them again. Remember, 'if it's worth writing down, it's worth writing legibly'.

Emphasis

Emphasis can be achieved by the following devices:

1. upper-case lettering;
2. underlining;
3. encasing the word;
4. colouring the words.

Diagrams

These must be large enough to allow the audience to see the details with the labelling written at the periphery and arrows used to pinpoint the component.

Labels should not be written on the diagram itself, since they obscure the detail. Diagrams that have to be reproduced regularly are best done using a template. This is then simply drawn around during the class, and provides a quick way of producing an accurate diagram.

Erasing

Whiteboards are cleaned either by using a damp cloth or a dry one, according to the type of board. It is important that the correct type of pen is used; it is frustrating on entering a classroom to find that permanent markers have been used to write on boards intended for dry-markers, as such writing is difficult to remove.

The whiteboard plan

This is a very useful idea for structured teaching sessions and consists of a replica of exactly what the board will look like when the teaching session has been completed. More than one may be required if the teaching session involves a great deal of material, but if the key points only are written, then one plan should suffice. It is important to leave a margin at the side of the board for impromptu explanations and the plan should indicate the indentations and use of colour. A plan ensures that the whiteboard work is of a high standard and has been carefully thought out for maximum impact.

Table 9.1 gives a checklist for effective use of the whiteboard.

Table 9.1

Checklist for effective use of whiteboard

A.   Before the teaching session
1.   Devise a whiteboard plan.
2.   Clean the board.
3.   Ensure that sufficient pens are available, in a variety of colours.
4.   Check for glare spots by walking around room.
5.   Check visibility using a sample heading, and viewing from rear of room.
B.   During the teaching session
6.   Adhere to whiteboard plan; use margin for impromptu explanations.
7.   Use appropriate lettering.
8.   Emphasize by upper case, underlining, colour, encasing.
9.   Write slowly enough to be legible.
10.   Stop talking when writing.
11.   Allow everyone to see, by using pointer from a distance.
12.   Erase only when more space required, or when material will cause interference with subsequent points.
13.   Check with students before erasing.
C.   End of teaching session
14.   Use whiteboard material as a summary.
15.   Erase completely for next lecturer.

USING FLIPCHARTS

Flipcharts are simply large notepads which can be mounted on a stand or over a whiteboard, and marker pens are used to write or draw. When a sheet is completed, it is simply folded over, revealing a clean one. Material can be prepared in advance and revealed at the appropriate time. The guidelines for positioning, illumination and lettering are as for whiteboards. Erasing is not an issue, as the sheets are simply discarded when finished with.

USING AN OVERHEAD PROJECTOR

The overhead projector (OHP) is one of the most useful and versatile of educational media, consisting of a machine that projects large images of clear acetate sheets, called overhead transparencies, onto a screen. The overhead projector is designed for use in daylight, which saves the inconvenience of blackout, and has the advantage over the whiteboard, in that the teacher faces the audience whilst using it. Transparencies can be prepared from a variety of sources:

1. hand-written/hand-drawn by teachers;
2. computer-generated by teachers;

3. produced by teachers using a photocopier

4. produced by commercial publishers.

Overhead projection has another advantage over the whiteboard, in that transparencies can prepared in advance of the teaching session. They offer the facility for step-by-step presentations, using revelation technique or overlays. On the downside, though, there may be some glare from the bright light of the projector and the noise of the projector fan can be distracting. During the session, it is important to make full use of the 'Off' switch, and this should be done whenever a transparency is changed and also if the teacher needs to give a detailed explanation regarding one of the points on the transparency. Switching off the machine will focus the students' attention back to the teacher.

Setting up the overhead projector

In my experience as an assessor, the most common problem encountered by new teachers is how to correctly set up the overhead projector.

The screen

Screens are either fixed or portable, the former being more common in higher education teaching rooms. If using a portable screen, the height of the screen can be adjusted by sliding the vertical supporting rod up or down. The bottom edge of the screen should be no lower than head level of the audience and it should be tilted forwards to prevent the 'keystone' effect, indicated by the image being wider at the top than the bottom. Although the projector is designed for use in daylight, strong sunlight or artificial light shining directly on the screen may bleach out the image, so, if possible, the lights nearest the screen may be switched off, or blinds drawn. It is often useful, if the screen is portable, to place it across the corner of the room, as this will also permit full use of the whiteboard without obstruction from the screen.

Image size and focusing

The projected image should fill the entire surface of the screen; if it is smaller or larger than this, the projector should be moved closer or further away until the image size is correct. The projector is focused by turning a knob on the neck of the projection head. At the commencement of the teaching session, the teacher should take a minute or two to set the correct image size, and also focus the image by placing a pencil on the projector table and turning the focus knob until the image is sharp.

Teacher's position

The decision as to whether the teacher wishes to stand or sit will depend upon the nature of the session and the size of the audience. From the students' point of view, the perceived agenda for the session can be influenced by the position adopted by the teacher. A teacher who is standing tends to be perceived as being in a declamatory or telling mode, which implies a more one-way teaching encounter. When the teacher is seated, however, there is a different social perception of the session; sitting on the same level as the students implies a more discursive, interactive encounter, which may encourage students to contribute more freely.

Whether standing or sitting, I prefer to have the overhead projector on my right-hand side, but the main criterion is that each member of the audience has an uninterrupted view of the screen image.

Creating transparencies for overhead projection

Computers are by far the best way to design professional transparencies, and a range of software is available which enables the production of sophisticated transparencies without having to be a computer expert, e.g. Microsoft® PowerPoint, discussed later in this section. If this facility is not available, they can be made by photocopying from paper originals, or by writing or drawing directly onto the acetate sheets.

Hand-produced transparencies

Pens specially designed for overhead projection are available in either water-soluble or permanent forms, the latter being much more durable if the acetate is to be used a number of times. Permanent ink can be erased by using spirit-based products, whereas soluble ink needs only a wipe with a damp cloth.

When designing acetates, the lettering should be no less than six millimetres in size and it is useful to use lined paper underneath the acetate so that the lettering is kept even. One of the golden rules of making transparencies is to keep them simple, preferably expressing a single concept only, on any one acetate. It is tempting to be economical with acetates by overcrowding them with masses of writing, but this is very bad for the students, who have to cope with trying to write down all the information before it is removed. It is also important to leave a margin at each end of the acetate, or it may be too big for the image area and suffer loss of letters or words at the periphery.

When drawing lines of different colours that are very close to each other, it is a good idea to draw one line on one side of the acetate and then turn it over to draw the other; this prevents smudging or blurring of colours. Colour can be added at the end of the preparation by the use of coloured adhesive film, producing excellent results on such things as pie diagrams and bar charts. Transparencies can be mounted on cardboard mounts specially designed for the purpose and these provide a safe system for storage as well.

Using transparency overlays and revelation technique

Presentation of ideas can be extended by the use of revelation and overlay techniques.

Overlays

Overlays consist of two or more transparencies which build up a concept or diagram. They are constructed by taping a base transparency to a cardboard mount and then taping the overlay transparencies to this, ensuring that the alignment is accurate and that only one side of each overlay is taped. Presentation commences with the base, and then each overlay is hinged into place to build up the transparency. If the order of overlays is fixed, then they should all be taped on the same side of the mount. If the order can be varied, then each can be taped to one of the four sides of the mount and this allows the student's contributions to be added as they arise.

Revelation technique

For this technique, the transparency is covered with a sheet of paper, which is then progressively removed to reveal each point. I find it useful to use two sizes of paper as a mask; an A4 size sheet for the initial coverage of the transparency and a small one for the last two or three points. The small mask will conceal the final points effectively, but unlike the larger sheet, will not fall off the projector if the teacher moves his hand. If points need to be added to a transparency but the teacher wishes to keep it for further use, then an acetate roll can be attached to the machine and the original transparency slipped beneath it. The teacher then adds the points on the acetate roll, leaving the original unmarked.

Projection of silhouettes

The overhead projector will project a silhouette of any solid object on to the screen, such as the shape of an organ, or of instruments and drains. For example, the teacher could drawn an outline of a leg onto acetate and then add cardboard silhouettes of the two fragments of a fractured femoral shaft to indicate the displacement and the effects of reduction.

Projection of X-rays and scans

Provided that the lamp is bright enough, any good-contrast X-ray should project onto the screen. An object can be then added, such as a femoral head prosthesis or intercostal drain, to indicate the position in relation to the X-ray structures. Table 9.2 shows a checklist for using the OHP.

DESIGNING AND USING HANDOUT MATERIAL

Handouts are a common strategy in higher education and consist of a sheet or sheets of paper given to each student for permanent use.

Purposes of handouts

The purposes of handouts can be summarized, as follows:

Table 9.2

Checklist for effective use of overhead projector

A. Before the teaching session
1. Position screen so that everyone can see it, with lower border level with heads of audience.
2. If available, use tilting screen to avoid keystone effect.
3. Obtain correct image size by moving machine backwards or forwards in relation to screen.
4. Focus image sharply.
5. Place masking sheet to hand.
6. Place transparencies in correct order.
7. Check table and head for dust, and wipe if necessary.
8. Ensure that a spare lamp is available in case of blow-out.

B. During the teaching session
9. Switch off when:
   (a) placing transparency on table;
   (b) removing transparencies;
   (c) point has been explained.
10. Use pointer to indicate, preferably on the transparency rather than screen. Avoid use of fingers.
11. Use mask to reveal points in a step-by-step fashion when required.

C. After the teaching session
12. Do not move the machine while lamp is hot, and never disconnect from mains supply whilst fan is operating.

1. *To provide information.* Handouts can be given to provide information to the students, such as teaching session objectives, facts or statistics and diagrams and charts.
2. *As a lecture guide.* If the lecture structure is particularly complex, it may be given to the students in the form of a handout that they can follow, adding their own notes.
3. *References and further reading.* If a lecture contains many references, it is useful to record them on a handout so that the exact details are correct. Further reading can also be suggested.
4. *Assessment and questioning.* Handouts in incomplete form are commonly used to assess learning during the course of a teaching session. In addition, handouts may be given containing written questions for evaluation at the end of a session.
5. *Worksheets and assignments.* The student is required to complete the instructions on the sheet, which may require information to be sought or problems to be solved. It is commonly assumed that worksheets should be handed in to the teacher for assessment on completion, but the real role of a worksheet is to put the students in the position of having to gain certain knowledge or skills. These can then be assessed using the conventional methods of assessment, rather than trying to mark the wide variety of responses made to a worksheet.

Bligh (1998) provides a useful summary of research studies relating to the effectiveness of handouts, and concludes that, on balance, it is helpful to provide handouts for students.

Design of handouts

Students should be encouraged to file handouts, so it is helpful to use paper with punched holes for ease of filing. The actual layout of text and diagrams will depend upon the nature of the topic, but in general they should not be overcrowded with text. Handouts can be designed in a very professional way by using desktop publishing computer packages, which have the advantage of novel designs such as newspaper columns or magazine format.

Student-teachers often ask 'What is the best time to distribute handouts?'; there is no single answer to this, as it depends upon the purpose of the handout. Some lecturers will only distribute them at the end of the lecture, because they feel that giving them out during the lecture will distract the students' attention away from what the lecturer is saying. The problem here is that if the handout is given at the end, it has no current relevance for the student and will probably end up being filed without first being read. Given that higher education students are adults, they should be able to use a handout during the session, provided that the lecturer makes reference to the handout at appropriate points. This is even more effective if the handout is designed with spaces for students to insert any further points gleaned from the lecturer.

Methods of reproducing material

In the higher education sector, large-scale reproduction of items such as student handbooks is done by a central printing service. Small-scale reproduction usually consists of photocopying; however, copies are relatively expensive and expenditure on photocopying needs careful monitoring.

Copyright

Copyright laws are designed to protect authors from the wholesale copying of their works, a very real need in view of the ease with which modern copying machines can reproduce materials. However, copying is an important aspect of good teaching, and the licensing scheme operated by the Copyright Licensing Agency (CLA) allows copying without permission within clearly defined limits. In higher education institutions the licence enables teaching, administrative and technician staff, librarians and all students to copy for any one course of study in one academic year. It is a condition of the licence that the number of multiple copies of any one item of copyright material shall not exceed the number needed to ensure that the tutor and each member of a class has one reproduction only. The CLA produces *Guidelines for Users of the CLA Licence*, and copy must be kept beside the copying machine. Information on copyright can be found in the CLA website pages on http://www.cla.uk

USING THE SLIDE PROJECTOR

Slide projection is used for showing still pictures to an audience using 35 mm slides. In order to obtain a clear image it is necessary to operate slide projectors in darkness.

Setting up and using slide projectors

As with all equipment, the slide projector should be set up before the teaching session and carefully positioned so that every member of the audience can see the screen. Image size is dictated by the distance of the projector from the screen – the further away it is, the larger the image. The size of the group should determine how large an image is required, and the slides should be inserted with the teacher standing at the rear of the projector and facing the screen. Each slide should be held up to the light so that it is seen and read in the normal manner and then it should be turned upside down before being inserted into the projector. If the projector has an automatic feed the magazine should be filled using the same technique. The projector should then be switched on and the picture focused sharply.

If a remote control lead is being used, then it should be tested and then positioned at the teacher's station. Blackout facilities should be operated before the class begins and the lights switched on, as this causes less disruption than doing it during the teaching session. If the slide sequence is spread over different parts of the teaching session with verbal exposition in between, it is convenient to place an exposed black slide between each of the sequences. This saves the teacher having to keep switching the projector on and off, particularly when teaching in a lecture theatre with a separate projection room.

Slides

Slides can be obtained commercially, or teachers can make their own slides using any modern 35 mm camera with a close-up facility. When purchasing film for slides it is important to obtain film for transparencies and not the ordinary film for colour prints. Table 9.3 shows a checklist for slide projection.

Table 9.3

Checklist for effective use of slide projector

A. **Before the teaching session**
1. Position screen for maximum visibility.
2. Align projector so that required size of image is obtained.
3. Focus sharply using a slide.
4. Attach the remote lead if required, and position control near teacher's position.
5. Check blackout. If curtains are used, close them at beginning of teaching session and put on lights.
6. Insert slides if automatic projector, standing behind the projector and turning each slide upside down before inserting into magazine.
7. If more than one sequence of slides is required during the teaching session, insert an exposed black slide between each sequence to prevent continually switching projector on and off.

B. **During the teaching session**
8. Switch off lights when showing slides.
9. Use a pointer on the screen.
10. Use remote control lead to re-focus and change slides

C. **After the teaching session**
11. Remove all slides, including the last one in the 'well'.
12. Don't move projector until lamp is cool.

USING AUDIO-CASSETTES

Audio-cassettes can be a useful resource in teaching, provided they are used appropriately. They are used extensively for data collection in research, and are useful because a transcript of the material can be taken for analysis. The use of audio-cassettes for long periods during lectures or small-group sessions can become very boring, but it is useful to use 'trigger-tapes' to stimulate discussion. Audio-cassettes are also useful for capturing the feelings and experiences of patients, which makes it a good medium for adding interest to sessions on nursing care.

Sources of audio-cassette recordings

Audio-cassette recordings can be taken 'off-air' from radio and television programmes, or used with the integral microphone. The purpose of making an audio-cassette recording is to capture specific content and make it available to an audience. This does not imply, however, that the quality of the recording is irrelevant, for, indeed, it is very important to ensure that it is of the highest technical quality if people are going to listen to it without distraction. A little attention to the technical points can make all the difference between a good recording and a poor one.

Universities have professional recording studies for audio and video, but teachers may wish to make their own audio recordings.

Making amateur audio recordings

When reading a script for a recording session, the teacher should be sitting comfortably at a table, with the integral microphone high enough to avoid having to lower the head to speak. The script must not intervene between the face and the microphone, and to prevent the rustling of paper being detected, it is useful to enclose each sheet in a polythene sleeve so that it glides noiselessly to one side.

Recording requires an assistant to switch the machine on and to monitor sound levels. It is important to position the cassette recorder at some distance from the microphone so that amplifier hum is not picked up. If the cassette recorder does not have automatic recording level, the sound level must be monitored by watching the 'VU' indicator on the recorder, ensuring that this does not exceed 0 VU during the recording. On the other hand, it is important to record the signal at a high level, so the level should approach 0 VU but not exceed it.

Teachers who are new to recording often feel nervous or embarrassed and this makes their delivery stilted. It is a good tip to have someone sitting opposite the speaker, behind the microphone, to whom the speaker addresses his words. This often makes the tone more natural and conversational.

It is worth mentioning that poor quality recordings may result not only from technique, but from badly maintained equipment. The heads on the recorder should be cleaned weekly with head-cleaning fluid and demagnetization should be carried out at monthly intervals using a tape-head demagnetizer.

USING VIDEO-RECORDINGS IN TEACHING

Video is now firmly established as a aspect of the entertainment industry, and video-recorders have become a standard feature in most households. Their use in education is similarly established for a wide range of applications.

Pre-recorded videos

Pre-recorded videos are available either as off-air recordings of television programmes, or as commercially-produced videos; both form an important component of library stock in higher education. The use of pre-recorded videos in teaching needs careful thought; lecturers must brief students in advance so that the students understand its purpose, and can jot down relevant notes. Equally important is debriefing after the video, to share students' impressions and conclusions.

Making video recordings

Video cameras allow teachers and students to make their own video recordings, and this enables the reality of society or the workplace to be brought into the classroom, providing authentic material for discussion and analysis. However, students require careful briefing about the use of video cameras in the hospital or community; permission has to be sought from appropriate authorities, and the public may resent the invasion of privacy.

Closed-circuit television

A less commonly used form of television in education is closed-circuit television; this does not involve recording, but relays live events to other parts of a building via slave monitors. It is useful for observing events where large numbers of observers would be obtrusive or over-crowded, such as in the operating theatre, or for observing interviews without affecting the interaction between participants.

Videoconferencing

Videoconferencing facilities are an increasingly-common feature of university campuses, and utilize live video-links between geographically separated campuses. The facility enables groups of students and staff to interact, who would otherwise have to travel long distances to meet together, and can be used for all kinds of meetings. For example, students who live at a distance from a campus are able to register for a programme that is taught at another location; they then participate in the teaching and learning experience by means of videoconferencing. This can help to ensure the viability of programmes that recruit small numbers, by opening it up to students at a distance. Videoconferencing is also useful for conducting tutorial group meetings on programmes where students live in geographically distant locations.

USING MICROSOFT® POWERPOINT FOR PRESENTATIONS

This is one of the newest forms of visual presentation, and is beginning to replace the overhead projector as the medium of choice for presentations to both large and small groups. *Microsoft*® PowerPoint is a graphics package that is part of the *Microsoft*® Office computer software, and it enables the teacher to produce highly sophisticated slides or overhead transparencies for presentations. It can also create handouts and teacher's notes, and is relatively straightforward to use if the teacher has basic computer skills.

Creating a PowerPoint presentation

PowerPoint has a facility called Autocontent wizard that already contains suggested content material for a variety of presentations such as company meetings, a project overview, a business plan, publicity flyers, etc. If this pre-determined content is not appropriate, the teacher can select a design template; these consist of a background design for the presentation, onto which the text is added by the teacher. There is a bewildering choice of design templates, including 'Dad's tie', a vertical design at the left hand margin of the slide, similar to a garish man's tie, and 'Fans', a helical arrangement of fans along the left-hand edge. A blank presentation is also available, containing neither suggested text nor design template, but with AutoLayout; this allows the teacher to place text in a given pattern according to her choice of autolayout.

Slides can be animated to make text fly in from the right or the left, or simply designed for a gradual revelation of key points. When the teacher has completed the slides, there is the option of seeing them all by simply clicking on the 'Slide Show' button on the title bar on the *PowerPoint window.*

Making a PowerPoint presentation

PowerPoint can produce either a slide show for projection onto a full-size screen, or transparencies for overhead projection. It is well worth preparing both options when considering a *PowerPoint* presentation, so that you have OHP transparencies to fall back on if the technology goes wrong! The most common method is a presentation by the teacher, who is in complete control of the technology. One of the disadvantages of *PowerPoint*, however, is that it requires a darkened classroom for optimum visibility, and this can cause problems with students' note-taking during the presentation.

COMPUTER-ASSISTED LEARNING

Computer-assisted learning (CAL) is a general term used to cover a wide variety of teaching applications; for example, it includes learning material posted on the WWW to allow students to prepare for tutorials, retrieval of on-line reports and databases, e-mail noticeboards, and courseware (CTI, 1998).

Courseware

Courseware, i.e. teaching materials, for CAL can use a single computer or in combination with a range of other media as in multimedia CAL. With a single computer approach, the teacher either develops appropriate courseware or it is purchased from manufacturers of educational media. The courseware is selected by the student and loaded into the computer, where it forms the learning experience for the student in whichever mode is appropriate.

Computer-assisted learning is only as good as the courseware that goes into it, but computers do have the potential to produce high-quality graphic displays, data storage and retrieval and a host of other effects that would be almost impossible for the individual teacher to emulate in standard teaching situations. Single-computer CAL does have limitations and these can be overcome by the use of multimedia CAL, which consists of a range of media that is used in the same instructional program, e.g. sound, pictures, video.

CAL and independent learning

CAL is particularly useful for independent, self-managed learning; students using a computer can take the material at their own pace, referring back to previous sections as and when they deem necessary. They can answer the questions posed by the program in total privacy, without the embarrassment of having their lack of knowledge exposed in front of a group of peers. CAL can help foster the intuitive kind of thinking that is important for discovery learning, by presenting problem-based information about which the student has to make hypotheses and subsequently checking her answers against the computer.

CAL can accomplish a number of other teaching functions, such as presentation of information on new topics, follow-up activities, revision, diagnostic and remedial teaching, in fact most of the activities normally associated with classroom teaching. The great advantage of CAL is that it can offer high-quality instruction that eliminates such variables as poor preparation and presentation by the teacher, problems of timing, fatigue, boredom and loss of attention. Of course, the last three can happen in any medium, but at least with CAL the student can switch off and go for a walk to restore her concentration.

Advantages and disadvantages of CAL

Claims about the advantages of CAL over conventional classroom teaching are summarized by Hartley (1998):

1. learning is individualized and self-paced;
2. feedback on students' responses is instant;
3. programs are written by experts, and have undergone rigorous testing before publication;
4. it is cost-effective.

However, Hartley points out that these claims may not be justified, as students may not have control over the pace of their learning, and the quality of some programs is questionable.

THE INTERNET AND WORLD WIDE WEB

The term *internet* is shorthand for 'international network of computers', a network of computers across the world that are connected by high technology telephone lines. Some companies charge a subscription fee for internet access, but there is now a growing market of providers who offer free access. Telephone calls to access the internet are normally charged at the local call rate, which makes browsing the internet relatively inexpensive if used sensibly. The internet, usually abbreviated to the net, provides the user with access to almost limitless amounts of information, and also allows them to communicate with other internet users anywhere in the world.

The internet has three main aspects: email, the world wide web, and newsgroups.

Electronic mail (email)

Electronic mail or email has brought about a revolution in the way teachers and students in education communicate with each other. Email allows a message to be sent to individuals anywhere in the world, who will receive it instantaneously. The same message can be sent to many people at the same time, at the cost of only a local telephone call. Although email is available on the internet, it can also be used with any computer that has the appropriate software and a telephone modem. The system is very easy to use; you simply type out your message, select the address(s) of the recipient(s), and then click on the 'send' button on the computer. One of the advantages of email is that the sender gets an acknowledgement that it has been delivered; also, a record is kept of both outgoing and incoming mail, a valuable reference source for later queries. It is also very secure, as a password is required for entry.

Tutoring via email

Email has proved to be extremely useful for maintaining tutorial contact with students; it bypasses that bain of tutor's lives, the answering machine (voice mail), allowing the tutor to leave a message without the need to ring back later. Messages can be sent at any time, day or night, and do not disturb the recipient as a telephone call would. Email is particularly useful for tutor's comments on draft assignments, facilitating a very quick turnaround of feedback to the student.

One of the exciting innovations in email tutoring is computer-mediated-tutoring (CMT), also termed computer-mediated-conferencing (CMT), a type of computer conferencing that allows students and tutors to discuss issues in a 'virtual group', but does not take place in real-time. Hence, a tutor may initiate activities or ideas onto the server, and the students in the virtual group can respond at any time of the day or night. Students and tutor may initiate and respond to each others' inputs just like a live seminar, but with the advantage of not having to be in the same place at the same time. CMC is discussed further in the context of open and distance learning, in Chapter 11.

World wide web

Usually referred to as the web or WWW, this consists of documents published on the internet, and linked to other documents via 'hypertext links'. The web is organized into web sites, i.e. collections of documents relating to a specific topic, and web pages, i.e. single documents about some aspect of the site topic (Kennedy, 1998). The web sites offer information on an astounding range of topics, and almost anything can be purchased from the online shopping stores using a credit card. There are also entertainment sites for computer games, music, art, etc.

Surfing the web

Teachers in nurse education will normally use their university's internet service to access the web, but many teachers will also have their own internet facilities at home. When you click on the internet browser icon on the computer, the first page to appear is the home page. This is the base from which you can explore (surf) the web sites, and like all web pages, contains links to other pages in the form of hypertext. Text which contains links is normally in a different colour, or underlined, and when the mouse cursor moves across a link it changes shape from an arrow to a pointing hand. To follow the link you click on the mouse and the new document appears, and these can also be downloaded and saved into your computer.

Web site addresses for nursing and higher education

If you already know the address of the internet site you require, you simply key in (type) this into the appropriate box, click on the mouse, and the appropriate page appears. Table 9.4 gives a list of web addresses that are relevant to nursing and higher education.

INTRANETS

Intranets operate in much the same way as the internet, but within an institution's own internal computer network (inter = between; intra = within). Hence, intranets are not accessible by the community at large. There is a wide variety of information contained on an intranet, including teaching and learning materials in the form of journal articles, lecture handouts, assignments, revision tips, etc. Intranets are particularly useful for students studying at a distance from the main site, as they can easily access the materials without the need to travel.

ONLINE CAMPUS

This is a web-based, virtual university campus that supports students on their programme of studies (Ryan and Culwick, 1997) and it requires

United Kingdom Central Council for Nursing, Midwifery and Health Visiting (UKCC)	http://www.ukcc.org.uk	
English National Board for Nursing, Midwifery and Health Visiting (ENB)	http://www.enb.org.uk	
Department of Health (DOH)	http://www.open.gov.uk/doh	
Quality Assurance Agency for Higher Education (QAA)	http://www.qaa.ac.uk	
Department for Education and Employment (DfEE)	http://www.dfee.gov.uk	
Committee of Vice-Chancellors and Principals (CVCP)	http://www.cvcp.ac.uk	
Computers for Teaching Initiative (CTI)	http://www.cti.ac.uk	
Institute for Learning and Teaching	http://www.ilt.ac.uk	

Table 9.4

Web site addresses for nursing and higher education

students and staff to have access to the internet and an internet browser. The online campus consists of three aspects:

1. *A discussion forum.* Any registered student may contribute ideas, ask questions, seek advice or share experiences, and teachers can set up student activities in relation to their own courses. Students can respond to each other's contributions and to those of the teachers, thus providing an environment similar to a face-to-face discussion.
2. *An electronic resource centre.* This contains copies of teachers' resource files to help students with their programme work, and also links to other web sites and pages.
3. *Student common room.* This is an area to which teachers do not have access, and provides a point of informal social contact and chat. It is particularly useful for students on open and distance learning programmes who do not have regular face-to-face inter-action with a group.

REFERENCES

Bligh, D. (1998) *What's the Use of Lectures?*, 5th edn, Intellect, Exeter.

CTI (1998) *Communication and Information Technologies for Teaching and Learning In Higher Education*, CTISS, Oxford.

Further Education Funding Council (1998) *The Use of Technology to Support Learning in Colleges*, National Survey Report, FEFC, Coventry.

Hartley, J. (1998) *Learning and Studying: A Research Perspective*, Routledge, London.

Kennedy, A. (1998) *The Internet: The Rough Guide*, 4th edn, Rough Guides, London.

Ryan, M. and Culwick, G. (1997) Creating a virtual integrated learning environment (VILE), in *ED-MEDIA and ED-TELECOM 97 Proceedings*, T. Muldner and T. Reeves (eds), Calgary, AACE, Virginia.

Severs, M. and Pearson, C. (1999) *Learning to Manage Health Information: A Theme for Clinical Education*, NHS Executive, Bristol.

10 COURSE AND PROGRAMME MANAGEMENT

The management of an educational programme requires a clearly-defined management structure and capable, motivated and well-organized individuals if the quality of the student experience is to be maintained. The role of programme leader is pivotal, and the academic and administrative responsibilities of the role are normally acknowledged by a certain amount of 'easement' from teaching duties, and possibly a temporary promotion while the post is held, depending on the size of the programme.

Within the higher education sector, there are a number of terms used to describe the formal process of study undertaken by a student under the auspices of a higher education institution, depending upon the academic information system in use in a given institution. A guide to current terminology of the Banner academic information system used within the University of Greenwich is given in Table 10.1.

Hence, what the person in the street would call a *course* is now termed a *programme*, and I will use this term throughout the rest of the chapter.

Table 10.1

Terminology relating to formal study

Definition	Previous Name(s)	Latest Name(s)
A period of formal study leading to an academic award	Course; pathway	Programme
A self-contained sub-component of a programme	Module; unit	Course

MANAGEMENT AND LEADERSHIP

The terms *management* and *leadership* are often used synonymously in describing the organization of programmes in higher education. However, it is useful to consider them as complementary systems, both of which are important for the achievement of the institution's objectives. Taking Kotter's (1990) analysis as his starting point, Ramsden (1998) discusses the differences between these two concepts.

Management is not some unnecessary bureaucratic process: 'it is the essence of rationality. Managers plan, organize, staff, and solve problems. Management is about "doing things right"'. This contrasts markedly with leadership: 'effective leaders produce "constructive or adaptive" change to help people and firms to grow. They establish direction, align people, and motivate them. Leadership is about "doing the right thing"'. Ramsden goes on to argue that, in periods of major change, strong leadership is required to help people adapt but, equally, strong leadership without strong management 'is a characteristic and disruptive failing of innovative courses in traditional academic contexts'.

The programme leader is, in relation to the programme management team, *primus inter pares*, first among equals. Whilst there is normally no line management function between the programme leader and colleagues in the team, s/he is formally defined as the team leader. The terms formal and informal leader are often used to distinguish types of leader; the role of programme leader is one of formal leadership. On the other hand, an informal leader is one who most closely embodies the group's norms. The formal leader is often described by the term *headship* to signify the nature of the leadership position, but it is not necessarily the formal leader who has most power in a group.

It is probably fair to say that there is no such thing as an ideal leadership personality or style; leadership is very much dependent on relationships within the group and the particular purpose for which the group exists. An individual may be an effective leader in one setting but of little use in another; it would be hard to imagine an army officer, who is a capable leader of his men, functioning effectively as leader of an encounter group because of the very different style and context in which it operates.

McNay (1998) offers a triangular model of leadership, consisting of three elements: inspiration, organization, and education. Leadership can be based on one of these elements, or a combination of them. For example, leadership based on inspiration requires vision and entrepreneurial flair, but it also needs organization in order to be implemented successfully. Leadership based on education is about changing the way people think. McNay points out that leaders need to be in touch with the context of their followers:

'it is no use leading if the gap between you and your followers is such that they cannot see you and you cannot see them in order to give them support or even understand their situation. Empathy is a necessary condition for good leadership'.

A classic study of leadership that formed the beginning of experimental approaches to social groups was that by White and Lippit (1960). They used real-life groups of boys who attended an after-school club to carry out model-making and other handicrafts. The boys were allocated to three groups, each led by an adult who adopted a predetermined style of leadership:

1. In the 'autocratic' groups, the leader imposed work on the boys, remaining friendly but aloof from them.
2. In the 'democratic' groups, the leader discussed the work with the boys, and functioned as part of the group, allowing them to decide what to do.
3. The 'laissez-faire' groups were left to their own devices to do

what they wished, with the leader offering no help unless requested.

The results of the different styles of leadership were evaluated after several weeks with striking differences being found. The autocratic groups showed aggression towards the leader or to a scapegoat within the group and were resentful and hostile. The work rate was good, but dropped off when the leader left the room. In contrast, the democratic groups were more cohesive, the leader was popular, the work was better and they continued to work when the leader was absent. The laissez-faire groups did very little work, showed some aggression and were uncontrolled whether or not the leader was present. This study is often quoted as supporting the superiority of democratic leadership and the importance of self-imposed discipline.

TEAMWORK

Teamwork and co-operation is essential if programme management is to be effective. Not everyone is a natural team leader, and the skills of team work may have to be learned. Atkins and Katcher (1996) propose that good team work depends upon the leader's ability to take into account individual team members' operating styles. According to these authors, individuals' behaviour is oriented through four fundamental patterns of behaviour, although only one or two will be dominant in a given individual.

The four behaviour patterns

The four behaviour patterns are simply the ways in which individuals operate in their environment, and no one pattern is good or bad. The following descriptors refer to individuals' characteristics for a given dominant behaviour pattern.

1. *Supporting/giving-in*. Individuals for whom this is their dominant style tend to be good team members, being co-operative, open to ideas, and with high standards.
2. *Controlling/taking-over*. When this is the dominant style, individuals tend to be self-confidence, persuasive and competitive. They are initiators of action, and require little supervision.
3. *Conserving/holding-on*. Individuals with this dominant orientation are reliable, methodical 'plodders' who consider all the angles before undertaking a task.
4. *Adapting/dealing-away*. Individuals for whom this is their dominant style tend to be popular people who enjoy being in the spotlight, and who exhibit sensitivity to the needs of others. Their enthusiasm can motive other workers, and flexibility is a characteristic.

The team leader needs to assess the orientations of each team member in order to individualize her management approach to their particular dominant orientation.

PROGRAMME MANAGEMENT STRUCTURES

Programme management structures consist of the programme leader, the programme management team, and the programme committee. The basic structure of programme management applies to all programmes regardless of the number of students and the pattern of attendance. However, very large programmes will require one or more deputy programme leader roles to cope with the greater administrative workload.

The programme leader

The key role in relation to programme management is that of programme leader, who is responsible for the day-to-day running of the programme. The typical responsibilities of the role are shown in Table 10.2. These responsibilities are discussed later in this chapter.

1.	Preparation of validation documentation, and liaison with appropriate validation personnel
2.	Preparation of the definitive programme document
3.	Preparation of a student handbook for students on the programme
4.	Oversight of recruitment and selection and induction of students, in conjunction with the admissions tutor
5.	Organizing the staffing, timetabling, and rooming for the programme
6.	Organizing the teaching, tutoring, and pastoral care of students on the programme
7.	Liaison with placement co-ordinators for practice placements
8.	Liaison with appropriate personnel regarding examinations and assessments
9.	Preparation of pass lists for boards of examiners, in conjunction with the chair
10.	Programme monitoring and production of the annual programme monitoring report
11.	Academic leadership of the programme

Table 10.2

Typical responsibilities of a programme leader

Staff development for the role of programme leader

The 'sharp-end' role of programme leader can be one of the most rewarding in education, as the incumbent has considerable scope to influence the development of the programme and the students' experience of it. The role of programme leader may be undertaken by academic staff of varying grades and is not necessarily linked with formal positions of seniority nor with line-management responsibility. It is common to find that the role is held for some three to five years before being assigned to another member of the academic staff. This helps to avoid complacency and the danger of becoming stale, and encourages new ideas and approaches.

Staff development is an essential pre-requisite for a new programme leader, and commonly takes the form of an overlapping appointment with the previous post-holder, so that both the outgoing and the incoming programme leaders work together on the programme for a period of some three months. This preceptorship system allows the incoming leader to 'shadow' the outgoing one, and to learn the requirements of the role before taking full responsibility for programme leadership.

The programme management team

This normally consists of the programme leader and a number of colleagues teaching courses on the programme, according to the number of students on the programme. The role of the programme management team is to assist the programme leader in the day to day operation of the programme.

The programme committee

The programme committee has representation from a range of key people involved in either the delivery of the programme, or its consumption. The typical composition of this committee is given in Table 10.3, and the role of the committee in Table 10.4.

Table 10.3

Typical composition of a programme committee

Programme Leader (Chair)
Representatives of staff teaching the course
Representative from library/resources
Normally one student from each year of the programme

Earlier in this chapter, the roles of the programme leader were identified. In the following section, the range of roles will be explored.

Table 10.4

Role of the programme committee

1.	Develop new courses (i.e. modules) as required
2.	Review and develop teaching and learning strategies
3.	Review and develop assessment strategies
4.	Review programme recruitment
5.	Monitor student progress
6.	Assist the course leader with preparation of annual programme monitoring report
7.	Provide a formal route of communication between teachers and students
8.	Address issues raised by the programme leader, senior managers or relevant committees

PREPARING FOR A PROGRAMME VALIDATION EVENT

When a new programme is being planned, one of the earliest decisions should be the identification of the programme leader designate. This individual will take the leading role in the preparation of the documentation that will go to validation, as well as the administration of the curriculum team that is planning the new programme. The programme leader designate will need to liaise with the academic registry over such issues as external professional membership of the validation panel, and deadline dates for submission of documentation to the university and the professional nursing body that will conjointly validate the programme.

Validation is discussed in detail in Chapter 12.

STUDENT ADMISSIONS

It is common in higher education for departments to have admissions tutors who are responsible for admissions procedures for one or more courses or programmes. They liaise closely with the programme leader and the academic registry, and their role involves making arrangements for recruitment and selection of students.

There are two categories of student who can access courses (i.e. units/modules): registered students and associate students. Registered students are those who have registered with the institution to undertake a programme leading to an academic award. Associate students, on the other hand, simply undertake one or more courses that they need for some specific staff development purpose, e.g. counselling skills or research. They receive the appropriate credit for the course on successful completion, but they do not register for an academic award.

Admissions regulations

Each programme will have its own admission regulations within which recruitment and selection will operate. One very important aspect of this is equal opportunities, in that recruitment and selection processes must be compatible with the equal opportunities policy of the institution. Admissions regulations normally contain a statement on equal opportunities, and the following is a typical example:

> *'This institution operates an equal opportunities policy and invites applications from suitable candidates regardless of race, gender, age, disability, religion, political affiliation, or sexual orientation'.*

Another important aspect is that of access. Programmes will vary in their degree of openness of access according to the nature of the programme and the ideology of the institution. For example, pre-registration programmes at degree level would normally have specific admission requirements such as a minimum of five GCSE passes, whereas post-registration programme requirements tend to be more general, e.g. a minimum of two years' post-registration experience in nursing or midwifery. Some programmes may have completely open access, with candidates being required solely to demonstrate that they can benefit from undertaking the programme.

Publicity and recruitment

Students find out about programmes from a variety of sources such as the institute's prospectus, recommendations from friends, direct marketing by the institution, such as mail-shots, careers advisors, and advertising in journals and newspapers.

Desktop publishing (DTP) enables departments to produce sophisticated publicity materials in house for mail shots and other distribution. Advertising can reach much greater numbers of people, but the cost is relatively high

Programme enquiries from prospective candidates are dealt with by the registry, who send out an information pack about the programme, including an application form. The information is compiled by the programme leader, and it is helpful to give the candidates as much information as possible to assist them in making a decision about the suitability of the programme for their own needs. It is helpful to include a document of the form *Your Questions Answered* in the programme information pack, containing answers to all the likely questions that a candidate might have about the programme. If the selection procedures involve a face-to-face interview, this type of document makes the interview much more efficient by cutting down information-giving, thus allowing the interviewer more time to focus on the candidate. The key questions that could be addressed are given in Table 10.5.

Table 10.5

A typical 'Your Questions Answered' document

What are my existing qualifications worth?
What are core units?
What are option units?
How is the programme assessed?
What tutorial support will I receive?
When does the programme run?
How many units can I take at one time?
How much does a unit cost?
How long will I take to complete the programme?
How can I get credit for experiential learning?
What will my interview be like?

The selection interview

Interviews are a standard technique for selecting pre-registration students in nursing and midwifery, whereas for post-registration programmes an employer's recommendation may be considered sufficient grounds for access to the programme. Although interviewing has been the subject of widespread criticism on the grounds of the subjective nature of the decision-making process, the technique is well-established in health care education generally. Ideally, an interview should give the candidate and the institution the opportunity to explore the match between the candidate's needs and the given programme under consideration, and also to clarify any questions or issues on which either party is unclear. In reality, it can easily become an ordeal for the candidate if the style of the interview is that of an inquisition, so interviewers need to be aware of the basic requirements for conducting interviews.

Preparing to interview

Wherever the interview is held, there are certain requirements that must be met, namely privacy and freedom from interruption. This implies the cancellation of all incoming telephone calls for the duration of the interview and the use of 'Do Not Disturb' signs on the door. An informal arrangement of room, with no desk intervening between the candidate and the interviewer – and using chairs of the same height –

attempts to make the interview appear as normal as any other social meeting, so that the candidate feels at ease.

There is no consensus of opinion with regard to the number of interviewers present, but if one agrees with the aim of the interview as outlined above, then it becomes obvious that the more people who are involved, the less 'normal' the situation becomes from the candidate's point of view. This might imply that a single interviewer is best. On the other hand, if two interviewers are present, one can observe the candidate closely whilst the other is engaged in conversation.

Courtesy is the watchword for interviewing, however challenging and probing the interview becomes. Candidates should be given an indication of the time of their interview, and the availability of refreshments made clear. It is the responsibility of the interviewer to have read the candidate's application form thoroughly before the interview, so that the impression gained can be extended and modified according to the candidate's response. It is debatable whether or not the interviewers should have access to references prior to the interview; there is the possibility of a positive or negative halo effect if they are seen beforehand.

Conducting the interview

There are a number of approaches or plans for interviewing; two of the better-known ones are considered here.

The seven-point plan

This classic plan for interviewing was formulated by the National Institute of Industrial Psychology (1970) and this is still cited extensively in the literature of interviewing. It consists of seven main headings not ranked in any particular order. The headings are really questions that the interviewer(s) ask themselves when conducting the interview.

1. *Physical make-up*. This deals with any physical defects or health problems that might affect job performance. In addition, it includes appearance, manner and speech.
2. *Attainments*. This involves education attainment as well as occupational training. Consideration should be given to achievement in relation to circumstances, rather than in isolation. For example, a candidate may have obtained five GCSE passes despite lack of interest by parents.
3. *General intelligence*. This is a difficult concept to measure without using specific tests, but an idea can be gained by noting the candidate's use of language and ability to formulate responses.
4. *Special aptitudes*. Aptitude is best measured by specific aptitude tests.
5. *Interests*. These give an overall indication of the candidate's breadth, and when taken into account with other aspects, may help in coming to a final decision.
6. *Disposition*. This concerns personality, character and temperament, and may indicate qualities of self-reliance, etc.

7. *Circumstances*. This involves the candidate's background and opportunities.

The Fear method

This method consists of a number of stages (Fear, 1978), of which the main ones are outlined below.

1. *Helping the candidate to talk spontaneously*. This is designed to ensure that the candidate feels at ease, and so will volunteer information freely. It is facilitated by use of social skills such as pleasant greetings, facial expression, use of small-talk and giving encouragement by minimizing reactions to unfavourable revelations.

2. *Exploratory questions*. These are used to prompt candidates from time to time, to encourage them to reveal more information. Comments are usually more effective for stimulating conversation, and they are less like interrogation. The main skill in using these is to keep the candidate at the centre of attention, with the interviewer remaining unobtrusive.

3. *Controlling the interview*. Control is a delicate mechanism, for if it is overused the candidate will become less spontaneous. An interview guide sheet helps to keep the interview going in the right direction, but skill is required in its use.

4. *Interpretation*. Every statement which is made by the candidate is interpreted by the interviewer, and it is through this process that a picture is built up. It is useful to make a mental list of assets and liabilities during the interview. These should be so well documented in the interviewer's mind that they can be written down when the candidate leaves the room.

Making a decision

After the interview has been concluded, a decision must be reached as to whether or not the candidate is acceptable. This is done by weighing the positive and negative aspects, including the results of any special tests, such as aptitude or trainability tests. The information is then conveyed to the registry, who send out the standard letters that either offer a place on the programme, or reject the candidate's application. Once the target recruitment figure has been reached, the registry is instructed to notify any further applicants that the programme is full.

ORGANIZING THE TIMETABLING, ROOMING AND STAFFING

Once a decision has been made to run the programme, it is necessary to undertake timetabling and rooming. As part of the programme planning process the pattern of attendance will have been established, including semesters, day(s) and times. Most institutions have a central system of room booking, and it is important that the programme leader is able to make a case for any special requirements such as lecture or laboratory space. Evening sessions require the availability of late catering facilities, but this may not be cost effective if only small numbers of students are involved.

A programme leader would not normally have direct responsibility for allocation of staff, rather, he or she needs to make the teaching staff and technician requirements known to the appropriate senior manager. The staffing requirements for a given programme are largely determined by the amount of resource that is generated by the student numbers, and this will vary according to the funding arrangements of the programme in question. The financial pressures in higher education have led to a progressive reduction in the amount of face-to-face teaching students receive.

The apportioning of the available hours needs careful consideration by the programme team, as it is important to strike an appropriate balance between face-to-face teaching and individual tutorials.

It is common practice in some programmes that unit teachers are required to keep two meetings free of normal unit content, to enable them to undertake individual tutorials on the assessment requirements of the unit during this class time. This ensures that every student has the opportunity to discuss assessment ideas with the unit teacher on at least two occasions during the course of the unit.

INDUCTION OF STUDENTS

The first stage in the induction of students is the mailing of joining instructions for the programme. These should contain details of the date, time and venue of the induction meeting of the programme. The joining instructions should also contain details of the induction programme, and a typical example is shown in Table 10.6.

BSc Honours degree in Nursing Studies (Post Registration)		
Date:	23 September 2001	
Venue:	Williams Lecture Theatre, Hardy Hill Campus, University of Melchester	
Programme:		
1400	Welcome and introduction to programme	Programme leader
1410	Outline of units for first semester	Unit leaders
1500	Registration	Registrars
1600	Resources for learning	RFL team
1630	Individual consultations, issuing of student handbook	Programme team

Table 10.6

A typical student induction programme

At the induction meeting, students are issued with their own copy of the *Student Handbook* for the current academic year. This handbook is of major importance to students, since it sets out the regulations and procedures for all aspects of the programme. Typical contents of a *Student Handbook* are shown in Table 10.7

One of the problems that arises within modularized programmes is

Table 10.7

Typical contents page of a student handbook

BSc Honours degree in Nursing Studies
STUDENT HANDBOOK 2001/2002
Contents
1. Introduction to the programme
2. Summary of key information
   (a) Semester dates 2001/2002
   (b) Assessment handing-in deadlines
   (c) Procedure for handing-in assessments
   (d) Return of marked assignments
   (e) List of courses for 2001/2002
   (f) Tutorial arrangements
3. Key personnel
4. Aims of programme
5. Programme structure and process
6. Accreditation of prior learning
7. Assessment regulations
8. Board of Examiners
9. Programme committee
10. Quality assurance
11. Equal opportunities policy

Appendices
A: Grounds and procedures for appeal: the University of Melchester
B: Statement on cheating and plagiarism: the University of Melchester
C: Course specifications
D: APL Tariff for nursing and midwifery qualifications

the very wide range of option units from which students choose their programme of study. There is great potential for chaos if the organization of choices is left until the induction day, as it is virtually impossible to negotiate with each individual on the day. It is preferable to send out a questionnaire to both new and continuing students before the end of the previous academic year, to ascertain their unit preferences, so that they can be allocated to units in advance of their arrival. There is still some opportunity for students to adjust their preferences on the induction day, but there should be relatively few who need to do this.

Another idea which may prove useful during the induction programme is to distribute a *Guide to Successful Study and Assessment*. Regardless of whether the programme is pre- or post-registration, students often experience difficulty in adjusting to the level of work required for a diploma or degree course, and also in organizing their study effectively.

Some post-registration students have not undertaken formal study since their initial qualifications many years ago, and often experience great difficulty, especially in relation to the writing of assessment work. A written guide can help these students to approach their studies more effectively, and the contents of such a guide are given in Table 10.8.

TAKING A REGISTER OF ATTENDANCE

The programme leader is responsible for the day-to-day running and trouble shooting of the programme and this involves a variety of tasks. For example, attendance registers must be available for unit teachers to complete at each meeting of the unit, since it is common to find that

Introduction
1. Studying at honours degree level
2. Planning your studies
3. Undertaking a unit
    (a) Pre-reading and follow-up reading
    (b) Note-taking
    (c) Participation in unit activities
    (d) Choosing a contract unit
4. Application to professional practice
5. Planning your assignments for unit assessment
6. Reading for your assignment
7. Writing your assignment
    (a) Designing the structure
    (b) Achieving the right level
    (c) Editing for the final draft
    (d) Handing-in the assignment
8. Making the most of tutorials
9. Tackling the research project
10. Further reading

Table 10.8

Contents of a Guide to Successful Study and Assessment

programmes have a percentage attendance requirement regulation. In order to pass a unit, students have to attend a certain percentage of classes, e.g. 75 per cent, and the unit registers provide evidence of this attendance. Programme leaders usually offer a personal tutorial service to students which complements any unit specific tutorials offered by the unit tutors. At these tutorials, the programme leader can advise students on general aspects of the programme such as accreditation of prior learning, and deal with requests for extensions to assessment deadlines, and other programme issues.

PROGRAMME COMMITTEE MEETINGS

Meetings can be the bane of most nurse teachers' lives if the conduct is not well regulated, especially where one or two individuals are allowed to go on and on without any attempt by the chairperson to check them. Meetings are extremely costly in terms of the time occupied by individuals; a meeting lasting one and a half hours with fifteen members of the teaching staff is extremely costly in staff salaries. It can be seen that a poorly managed meeting is extremely wasteful of resources, as well as acting to de-motivate the members present.

The principles of running an effective meeting are straightforward, and involve adequate prior planning, effective group and leadership skills and a good sense of timing. Most committees need a secretary to take minutes and it is worth considering the use of a member of the non-teaching staff for this as they tend to be more efficient at recording proceedings and might even enjoy the chance to be involved in something different from the day-to-day administration.

The importance of prior planning

The chairperson is responsible for requesting agenda items from members of staff and subsequently drawing up the agenda in an appropriate order. All substantive items on the agenda should be accompanied by a paper addressing the item, so that members of the committee are given the opportunity to read and digest the issues in good time before the day of the meeting. Only rarely should the chairperson allow tabled items to be included, since this precludes the proper study of such items prior to the meeting.

The room in which the meeting is to be held needs to be booked in advance and made ready for the meeting. It is good practice to ensure that tables are available, plus note-pads and pencils for each committee member. It is also important to provide glasses and jugs of water, and to maintain a no-smoking rule at all committee meetings. The latter point is extremely important, since every individual should have the right to conduct his business in an atmosphere that is conducive to discussion and thinking. Some chairpersons choose to take a vote on whether smoking should be permitted, but this should not be a subject for democratic voting: only one objection should ensure that the no-smoking rule applies.

Effective chairmanship

The role of the chairperson is to ensure the smooth running of the committee and to make an accurate recording of the business that takes place. Chairpersons differ in the degree of formality they prefer; on the one hand they may insist that all the correct procedures and formalities are observed, such as raising the hand before being given permission to speak and addressing all comments through the chair. Alternatively, some chairpersons allow a degree of informality by letting discussion flow more spontaneously rather than insisting on each remark going through the chair. This can make the meeting less rigid and more interesting, but there is always the danger of total confusion if everyone tries to make a point at the same time.

A good sense of timing is crucial to the effective running of meetings; so often a great deal of time is spent on the first one or two items, leaving little time for the rest of the agenda. An effective chairperson will allocate a block of time for each substantive item, and should be prepared to move on, even if discussion is still proceeding. Some people may feel that this is undemocratic, yet it is no more undemocratic than allowing one item to dominate the agenda at the expense of all the others. One major facet of committees is the system of voting, in which members vote for or against a particular motion. This ensures a democratic system in which the majority decision carries the motion, but its use needs careful consideration. The chairperson needs to ensure that voting is reserved for crucial issues in which there is genuine division of opinion about the merits of a motion.

EXAMINATIONS AND ASSESSMENT

One of the most important aspects of the programme leader's role is the administration of examinations and assessment. S/he is responsible for a range of assessment-related issues, including drawing up results lists for boards of examiners in conjunction with the academic registry and the chair. This aspect is discussed in detail in Chapter 8, Assessment of Learning.

PREPARATION OF THE ANNUAL PROGRAMME MONITORING REPORT

The main formal mechanism for quality assurance of programmes is the annual programme monitoring report. This is prepared by the programme leader in consultation with the programme committee, and an example of typical aspects for inclusion is given in Table 10.9.

1. Cohort analysis and statistics on students, including admissions, progression, examinations and withdrawals
2. Overall view of the delivery of the programme, including an analysis of students' evaluations
3. Response to the external examiners' reports
4. Examples of good practice in teaching and assessments
5. Views of employers about the programme, where appropriate
6. Action plan for the next academic year, including identified personnel and timescale for implementation

Table 10.9

Typical aspects included in the annual programme monitoring report (AMR)

The annual monitoring report (AMR) goes to the faculty board, where issues raised by the report are discussed. Some institutions use a scrutineer system, in which a member of staff from another department in the faculty acts as a scrutineer of the report, offering the programme leader advice about aspects of the report. Subsequently, the scrutineer leads the discussion at faculty board about the monitoring report.

Annual programme monitoring is addressed further in Chapter 12.

REFERENCES

Atkins, A. and Katcher, A. (1996) *Strength Management, Strength Development: General Applications Workbook*, The LIFO Organization, Sherborne.
Fear, R. (1978) *The Evaluation Interview*, McGraw Hill, New York.
Kotter, J.P. (1990) *A Force for Change: How Leadership Differs from Management*, Free Press, New York.
McNay, I. (1998) *Organisation Culture, Leadership and the Role of the Senior Management Team in Universities*, Inaugural Lecture, University of Greenwich, London.
National Institute of Industrial Psychology (1970) *The Seven Point Plan*, NIP, London.
Ramsden, P. (1998) *Learning to Lead in Higher Education*, Routledge, London.
White, R. and Lippit, R. (1960) *Autocracy and Democracy*, Harper and Row, New York.

11 OPEN, DISTANCE AND FLEXIBLE LEARNING

The educational literature is replete with definitions of open, distance and flexible learning, but no consensus has yet emerged. To be fair, the terms are difficult to pin down because they have more than one meaning; for example, open learning is considered to be both an educational philosophy and a method of delivering teaching. However, it is useful for teachers to have an understanding of the similarities and differences between the terms, and the following section attempts to address these.

DEFINING OPEN, DISTANCE AND FLEXIBLE LEARNING

It is helpful to consider higher education as having four main modes of delivery, as shown in Figure 11.1.

Figure 11.1

Modes of delivery in higher education

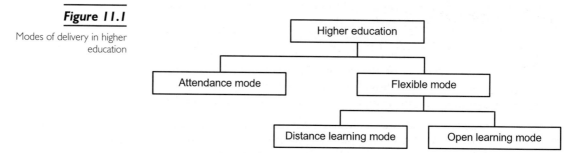

The left-hand box on the diagram shows the traditional delivery pattern in higher education, i.e. students attend the university for their teaching. The right-hand box shows the flexible mode of delivery, a broad category that includes both the distance learning mode and the open learning mode. Given the considerable degree of overlap between the three concepts, it may be helpful to identify the critical attributes that each must possess in order to warrant its title.

Distance learning

In order for a programme to count as distance learning, a significant proportion must be delivered on the basis of a wide geographical separation between the student and the teaching institution responsible for the programme. Distance is normally defined in terms of a student who is more than one hour's travelling time from the institution. Distance, however, is not the only critical attribute; distance learning is invariably delivered by means of text-based learning materials and information and communication technology (ICT), e.g. email, Internet, video, etc. The Quality Assurance Agency (QAA) defines distance learning as

> *'a mode of provision of higher' education that involves student learning resources being transferred to the student's location rather than the student moving to the location of the resources' (QAA, 1998).*

Open learning

In order for a programme to count as open learning, there must be a significant element of openness in comparison with traditional attendance programmes. By 'openness' we mean a minimum of restrictions on such things as students' access to programmes, the teaching and learning methods used, the assessment methods, the venue for study, and the timing of study. In reality, absolute openness does not exist; open learning programmes fall somewhere on a continuum, from more or less closed to more or less open. There will always be some kind of restrictions imposed upon students in higher education by virtue of validation requirements, quality assurance requirements, and other institutional imperatives.

Open learning as a philosophical stance

Open learning is also a philosophical stance, whose adherents espouse a range of beliefs about the educational process. Hull (1998) includes the following:

1. the centrality of student autonomy and self-direction;
2. focus on the process of learning rather than the content;
3. an emphasis on enquiry, reflection, evaluation and action;
4. student ownership of learning, assessment, and reflection processes;
5. the integration of theory and practice.

Open learning students normally study at a distance from their educational institution, and their studies utilize text-based learning materials and information and communication technology, e.g. email, internet, video, etc.

Flexible learning

Flexible learning is the most generic member of the triad of terms, as it covers any strategy that helps to reduce restrictions on students' learning opportunities. It therefore subsumes open learning and distance learning, since both these approaches confer a greater or lesser degree of flexibility upon programmes. Flexible learning also applies to methods used with traditional attendance mode programmes, such as the inclusion of resource materials for self directed study as part of a course.

Another way in which the term flexible learning is used, is to indicate programmes on which students can combine different modes of study; for example, some courses (modules) could be studied by attending classes at the university, and others by distance learning, using appropriate study materials. The English National Board for Nursing, Midwifery and Health Visiting (ENB) define flexible learning in post-registration nurse education as

> *'an approach which seeks to improve provision to achieve a number of explicit purposes which are concerned with access, availability, self-direction of the learners, relevance and meeting learners' needs and the needs of other stakeholders' (ENB, 1996).*

Relationship between open, distance and flexible learning

The relationship between distance learning, open learning and flexible learning is summarized in Table 11.1.

Table 11.1

Relationship between open, distance, and flexible learning

1. Open learning may involve learning at a distance, but this is not a requirement; attendance mode programmes may well have many characteristics of open learning.
2. Distance learning programmes may involve an open learning approach, but this is not a requirement; distance learning programmes may offer little or no opportunity for students to control aspects of their programme.
3. Both distance learning and open learning programmes come under the heading of flexible learning, as they offer opportunities for student control over elements of the programme.
4. Flexible learning may involve both distance learning and open learning, but this is not a requirement; attendance mode programmes may well have elements of flexibility within them.

THE CONTEXT OF OPEN, DISTANCE AND FLEXIBLE LEARNING

Although the origins of flexible learning can be traced as far back as the turn of the century in the work of writers such as John Dewey, the humanistic educational culture of the 1960s and 1970s provided the real thrust for its further development. The writings of Carl Rogers on client-centred therapy, and its corollary student-centred learning, emphasized the pre-eminence of student empowerment and autonomy, and these ideas found fertile soil in those educators wishing for a more humanistic approach to teaching and learning. During this period there was also a growing interest in the opening up of access to further and higher education using alternatives to traditional entry qualifications, and also flexible methods of delivery. The best known UK example of a mass, open access, distance learning scheme originating at this time is the Open University.

Race (1993) cites a number of reasons for the move towards flexible learning in higher education, including:

1. increasing competition between institutions;
2. greater availability of curriculum packages;
3. increasing class sizes;
4. greater numbers of mature and non-traditional entry students;
5. the perception that students in higher education are over-taught;
6. the need to foster students' ability to manage their own learning.

In addition to these general factors, the 1980s found nurse education experiencing severe resource constraints on continuing professional education, with employers placing limitations on the amount of funding available for attendance at courses, and reduced opportunities for study leave. The creation of the NHS internal market gave employers a much greater say in the kind of continuing education provision they required for their nursing staff, including more flexible approaches to course delivery.

DELIVERY SYSTEMS FOR OPEN, DISTANCE AND FLEXIBLE LEARNING

Open learning can be operated in a number of different ways and it is possible to identify four types of system currently in use in UK further and higher education (FEU/Open Tech, 1986):

1. *Flexible learning workshops*. In this system, students have access to learning materials within the institution, plus tutorial support as and when they need it. Thus, students can make appointments to visit the workshop, or simply drop in as required.
2. *Local systems*. Here the students are within reasonable travelling distance from the institution, and correspondence materials are supplemented by telephone communication and group seminars as required.
3. *Remote systems*. In the case of students who live at a significant distance from the institution, correspondence material is the main vehicle for tuition, but there may be residential blocks or weekends.
4. *Sub-contracting systems*. In this scheme, students are registered with the main provider institution, but can attend another institution that is close to their home for tutorial or other contact.

Flexible learning workshops

Flexible learning workshops allow students to drop in at a time convenient to them in order to study from specific learning resources, with the additional facility of tutorial guidance if required. Access to the learning workshop may constitute part of a student's normal timetable or simply be available for any learner when he or she happens to require its use. The notion of a learning workshop is different from the commonly encountered resource centre in that it offers more than simple access to learning materials. The tutorial backup needs a more sophisticated system of organization, with a nurse teacher designated as manager of the workshop; the role of the manager is to maintain records of the use of materials, to monitor the functioning of all aspects of the provision and to call upon the appropriate teaching staff to supplement students when required.

There are important differences in the role of workshop tutors from the everyday role of a nurse teacher. In a workshop, the tutor is engaged in a one-to-one role as facilitator and consultant and therefore needs the skills of negotiation and diagnosis to be effective in this role. The tutor must be able to use the learning materials available in the workshop, and effective management also involves the selection of materials for study. The manager needs to work closely with the library and media resources staff who can provide help with both the classification of materials and with one-to-one support of students.

Kelly and Keeley (1992) describe the development of a flexible learning unit (FLU) for continuing education in nursing using the concept of a 'drop-in centre', which is situated close to a nursing library. The centre offers information, resources and guidance, and the opportunity for personal contact with centre staff. The FLU uses only commercially-produced, off-the-shelf materials that have undergone rigorous testing.

Remote systems

One of the earliest UK examples of a national remote system is the Open University, which offers undergraduate and postgraduate programmes in a wide range of subject areas. There is also an element of sub-contracting within the Open University, with students having access to local educational institutions for tutorial, computing and other support.

Another example of a remote system is the Postgraduate Diploma in Higher Education programme offered by University of Greenwich School of Post Compulsory Education and Training. This programme of initial teacher training for nurse teachers is at master's degree level, and delivered by distance learning. This programme recruits students from across the UK.

Sub-contracting systems

The University of Greenwich School of Post Compulsory Education and Training is involved in one of the largest sub-contracting systems of flexible learning for nursing within the UK. This is the University of Greenwich/Macmillan Open Learning Scheme, a partnership between the university and Macmillan Publishers (now Emap Healthcare Open Learning) to provide academic awards for nurses and other health professionals. The programmes within the scheme are delivered by means of text-based open learning materials, and students receive support within a local university department of nursing. The scheme is discussed in detail later in this chapter.

Selecting, designing and writing materials for open, distance and flexible learning

The introduction of flexible learning into a course or programme can be done in three ways (Race, 1993):

1. by using existing materials that match the requirements, e.g. commercially-produced materials such as those from the Open University;

2. by adapting existing materials so that they match the requirements;
3. by writing new materials to the required specification.

There are clearly advantages and disadvantages with each of these approaches; the use of existing materials means that flexible learning can be introduced quickly, without the need for extensive materials development, but if such materials do not exactly meet the requirements of the course or programme, it may be better to adapt existing materials. The writing of new materials requires a major resource investment, including staff development costs, design and production costs, and copyright payments. There is also a considerable lead-in time before the materials are ready for use by students.

Selecting existing materials

A wide range of flexible learning materials is available within higher education and nursing. For example, the Open Learning Foundation (OLF) offers materials and services to help universities implement open learning. The OLF service includes the following:

1. provision of entire open learning programmes e.g. Diploma in Social Work (DipSW);
2. development of open learning packages for universities and other education and training organizations;
3. teaching and learning materials, and other publications;
4. advisory service to institutions.

The Open Learning Foundation also operates a nursing credit scheme to enable nurses to meet the UKCC PREP requirements, and the scheme is linked to a series of materials called Healthcare Active Learning. The web site address for the Open Learning Foundation is http://elgar.tvu.ac.uk/olf

Designing materials

The design of flexible learning materials will depend to some extent on their proposed use:

1. They may comprise the teaching and learning material for an entire programme of study.
2. They may be a sub-component of a programme, e.g. a single course (module) on health promotion.
3. They may be entirely free-standing and generic, i.e. not related to a specific programme of study. For example, a flexible learning package on intravenous drug administration.

Whilst there is no hard and fast rule about the design of flexible learning materials for each purpose, a useful rule of thumb is that materials for an entire course commonly follow the 'Reader and Study Guide' format, whereas those for a single element normally comprise the 'learning package' format.

Reader and study guide format

Most programmes of study in higher education are now modular in design, i.e. the components of the programme are broken down into discrete, self-contained units of learning. The 'Reader and Study Guide' format has two sets of flexible learning materials for each course (module), a Reader and a Study Guide.

Reader

The Reader can be thought of as the content of the course, i.e. what the teacher would normally teach in a classroom; hence, the Reader could contain extracts from the relevant literature and/or text written by the teacher. The text may be supplemented by pictures and other graphic material.

Study Guide

The Study Guide is a substitute for the teacher, in that it contains the kinds of learning activities that teachers would normally use in a classroom, e.g. questions, problem-solving exercises, analyses, etc. The Guide is designed to relate to each of the sections in the Reader, so that students are asked to study a particular section of the Reader, and are then required to carry out the appropriate activity in the Guide. Table 11.2 shows an example of a Study Guide activity that I designed for a distance learning programme for nurse teacher training at the University of Greenwich.

Table 11.2

Example of a study guide activity (University of Greenwich School of PCET)

Task 2.6: Learning Contracts
For the purpose of this task, you will be both student and teacher! This task will give you an idea of the relative difficulty of each stage of the contracting process, from the point of view of both student and teacher.
(a) Firstly, identify an area of teaching about which you would like to learn more (e.g. use of information technology; disruptive students, etc).
(b) Secondly, using Table 2.5 in the Reader, follow Knowles' stages in developing a learning contract as far as Step 5. (Steps 6 and 7 are about implementation, so you can omit these.)
Step 1.   Diagnose your learning needs for the area about which you would like to learn more
Step 2.   Write your learning objectives (outcomes)
Step 3.   Identify the learning resources and strategies you will use
Step 4.   State the evidence that will demonstrate your achievement of the learning outcomes
Step 5.   State the criteria by which the evidence will be judged

Some authors like to follow the activities with a commentary, so that the student gets a basis for comparison between her/his response and that of the author. However, this may render the activity meaningless, as students may simply read the author's commentary rather than carrying out the activity for themselves.

The 'Learning Package' format

This format is commonly used for self-contained units of learning, and whilst there is no specific formula for writing a learning package, there are some points which can be helpful in clarifying the process. A learning package typically consists of a number of components

Rationale	This consists of an introductory statement describing the package and its purpose. It provides an overview of the type of material to be studied and the reasons for each study.
Target population	This identifies the level of programme, or level of experience at which the package will be most suitable. For example, the package may have been designed as a module on the Adult Branch of a DipHE Registered Nurse course, or it may be a component of a master's degree in nursing.
Prerequisite	If successful completion of the package is dependent on the learner having already achieved certain knowledge or skills, then this knowledge or skill is termed a prerequisite for the learning package. For example, a prerequisite for many nursing subjects will be a knowledge of normal structure and function.
Learning outcomes	If the package is linked to a particular module or unit of study, then the learning outcomes will be derived from this. If the package is generic and free-standing, then appropriate learning outcomes will need to be formulated for the package.
Choice of learning activities	If individuals differ in their learning styles, then it is logical to include more than one form of activity by which the learner may achieve the objectives. Activities such as reading, writing, listening, looking and doing should provide sufficient variety in one package to suit the needs of most individuals, who can then select the medium by which they learn best. Further variety can be introduced by the use of different media within these activities, for example the use of video and the Internet.
Optional activities beyond the package	Optional activities may be presented to the learner to enrich the learning experience, but which are outside the confines of the learning package. For example, one suggested activity from a package on 'Nursing the patient with a myocardial infarction' might be that the learner should take the opportunity to visit a patient who has suffered an attack and to discuss with the patient how the condition has affected him or her as a person. It is important that the package contains information about obtaining the necessary permissions to undertake the activity.
Tests	The tests provide feedback to the learner and also serve as a diagnostic tool. They can be divided into three types. (a) Prerequisite test. This tests the prerequisite knowledge that the learner must possess before commencing the package. (b) Pre-test. This tests the actual content of the package to determine whether or not the learner needs to proceed through the package. If the pre-test is completed successfully, the implication is that the learner already knows the content of the package and can proceed to a higher level of study immediately. (c) Post-test. This is used to test the learner's achievement of the objective following completion of the learning package. The post-test is very commonly used as a pre-test, the learner initially attempting the test without success and then retaking it after completion of the package. The learner is usually successful the second time and this provides feelings of accomplishment from having visibly learned to pass the test.
Guidance concerning the next step	Successful completion of the learning package should not be the final step; instead, the learner should be directed to the next component in the series, or given advice on the type of learning activities that they should now pursue.
Teacher's notes	A learning package should contain notes intended for the teacher. It may seem unusual to include these, but one must bear in mind that the intentions of the designer may not always be obvious to a teacher who has not been involved in the production. Such notes might contain details of the feedback received during the pilot study and guidelines for the interpretation of test scores.

organized in a logical sequence to help students achieve particular learning goals, and is shown in Table 11.3.

The list of components given in Table 11.3 can be considered as a basic list of 'ingredients' for a learning package, so it is useful to examine the 'recipe' for putting these components together. The decision to produce a learning package will commit the institution to a considerable amount of time and effort and if this expenditure is to reap its benefits, careful planning must be employed from the outset. Table 11.4 illustrates a planning sequence for producing an individualized

Table 11.3

Typical components of a flexible learning package

287

Table 11.4

Planning sequence for producing a
flexible learning package

Explore the need	Does a similar package exist already? Is a learning package an appropriate medium?
Explore the feasibility of developing a package	Is the development feasible in terms of finance, personnel, resources and time?
Decide the target population	Pre-registration, post-registration or both? CATS level?
Decide the learning outcomes	Are they already prescribed in the programme document, or do they have to be formulated specifically for the package?
Identify pre-requisites and co-requisites	Are there other packages/materials/units that should be studied first, or studied in conjunction with the package?
Decide the activities and media for the package	Reading? Writing? Information and communication technology? Experiential? Sequencing? Instructions?
Decide any optional activities	For example, interviews with patients/clients/staff in relation to the theme of the package
Write the rationale for the package	Write a description of the purpose and structure of package.
Decide format of pre-test and post-test if used	Teacher or student marked? Where will the answers be found?
Decide format of self-tests	How will student monitor his or her own progress through the package?
Decide content of teacher notes	Write any additional information that teachers might require, e.g. the theoretical assumptions underpinning the approach taken in the package.
Decide format of students' evaluation of the package	How will the user's opinion of the package be solicited?
Decide the contents list	Outline the sequence of content but omit page numbers until final draft completed.
Set production deadlines	Realistic, achievable deadlines, including time for any slippage, are needed.
Undertake draft production	Use Desktop Publishing (DTP) if available.
Undertake pilot study	Use a sample of the intended consumers, and obtain detailed feedback on all aspects of the package.
Modify draft package in light of feedback from pilot study	Note 'user-friendliness', clarity, interest and accuracy.
Produce final draft	(a) Text: DTP gives professional finish. Type of cover? Quality of binding? Size of print run? Copyright? (b) Information and communication technology media: include instructions to user on how to operate the media.
Put package into full use	Include system of monitoring students' use of package, plus evaluation by users.

learning package. This sequence follows a logical order of progression, with each stage designed to eliminate errors and omissions.

Writing the materials

The foregoing discussion on designing flexible learning materials seems to make the assumption that teachers can simply sit down and write materials for public consumption. This is very far from being the case;

effective authoring of materials requires considerable staff development, and even then some teachers may simply not have the necessary skills to write effectively for this medium. It can be an advantage, when writing flexible learning materials, to have had experience of publishing books or journal papers, because the writer will have been exposed to external criticism as part of the publishing process. Experience of writing books and articles, however, does not necessarily mean that the same style will be appropriate for flexible learning materials, as the target audience is quite different. Race (1989, 1993) offers some useful tips for writers, as shown in Table 11.5.

Table 11.5

Tips for writers (Race, 1989, 1993)

1. Write in a user-friendly way, i.e. address the students as 'you', and use 'I' for the author
2. Leave sufficient white space in the materials for the students to write their notes and comments
3. Include questions and answers, so that students' responses will highlight lack of understanding or errors quickly
4. Use headings and sub-headings to act as signposts for the students
5. Use short words and sentences rather than long ones
6. Include summaries, reviews and self-assessments
7. Use illustrations to help maintain interest and foster understanding
8. Use visual symbols (flags) to indicate activities such as a pause for reflection, or a tea-break

THE ROLE OF THE TUTOR IN OPEN, DISTANCE AND FLEXIBLE LEARNING

The skills required in tutoring students on flexible learning programmes encompass the generic tutoring skills discussed in Chapter 15 on tutoring and counselling. However, the nature of flexible learning is such that tutors' interaction with students on a face-to-face basis may occur infrequently, so alternative approaches to tutoring need to be developed.

Tutoring at a distance

Depending upon the nature of the programme of study, distance learning students may meet their tutors on a face-to-face basis every three or four weeks, or as infrequently as once or twice per semester. In either case, the main form of communication will be the telephone and postal service, or electronic forms such as fax and email. The additional roles of the tutor in relation to distance learning students include those described below.

Establishing initial contact with students

It is good practice to send out to students a personal letter of welcome, containing some background details about the tutor, and also the arrangements for contacting the tutor. An example of contact details is given in Table 11.6.

Maintaining regular contact

It is very important that tutors maintain frequent contact with distance

Table 11.6

Example of contact details for
distance learning students

ARRANGEMENTS FOR TUTORIAL CONTACT

Address
Michael Henchard
University of Casterbridge
City Campus
CASTERBRIDGE
Wessex CA3 5TH

Telephone and fax   01234 77777

email   M.Henchard@ucb.ac.uk

Ground rules for contacting me
(i)   You should feel free to telephone me at any time within the published term dates, including
      evenings and weekends. (N.B. During vacation periods I am required to fulfil my contractual
      obligations with regard to research and scholarly activity, and am therefore not contactable
      outside term time.)
(ii) Depending upon my availability, the following options will apply:
                      I will answer the telephone and speak to you
                                              or
                      The answering machine will invite you to leave a voice or fax message.
(iii) If you leave a message, I will endeavour to get back to you within 24 hours. This may not
      always be possible, however, depending upon professional and personal commitments
      pertaining at the time, although there should never be a long delay in my response to you.

If you have access to a fax machine you may prefer me to fax my communications to you.
Please let me have the fax number if you think this would be a useful method. The same applies
to email; if you have a convenient email address, let me have it and I will contact you via this.

students, as the latter's motivation can quickly fade if they feel isolated
and out of touch with their programme. Contact is likely to involve
postal, telephone and/or electronic forms of communication; my own
preference is for a combination of telephone and postal communications. It is helpful for students to have some communications in a
permanent form, so that they can be referred to again and again. I use a
series of postal communications in the form of 'Quinfomation' sheets
that highlight key aspects of the programme, such as tips on assessments, arrangements for teaching practice assessment visits, etc. This
paper communication is supplemented by telephone calls from time to
time to enquire about students' progress, and to offer advice on assessments, etc.

Facilitating student networking
One of the disadvantages of distance learning is that students may
feel isolated and alone, so it is important that the tutor encourages
students to network with each other. This can be done simply by
contacting each student to seek permission to circulate their contact
details to other students in the tutorial group. Student should be asked
to indicate whether or not they are happy to have their home contact
details circulated, or whether they prefer their work details to be circulated.

Openness versus emptiness
One of the common issues raised by tutors on open and distance

learning programmes concerns those students who make no attempt to respond to communications from their tutor once they have registered onto the programme. One viewpoint is that tutors are resources for the student, and if the student chooses not to use them, that is perfectly acceptable; in this case the student could simply enrol on the programme, and then submit the assessment at the end, with no communication in-between. This viewpoint seems to be compatible with an adult learning philosophy, in which the students are considered self-directing adults responsible for their own learning.

I would like to offer an alternative viewpoint. I believe there is a world of difference between encouraging student autonomy and self-direction, and simply letting the student decide if and when they will communicate with the tutor. In a flexible learning programme, it is the student's responsibility to demonstrate to the tutor that they are under-going the process of learning, including critical reflection and analysis of issues and experiences. This requires a certain amount of communication with the tutor in order to monitor the student's progress through this process. Indeed, one of the terms of reference of a programme committee is the monitoring of student progress, and this cannot be fulfilled without a certain amount of interaction between student and tutor.

My own opinion is that it is unacceptable for flexible learning students to simply register for a unit of study and then to have no further contact with the institution until they submit an assessment for marking. Even if the students feel they require no tutorial help with their studies, the tutor will require evidence of engagement with the materials and the literature, and of reflection upon these. The tutor is also required to challenge students' assumptions and conclusions, thus facilitating the development of the latter's critical abilities.

Computer-mediated tutoring

One of the most recent innovations in tutoring distance students is computer-mediated tutoring, which is defined as:

> *'the use of computers, telephone lines and specialist software to facilitate interaction between students and tutors irrespective of geographical location or time zone' (Ryan, 1996).*

This system uses Lotus Notes software to offer both electronic mail and conferencing databases; email can be used for one-to-one messages and questions, or for one-to-many notices and information. Computer conferencing allows students and tutors to discuss issues in a 'virtual group', but does not take place in real-time. Hence, a tutor may initiate activities or ideas onto the server, and the students in the virtual group can respond at any time of the day or night. Students and tutor may initiate and respond to each others' inputs just like a live seminar, but with the advantage of not having to be in the same place at the same time.

MANAGING OPEN, DISTANCE AND FLEXIBLE LEARNING

Flexible learning programmes requires specific management structures to ensure the quality of materials and the quality of programme delivery. The English National Board for Nursing, Midwifery and Health Visiting identify 21 core performance indicators (PIs) for effective management of flexible learning, covering three dimensions: preconditions, process and outcomes (ENB, 1996). The following structures are based upon my experience with flexible learning programmes.

Editorial board

An editorial board is an essential component of the management structure, and membership would normally consist of the flexible learning manager, the materials editor, the design and layout technician, and representatives of authors. The editorial board is responsible for the commissioning, production scheduling, and review process; commissioning may be done on the basis of payment to the author for the writing, or by including the writing as part of the teacher's normal timetable commitments. It is important that the editorial board maintains oversight of the production schedule, so that action can be taken if there is slippage of deadlines. One of the major quality assurance aspects of the editorial board is organizing the critical review process for materials.

Critical reading of materials

It is essential that all flexible learning materials are exposed to critical reading before the final draft is published. Critical readers should be sought both internally and externally, and should consist of both teachers and students so that the materials are criticized from both perspectives. A guide should be issued so that critical readers have a framework to which they write their critique, and resources need to be made available to pay for the critical reader's services.

Flexible learning administrator

Appropriate skilled administrative support is required to operate distance learning programmes, and this work best if the administrator role is a dedicated one solely to the flexible learning operation. The administrator is responsible for mailing of all flexible learning materials, for liaison with the academic registry over issues relating to flexible learning students, and in conjunction with the appropriate programme leader, organizing the receipt, marking and moderation of students' assessment work.

Structures for flexible learning on a sub-contracting basis

It is relatively common within higher education to find that flexible learning is delivered via a system of sub-contracting with other educational institutions. These partner institutions offer tutorial support, library and information and communication technology support, and provide a venue for students to meet from time to time. In this system, the following management structures are required.

Partnership liaison tutor

For flexible learning systems that operate on a sub-contracting basis, it is necessary to have an academic member of staff who is responsible for liaison with the partner institutions who provide tutoring and other support for students. This individual would visit each partner institution on a regular basis to monitor the quality of support provided for flexible learning students, and to offer advice and staff development to tutors within the partner institution.

Administrative manual

Communication between the parent institution and its partners is of paramount importance for maintaining the quality of the student experience. An administrative manual sets out all the procedures in relation to student support and documentation, and provides a basis for monitoring of the partner organizations.

Staffing issues

If the students' experience of flexible learning is to be a quality experience, it requires motivated, committed, and above all, flexible tutors. The staffing of such programmes raises issues not encountered within traditional attendance mode programmes.

Tutor availability outside the working day

One of the most sensitive staffing issues in relation to flexible learning is the availability of tutors outside the normal working day. The majority of students undertake flexible learning programmes because they are fully committed to their employment during the working day. There is therefore little point in offering a tutorial service between the hours of 09.00 and 17.00, rather, the students will want tutorial contact in the evenings or at weekends. To operate such a system requires a fundamental rethink of tutorial staff timetables if overloading is to be avoided. Ideally, flexible learning tutors should deal exclusively with such programmes, to avoid clashes between teaching times on attendance mode courses.

Tutors working from home

One way of facilitating tutorials for these programmes is to consider a system whereby tutors can use their home as their main work-base. It is relatively easy for staff to be linked electronically to the University via telephone, fax and computer, and this would enable tutors to offer an out-of-hours service to students without having to stay late at work. Some tutors may be happy to offer an evening and weekend service as an alternative to travelling to work every day, but there is the danger that they could end up working a full day at the institution, and then being available out of hours for distance students. There is a growing movement in society towards a working-from-home culture, but some employers feel uneasy about this development, given that employees have to be trusted to do their work without the direct supervision normally available in an institutional setting.

Meeting with students at home

In some systems, tutors of flexible learning students arrange individual and group tutorials in their own homes, as this is much more convenient for evening and weekend meetings, particularly if the tutor lives at some distance from the institution. Whilst this can be a very useful approach, tutors need to be aware of some of the drawbacks; once students are aware of the location of a tutor's home, tutors may be subjected to students 'dropping-in' without appointments. They may also be open to accusations by students of improper behaviour, and whilst this applies also to attendance mode programmes, a defence may be more difficult if these are alleged to have occurred in the tutor's own home.

Roll-on, roll-off programmes

Another operational implication is that of access to flexible learning programmes. Since flexible provision means that educational provision is available when the student wants it, entry to programmes is commonly on a continuous 'roll-on roll-off' basis, and this presents a challenge to institutional systems, e.g. the scheduling of examination boards, and the tracking of students.

Cost implications

The cost of development and production of flexible learning materials should not be underestimated; an editorial board is required, writers need to be commissioned; decisions about design and quality of the materials will influence cost, critical readers need to be commissioned, permissions to reproduce copyright materials that will be scanned into texts needs to be obtained; materials need to be piloted, all of which have very substantial cost implications. Materials will not remain up-to-date forever, and so review and updating will need to be scheduled every three to five years depending upon the nature of the materials. There are also costs involved in the necessary staff development for flexible learning tutors.

On the other side of the equation, there are potential savings to be made from the implementation of flexible learning. The following are examples of such savings:

1. Savings can be made on the use of paper materials by downloading the units onto the students' computers.
2. In comparison with attendance mode courses, flexible learning does not require classroom space nor is there a need for face-to-face class contact between teachers and students, both of which consume considerable resources.
3. By freeing up the tutors from heavy class contact, there may be

more time available for staff to undertake research, an increasingly important issue in the light of the research assessment exercise.

4. The use of high-quality textual and computer material can be a far more effective learning strategy than poorly-delivered lectures, and from a quality assurance point of view are much more open to public scrutiny than the latter.

QUALITY ASSURANCE ISSUES IN OPEN, DISTANCE AND FLEXIBLE LEARNING

Quality assurance is a crucial aspect of open, distance and flexible learning, particularly as it commonly takes place at a distance from the main institution. The Quality Assurance Agency for Higher Education (QAA, 1998) offers guidelines on quality assurance of distance learning, under five main headings:

1. programme design and approval;
2. programme management for assurance of quality;
3. delivery systems;
4. learner support;
5. student assessment and the maintenance of academic standards.

There are a number of quality issues that cause particular difficulties on distance learning programmes, including the following issues.

Library and CIT support

Student access to library and CIT support facilities is an important aspect for distance learning, since the flexible learning materials need to be supplemented by further reading and inquiry. Whilst the main providing institution can easily monitor the quality of its own libraries, it is more difficult when partner institutions' library provision has to be evaluated.

Student peer support

Open learning can be a lonely experience for distance learning students, so it is important that networking is set up to help them interact with their peers on the same programme.

Use of locally-based tutors

Institutions often employ associate tutors who live within the student' locality, so as to facilitate tutoring, but this can present difficulties in ensuring that they maintain good communication with the institution, and also with attendance at staff development activities.

CASE-STUDY: THE UNIVERSITY OF GREENWICH/MACMILLAN OPEN LEARNING SCHEME

The following case study is offered as a real example of a flexible learning programme for nurses, operated on a sub-contracting basis at a

Table 12.5

Categories of FIAC

Teacher talk	Indirect influence	1.	Accepts feeling: accepts and clarifies the feeling tone of the students in a non-threatening manner. Feelings may be positive or negative. Predicting and recalling feelings are included
		2.	Praises or encourages: praises or encourages student action or behaviour. Jokes that release tension, not at the expense of another individual, nodding head or saying 'uh huh'?' or 'go on' are included
		3.	Accepts or uses ideas of student: clarifying, building, or developing ideas or suggestions by a student. As teacher brings more of his or her own ideas into play, shift to category five
		4.	Asks questions: asking a question about content or procedure with the intent that a student answer.
	Direct influence	5.	Lectures: giving facts or opinions about content or procedure; expressing own ideas; asking rhetorical questions
		6.	Gives directions: directions, commands, or orders with which a student is expected to comply
		7.	Criticizes or justifies authority: statements intended to change student behaviour from non-acceptable to acceptable pattern; bawling someone out; stating why the teacher is doing what he or she is doing, extreme self-reference
Student talk		8.	Student talk-response: talk by students in response to teacher. Teacher initiates the contact or solicits student statement
		9.	Student talk-initiation: talk by students, which they initiate. If 'calling on' student is only to indicate who may talk next, observer must decide whether student wanted to talk. If he or she did, use this category
		10.	Silence or confusion: pauses, short periods of silence, and periods of confusion in which communication cannot be understood by the observer

1970). The observer has been trained to use the ten categories in Flanders system and these are shown in Table 12.5.

There are eight categories for teacher talk and only two for student talk and the underlying philosophy is that the better teachers use a more indirect influence.

When the lesson begins the observer starts recording the teacher and student behaviours on an analysis sheet, entering a tick in the appropriate category every three seconds, according to who is speaking and in what category. At the end of the lesson the data is analysed to show the interaction patterns during the session and a whole range of ratios can be calculated. One of the great drawbacks is that so much of the richness of the classroom is lost during the process of reduction into categories. In addition, it has been argued that the categories are too over-inclusive. For example, the category for teacher questions does not distinguish between the type and level of question.

Another problem is that the schedule contains only two pupil categories, which puts the emphasis very much on the teacher talk; this approach has been criticized by some commentators, as it overlooks the importance of pupil talk as a classroom variable.

The use of FIAC is really only suitable for the classical type of lesson in which the teacher talks at the class from the front; it is not readily adaptable for group work. In addition, in order to make the findings reliable, observers have to undergo training in the use of categories and this may impose artificial constraints on their perceptions.

The underlying philosophy of FIAC is that of the direct versus the indirect style of teaching; the former implying authoritarian ways and the latter much more freedom and choice.

Many may not agree with these categories, since Flanders equates direct with 'bad' and indirect with 'good' teaching style!

Ethnographic (participant) observation of teaching

An alternative observation strategy is that called 'ethnographic' or 'participant' observation; in this system the observer or researcher attempts to see things from the point of view of the students by involving themselves in whatever is happening in the classroom. The observer can ask questions, observe events, listen and so on, the idea being that more of the richness of the classroom environment can be captured. This is obviously a much more qualitative evaluation as opposed to quantitative.

Distinguished teaching awards

Thomas (1993) describes the introduction of the first UK distinguished teaching award in the University of Ulster. Nominations are sought from students, former students or academic staff, with self-nomination being precluded. Nominators have to rate their nominee on seven criteria, using a scale of 1–5. All full-time teaching staff who have a minimum of three years' service are eligible for the award, and nominations are considered by a selection panel consisting of representatives of the senate, the students and the convocation. The seven criteria are:

1. communicates subject matter effectively;
2. provides regular and useful feedback on students' course work;
3. communicates an enthusiastic interest in the field of study;
4. stimulates thinking and develops understanding;
5. challenges the students' intellect;
6. uses methods of assessment that reflect the students' understanding of relevant course material;
7. takes a personal interest in students and is willing to help.

QUALITY OF STAFF DEVELOPMENT

It is generally acknowledged that one of the major factors determining the quality of education is the quality of the staff delivering the programme.

Given the constantly changing nature of subject areas and education, it is imperative that staff continue to build upon and develop the knowledge and skills acquired during their initial teacher training.

Continuing professional development (CPD) is currently the favoured term, and has appeared in a number of different guises over the years, including staff development, continuing education, professional development, and lifelong learning. Regardless of the term used, the aim is to ensure that the knowledge and skills of the lecturer are kept up to date and remain relevant, both in terms of her subject and also her educational expertise. Awareness of the importance of CPD has received a significant boost recently with the publication of several significant reports and documents relating to it.

The Fryer Report

The Fryer Report (DfEE, 1997) spells out a ten-point agenda for lifelong learning in society, and the Government response is contained in a green paper The Learning Age: A Renaissance for a New Britain (DfEE, 1998a). Whilst no direct reference is made within the green paper to continuing professional development, the Government acknowledges the Fryer Report's call for the development of a new culture of lifelong learning, and identifies the benefits for individuals, businesses, communities, and the nation.

The Dearing Report

The terms of reference of the Dearing Report (Dearing, 1997) were:

> *'To make recommendations on how the purposes, shape, structure, size and funding of higher education, including support for students, should develop to meet the needs of the United Kingdom over the next 20 years, recognizing that higher education embraces teaching, learning, scholarship and research.'*

Recommendations 9, 13, 14, 15, 47 and 48 refer specifically to staff development, and three main aspects are covered:

1. the need for institutions to review, update and make available to all staff their policies with regard to staff development;
2. the need for institutions to review the impact of communications and information technology on the role of staff, and ensure that the necessary support and training is made available;
3. that an Institute for Learning and Teaching in Higher Education (ILT) be established for the purpose of accrediting programmes of teacher-training, the commissioning of research into teaching and learning, and the encouragement of innovation. All new full-time academic staff should undertake ILT-accredited teacher-training as part of their probationary period of employment.

Government response to the Dearing Report

In February 1998 the Government published its response to the Dearing Report, Higher Education for the 21st Century. Response to the Dearing Report (DfEE, 1998b).

The Government welcomed the recommendations on the need for

institutions to review and update their staff development policies, and to make these available to staff, and encouraged institutions to follow-up these recommendations. They also welcomed the recommendations on the need for training and support of both staff and students in communications and information technology, and identified the importance of the Institute for Learning and Teaching (ILT) in the kite-marking and development of these materials. With regard to the recommendations concerning the ILT, the Government stated that the Institute would be established by September 1998; its functions should be the accreditation of programmes of training for HE teachers, the commissioning of research and development into effective teaching and learning practice, and to stimulate innovation. The Government also considers that one way of improving the quality of teaching is to make available examples of outstanding teaching, on film, video or by broadcasting, and will invite the ILT to consider setting up a national system for this.

The ILT is discussed in detail later in this chapter (p. 324).

Teacher-training for higher education

The issue of accredited teacher-training was also welcomed:

'The Government's long-term aim is to see all teachers in higher education carry a professional qualification, achieved by meeting demanding standards of teaching and supervisory competence through accredited learning or experience.'

This aim was welcomed by many people inside and outside the higher education sector. Indeed, most members of the public would have been unaware of the fact that higher education lecturers can be employed as teachers without possessing a teaching qualification. However, some higher education institutions already require all newly-appointed lecturers to undergo teacher training as a condition of employment, the most common routes being a postgraduate certificate in education, or a postgraduate diploma. It is interesting to note that in this area, nurse education is leading the way; the UKCC has always required teachers of nurses to hold a recognized teaching qualification.

QUALITY ASSURANCE AT PROGRAMME LEVEL

Higher education is delivered via programmes or courses leading to academic awards, with each programme having a programme team responsible for its day-to-day operational management. Whilst team members are responsible for the quality of their own teaching on the programme, the team has collective responsibility for the quality of the programme curriculum.

Quality of curriculum

The first check on the quality of curriculum occurs at the validation event for the programme, and continues in the form of programme

Figure 12.1

Components of curriculum

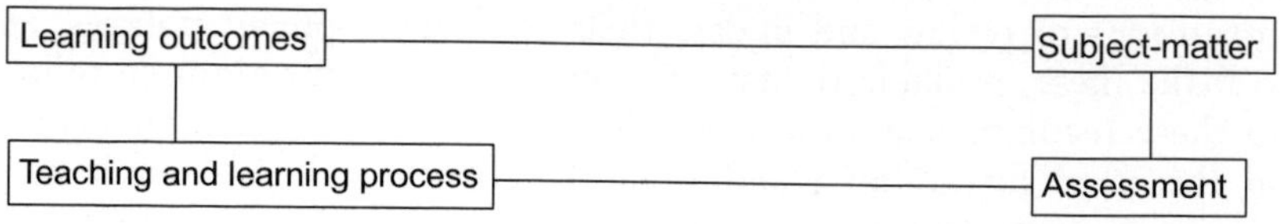

```
┌──────────────────┐                                    ┌──────────────┐
│ Learning outcomes │───────────────────────────────────│ Subject-matter│
└──────────────────┘                                    └──────────────┘
        │                                                       │
┌───────────────────────────────┐                      ┌──────────────┐
│ Teaching and learning process  │──────────────────────│ Assessment   │
└───────────────────────────────┘                      └──────────────┘
```

monitoring and programme review. The term curriculum encompasses four main aspects of educational provision, as shown in Figure 12.1. These four components are intimately related to each other and the model adopts a rational stance, in that the curriculum design is seen to begin with the formulating of student learning outcomes, and then progresses to decisions about what outcomes-related subject-matter should be included. Teaching and learning processes are then defined, e.g. lectures, laboratory work, etc. that will help the student to achieve the learning outcomes, and finally, the students' achievement of the learning outcomes is assessed using appropriate and relevant assessment methods.

Ashworth and Harvey (1994) offer the following criteria for a quality curriculum:

1. *Relevance*, relates to present and anticipated future needs;
2. *Aims and objectives*, explicit and carefully focused;
3. *Time constraints*, effective use of time for individual subjects and their arrangements;
4. *Content*, a body of knowledge which offers breadth and depth and is state of the art and well-balanced;
5. *Progression*, cumulative knowledge and skills which allows for planned progression;
6. *Sequencing*, coherent sequencing of subjects and subject matter;
7. *Integration*, different aspects of the curriculum allow for integrated working;
8. *Core skills*, relevant balance of all core skills;
9. *Accreditation*, appropriate accreditation of the programme from professional bodies, other colleges, NVQ, etc.

Programme evaluation

Programme evaluation needs to be distinguished from evaluation of teaching, the latter being just one component of the former. Although evaluation of teaching contributes useful information it is insufficient in itself as an indicator of course quality, since it does not cover other aspects such as organization and resources. Overall course evaluation is particularly important in credit schemes, where pathways consist of many units. In this case, unit evaluation will not provide evidence of the overall aspects of the pathway, so provision needs to be made for this before students leave the pathway. Institutions may have a standard format for course evaluation forms, or they can be designed specifically for the course in question. Table 12.6 shows an example of a course evaluation questionnaire specifically designed for a stress management course for GP referrals.

Table 12.6

Example of a programme evaluation from a stress management course for GP referrals

Dear Participant,

EVALUATION OF STRESS MANAGEMENT PROGRAMME

As the leader of the Stress Management Programme you have just completed, I would be very interested to know your opinion of the programme. This questionnaire is designed to evaluate the programme, and I would be most grateful if you could kindly take ten minutes or so to complete it, and to return it to me at the Health Centre in the envelope provided.

1. How adequate was the pre-course information?
2. How satisfied were you with the venue used for the programme?
3. How well-suited to your lifestyle was the time of day for the programme?
4. What are your feelings about the length of each session?
5. What did you feel about the social interactions within the group of participants on the programme?
6. What did you think about the overall standard of teaching on the programme?
7. What did you feel about the manner and approachability of the programme leader?
8. What did you think about the way in which the information was explained?
9. What did you feel about the exercises and activities you participated in?
10. How useful do you think the programme has been in reducing your level of stress?
11. Have you any suggestions about how the programme could be made more effective?

Thank you very much indeed for taking the time to complete this questionnaire.

Student evaluation of the curriculum

Evaluation of the programme curriculum by students is now established throughout the higher education sector, and forms an important aspect of educational quality assurance. Given that students are the most obvious consumers of higher education, it seems axiomatic that their opinions about the quality of their modules, units and programmes should be given serious consideration by the institution.

When designing student evaluation forms, institutions need to decide the breadth and scope of coverage; some institutions focus mainly on the quality of the teaching, whereas others include such aspects as the quality of pre-entry information, induction, tutorial support, etc.

The student satisfaction approach

The student satisfaction approach (SSA) to evaluation was developed by the University of Central England, and is a quality enhancement tool designed to improve the quality of the student learning experience (Harvey, 1999). The student satisfaction approach involves an institutional survey of students, and the approach claims to have a number of unique features:

1. students determine the questions in the questionnaire, via feedback from focus-groups;
2. focus is on the total learning experience of the students;
3. student satisfaction ratings are linked to importance ratings;
4. data is transformed into management information for action.

The survey is carried out on an annual cycle, and consists of four elements:

1. obtaining student views on which to base the questionnaire;
2. surveying a large sample of students;

3. producing a report that identifies areas for management inter-vention;
4. consultation to initiate action in response to student concerns and closing the loop by providing feedback of outcomes to students.

Quality of student assessment

Of all the aspects of the higher education curriculum, assessment is the area that is subject to the most rigorous quality assurance mechanisms. Whilst some of these mechanisms operate on an institution level, others operate at programme team level, hence the inclusion of the quality of assessment in this section. The Higher Education Quality Council (1996) offers the following principles in relation to the quality of student assessment.

1. Institutions should ensure that assessment rules, regulations and criteria are published in a full and accessible form and made freely available to students, staff and external examiners.
2. Assessment practices should be fair, valid, reliable and appropriate to the level of award being offered. Assessment should be under-taken only by appropriately qualified staff, who have been adequately trained and briefed, and given regular opportunities to update and enhance their expertise as assessors.
3. Boards of examiners and assessment panels have an important role in overseeing assessment practices and maintaining standards, and institutions should develop policies and procedures governing the structure, operation and timing of their boards/panels.
4. Institutions should have in place policies and procedures to deal thoroughly, fairly and expeditiously with problems which arise in the course of assessment of students. These should define the actions to be taken in the event of academic misconduct, and the grounds for student appeals against assessment outcomes.

Role of the external examiner in assuring the quality of assessment

The external examiner system plays a key role in educational quality assurance by bringing in an external, objective perspective to the assessment system. The role involves scrutiny of students' assessment work to ascertain if the standards are comparable with students on similar courses throughout higher education. In addition, the external examiner can comment on the consistency and standard of internal marking, and make suggestions for improvements to the assessment system. The role of the external examiner is discussed in detail in Chapter 8 (p. 243)

Ensuring quality of practice-based assessment

It is interesting to note that the rigour applied to ensuring the quality of written assessments is not nearly so apparent in the case of practice-based assessments in nursing. Assessment of practice is based upon observation of students in the workplace, and is largely the responsi-bility of qualified nurses based in the practice setting to which the student is allocated. Unlike written assessments, which constitute a single episode, practical assessment is a continuous process throughout the placement. The decision on whether to pass or fail a student will therefore be made on the basis of her/his overall progress during the placement.

Moderation of written work is based on the principle of sampling, i.e. the students' written work is only a sample of their knowledge, whereas practical assessment attempts to assess the total performance of the student during the placement. This suggests that the assessment of theory is based upon a different paradigm from that of practical assessment, the latter being more like staff appraisal than assessment per se. A moderator or external examiner cannot scrutinize the students' performance, nor moderate the assessor's judgement, because the assessment process has taken place over a period of several weeks. It is therefore very unusual to find that an external examiner has had any involvement in the practical assessment of student nurses, apart from scrutinizing the students' portfolio, and the assessment documentation produced by the assessor.

QUALITY ASSURANCE AT INSTITUTION LEVEL

So far in this chapter we have examined the role of the individual lecturer and the programme team in quality assurance. We now turn our attention to the institution's overall quality assurance system that impacts on all aspects of the work of the institution.

Aims, characteristics and spectrum of institutional quality assurance

It is essential that all the staff of the institution have a clear understanding of the quality assurance system, so this information should be available in the form of a quality assurance handbook or manual. This should include a statement of the aims and characteristics of the quality assurance system, and an example of these is given in Table 12.7.

In order to quality assure the totality of the educational experience of its students , the institution's quality assurance system must cover all aspects of its work, and not just the educational programmes. Table 12.8 illustrates the spectrum of institutional quality assurance, under the headings inputs, processes and outcomes. These can form the basis for the development of performance indicators, allowing comparison with other higher education institutions.

Programme validation, monitoring and review

There are three closely-related concepts involved in the quality assurance of programmes and courses, i.e. programme validation, programme monitoring and programme review.

1. Programme validation is the process by which a proposal for a new course or programme is examined to assess its suitability for inclusion in the institution's portfolio.

Table 12.7

Aims of a university's quality assurance system (University of Greenwich, 1999a)

Aims
Ensure that students have an appropriate academic experience
Assure the quality and standards of awards in principle and in delivery
Promote and enhance quality and stimulate curriculum development by requiring staff to evaluate their courses and programmes through the process of peer review

Characteristics
Rigorous, collaborative and developmental
Has the flexibility to meet the needs of the full range of awards in different stages of development, of different levels and lengths, and in different modes
Involves a wide range of appropriate staff within the University, and allows for the development of other staff
Promotes open, critical but not confrontational dialogue between teaching teams and those with formal responsibility for quality assurance
Enables a view to be formed of the health of the academic development, whether current or proposed
Facilitates maximum flexibility in the structure and organization of the University's academic portfolio

2. Programme monitoring involves the continuous ongoing appraisal of the course or programme by the Course Director and course team, and the production of an annual course or programme monitoring report for the institution.
3. Programme review is a periodic investigation to see if the course or programme is still meeting its objectives, and whether appropriate monitoring and evaluation is taking place.

Programme validation

The purpose of validation is to ensure that the course or programme is of a standard comparable to similar awards elsewhere within higher education. The peer-review procedure involves initial scrutiny by a panel of the course or programme documentation prior to the validation event, so that key issues can be identified and conveyed to the chair of the event for inclusion in the agenda for the meeting. During the event, the panel will engage the course or programme team in dialogue and debate on the issues identified, and at the end of the meeting a decision will be made on whether or not the course or programme should be approved to run. A report of the meeting and decisions is circulated to the course or programme team shortly after the event.

The composition of the validation panel should provide a rigorous examination of the course and the course team, thus ensuring the quality of the course. Membership is drawn from a wide range of individuals, including members from the proposing institution, subject experts from other institutions, members from the relevant industry or profession, and members with understanding of the processes of higher education.

Programme monitoring

This involves the continuous appraisal of the course or programme by the course director and course team, and the production of an annual or periodic monitoring report for the institution.

Table 12.8

Spectrum of institutional quality assurance

A. Inputs

1. College organization and policy	Quality of leadership Institutional philosophy Mission statement Vision Management structure Relationships with staff Financial management Staff development policy Public relations and publicity Equal opportunities policy Quality assurance systems	

2. Personnel	Teaching staff and library/support staff
	    qualifications
	    motivation
	    morale
	Staff-student ratio
	Staff development opportunities
	Individual performance review	

3. Library and support services	Adequacy of book stock and periodicals Opening hours Student support Information technology and media resources Secretarial and administrative support	
4. Enterprises	Teaching accommodation Halls of residence Security arrangements Ground maintenance Catering Car parking Recreation Child-care	
5. Students	Admission and access Entry qualifications Motivation	

B. Processes

6. Curriculum	Relevance Employer-focus Planning Validation, monitoring and review	
7. Teaching	Preparation Delivery Assessment Teacher-student relationships	
8. Research and consultancy	External funding Publication in refereed journals Citations Client satisfaction with consultancy	
9. Student guidance and counselling	Guidance and counselling by teachers Availability of a college counselling service	

C. Outputs

10. Student achievement	Assessment/examination success rates Employment rates Progress to further study Value-added	
11. Course monitoring/evaluation	Annual monitoring reports Quinquennial review	

Annual or periodic monitoring reports

The programme director and programme committee are responsible for the production of an annual or periodic monitoring report which is sent to the college or department faculty board or equivalent. The monitoring report is one of the key mechanisms for quality assurance, and provides data about a range of aspects of educational delivery. Table 12.9 gives the issues that annual or periodic programme monitoring reports should consider.

Table 12.9

Considerations for annual or periodic monitoring reports (University of Greenwich, 1999b)

1. Statistical evidence on student performance and progression
2. Quality-related issues at course, programme and, where appropriate, subject level
3. External examiners'/moderators' reports
4. Reports of professional bodies or other external agencies
5. Minutes of committees
6. Student feedback from a variety of sources (including the centrally-organized Student Satisfaction Survey)
7. University-wide issues raised by, for example, Faculty Quality Committee, Faculty Board, Academic Collaboration Committee, or Academic Council
8. Good practice, for example, in teaching, learning and assessment
9. Action taken as a consequence of the previous year's monitoring report
10. Actions undertaken or required as a consequence of the current monitoring report

Some institutions use a scrutineer system for monitoring. A scrutineer is a member of academic staff assigned to a particular course or programme, and who scrutinizes the monitoring procedure. There is dialogue between the scrutineer and the course director about the draft monitoring report and how it might be made more effective. The scrutineer also speaks to the report at the faculty board, and the system provides added rigour to the process of quality assurance.

Programme review

Review is a periodic investigation, usually five-yearly, to see if the course or programme is still meeting its objectives, and whether appropriate monitoring and evaluation is taking place. It follows a similar process to that of validation, including peer-review by a panel constituted in the same way as that for a validation event. However, there are three additional aspects required for a review event:

1. a critical appraisal of the strengths and weaknesses of the programme, including recommendations for changes in the light of the critical appraisal;
2. sample of current and past students is invited to attend to offer their opinions on their experience of the programme;
3. a sample of marked student assessments to indicate the standard of work achieved on the programme.

Internal quality audit

Internal quality audit is undertaken periodically by an institution to assure itself and others that its quality assurance systems are appropriate for maintaining the standard of its academic awards, and that its development activities are enhancing the quality of teaching and learning.

Internal quality audit covers the range of quality assurance mechanisms in the institution, including its validation, monitoring and review processes, the appointment of external examiners, the procedures of committees and boards, partnership arrangements, etc.

A useful model for internal quality audit is that of the English National Board for Nursing, Midwifery and Health Visiting.

ENB guidelines for educational audit

The English National Board for Nursing, Midwifery and Health Visiting has produced detailed guidelines for educational audit (ENB, 1993). There are seven audit areas and each is further subdivided into specific categories within which dimensions and focus are identified. Each area has a quality statement relating the area to the institution, and evidence of performance is described for each category.

Area 1: Efficiency
The quality statement is 'the institution demonstrates efficient management and utilization of resources', and there are seven categories:

- financial management;
- manpower;
- staff/student ratios;
- use of staff time;
- courses/programmes;
- learning resources; and
- accommodation.

Area 2: Effectiveness, goal achievement, fitness for purpose
The quality statement is 'the institution demonstrates a clearly identified purpose and progress in working towards its mission statement', and there are seven categories:

- organizational development;
- student academic development;
- student career development;
- student personal development;
- faculty academic development;
- faculty career development; and
- faculty personal development.

Note that the term faculty refers to staff.

Area 3: Effectiveness, resource acquisition
The quality statement is 'there is evidence that the institution is systematically analysing market forces and responding to identified needs', and there are three categories:

- income generation;

- market forces – students;
- market forces – faculty, community relations, and skill mix.

Area 4: Effectiveness, participant satisfaction

The quality statement is 'there is evidence that the institution is beginning to establish mechanisms to identify customer/consumer/staff satisfaction and acceptability', and there are five categories:

- students;
- faculty;
- higher education;
- region; and
- service providers.

Area 5: Effectiveness, social justice

The quality statement is 'the institution is committed to maximize accessibility to potential recruits, both staff and students', and there are seven categories:

- accessibility;
- equality of opportunity;
- availability;
- awareness;
- responsiveness;
- extensiveness; and
- appropriateness/relevance.

Area 6: Effectiveness, internal processes

The quality statement is 'the institution is committed to effective communication, effective course delivery and course development through efficient management information systems', and there are six categories:

- communication structures;
- human resources;
- evaluation styles;
- counselling support structures;
- management/leadership styles; and
- curricular policies.

Area 7: Effectiveness, practice placement

The quality statement is 'the institution is committed to the provision of effective clinical learning experiences to ensure the achievement of competencies to enhance the quality of patient care', and there are six categories:

- student learning experience/evaluation;
- academic staff perspective;
- service provider unit staff perspective;
- RHA purchaser/other purchaser requirements;

- environment; and
- quality assurance mechanisms.

A model for educational quality assurance in universities

Boyle and Bowden (1997) propose a model for comprehensive education quality assurance, the key principles and values of which are as follows:

1. The principal focus is on continual quality improvement.
2. Continual improvement is concerned with the quality of student learning, and the main process elements which influence student learning.
3. The key elements which influence the quality of student learning are related in an integrated and systematic way to provide a QA framework.
4. A necessary condition for QA is effective evaluation and evidence bases for actions and claims concerning quality and quality improvement.
5. The primary responsibility for QA should be invested in the group which has primary responsibility for achieving particular goals; where the goal is the facilitation of high quality educational programmes, this should be the academic programme teams.
6. Accountability is an important consequence, not the primary focus of QA.

EXTERNAL QUALITY MONITORING LEVEL

In this final level in the hierarchy of quality assurance, we turn our attention to those quality assurance agencies external to higher education institutions.

There is a wide range of such external agencies, including government agencies, accrediting bodies, and professional bodies, all of which exert considerable influence on the quality assurance mechanisms of higher education institutions.

In February 1998 the Government published its response to the Dearing Report, Higher Education for the 21st Century. Response to the Dearing Report (DfEE, 1998b). In Chapter 4 of the report the response includes recommendations about the Quality Assurance Agency.

The Quality Assurance Agency for Higher Education

Within the higher education sector, the Quality Assurance Agency (QAA) has been established which has taken over the functions of the now-defunct Higher Education Quality Council (HEQC).

Objectives of the QAA

In Quality Assurance: A New Approach, the Agency has set out its objectives (QAA, 1998):

1. There must be public confidence that quality of provision, and standards of awards in higher education are being safeguarded and enhanced.
2. Those who use, and those who pay for higher education must have ready access to reliable information about the performance of universities and colleges across the extensive and diverse range of programmes of study offered.
3. The Higher Education Funding Councils have statutory obligations to secure the assessment of the quality of provision they fund. Information must be provided, and quality assurance arrangements undertaken by the Agency in forms acceptable to the Councils.
4. A national quality assurance system must meet these needs in a manner that is effective, efficient and economical.

Institutional scrutiny and subject review

The QAA will provide independent verification of the quality of programmes of study throughout higher education, by a process of scrutiny of institutions and review of subject units. In order to avoid duplication of effort, it is intended that the scrutiny process should engage with the institution's internal validation and review cycle and also with any professional or statutory accreditation process, where relevant. The cycle will be six years in length, and in each year academic reviewers will review a number of programmes, culminating in reports on outcome standards and on quality of learning opportunities. There will be 42 standard subject units, e.g. medicine, psychology, archaeology, etc.

The Institute for Learning and Teaching

Earlier in this chapter, The Institute for Learning and Teaching (ILT) was introduced. Its aims are stated as follows:

1. enhance status of teaching in higher education;
2. monitor and improve quality of learning and teaching in higher education;
3. set standards of good professional practice for members, and in due course, all those with teaching and learning responsibilities.

On 8 February 1999, the ILT issued a consultation paper The National Framework for Higher Education Teaching (ILT, 1999). The consultation paper identifies five broad areas of responsibility associated with teaching in higher education:

1. teaching and/or support of learning;
2. contribution to the design and planning of learning activities;
3. assessment and giving feedback to students;
4. developing effective learning environments and student support systems;
5. reflective practice and personal development.

The paper also proposed a series of outcomes that academics would be expected to achieve in order to gain membership or associate membership of the Institute, but the results of consultation showed that a majority of academics were strongly opposed to these outcomes, so they were subsequently dropped. The ILT includes the following in its achievement intentions:

- criteria for peer-evaluation of teaching;
- promote recognition of quality in teaching in higher education;
- disseminate good practice;
- bridge between research and teaching practice;
- encourage diversity and cross-disciplinary activity;
- stimulate awareness of teaching as a professional activity.

The key areas of activity are:

1. Membership services:
   (a) publications in learning and teaching;
   (b) website: key issues in learning and teaching;
   (c) conferences/seminars: reduced rate or ILT-run;
   (d) networking opportunities;
   (e) occasional specialist publications;
   (f) access to information about ILT pathways and members.
2. Development and dissemination
   (a) linking into research databases and making them more accessible;
   (b) disseminating good practice in teaching and learning.
3. Accreditation for ILT membership.

This aspect is addressed in Chapter 21 (p. 555).

The English National Board for Nursing, Midwifery and Health Visiting

Higher education programmes that relate to practice within the professions are normally accredited by the relevant statutory or professional body, such accreditation often being a requirement for courses leading to entry to a given profession. Within the UK, all programmes leading to entry on the professional register of nurses held by the United Kingdom Central Council for Nursing, Midwifery and Health Visiting must be accredited by the appropriate National Board for Nursing, Midwifery and Health Visiting. There are four such boards, each being responsible for one of the four countries comprising the UK. In this section we will examine the English National Board for Nursing, Midwifery and Health Visiting (ENB) Standards for Approval of Higher Education Institutions and Programmes (ENB, 1997) and the ENB Quality Assurance Framework (ENB, 1998).

ENB Standards for Approval of Higher Education Institutions and Programmes

The Standards were published in October 1997 and mark a change of approach from the previous regulations and guidelines, towards measurable and achievable standards that are research-based or evidence-based where possible.

There are 18 standards, each having several criteria that further elaborate them. Table 12.10 shows example of the standard and associated criteria for Staff Development.

Table 12.10

Standard statement and criteria for staff development (ENB, 1997)

Standard 5: Staff development
Staff development strategy promotes the development of all staff
Criteria:
1. Staff development strategy is in place and is reviewed, monitored and evaluated annually
2. Training needs analysis informs the preparation of the staff development programme
3. The staff development programme promotes equity of opportunity

The ENB states that:

'all aspects of human, physical and learning resources, which are necessary for the creation of a stimulating teaching/ learning environment, are addressed within the standards.'

The standards are the means by which the quality of education provision is assured, and ENB education officers will use the standards for validation, monitoring and review of educational programmes.

The standards are underpinned by the following principles:

1. patient focused, i.e. improvement of patient/client care;
2. practice led, i.e. rooted in professional practice;
3. student centred, i.e. recognizes student individuality;
4. equitable, i.e. equality of opportunity;
5. appropriate, i.e. 'fitness for purpose';
6. effective, i.e. high standards and efficient resource use;
7. responsive, i.e. employment-focused and change-focused;
8. collaborative, i.e. partnership with major stakeholders;
9. accountable, i.e. 'open to scrutiny, explicable and defensible'.

The 18 standard statements are given in Table 12.11

The ENB Quality Assurance Framework

In 1998 the ENB launched its Quality Assurance Manual containing the Quality Assurance Framework (ENB, 1998) as a working manual for ENB education officers and institutions of higher education seeking institutional or programme approval by the board. The Framework uses an input–process–outcome model in which the board's standards for approval, monitoring and review are integrated, as outlined below.

Inputs

1. Institutional approval (5-year period of approval). Approval of the institution provides a *'judgement of organizational intent and its*

1. The policies and practices of the higher education institution meet the Board's requirements specified in this document and the curriculum guidelines.
2. The higher education institution works proactively with education purchasers to develop programmes which meet workforce requirements.
3. The head of the faculty/school/department providing nursing/midwifery/health visiting education participates in decision-making concerning strategic planning, organizational policy and budgeting.
4. The staff resource supports the delivery of each nursing/midwifery/health visiting programme at the stated professional and academic level.
5. Staff development strategy promotes the development of all staff.
6. The research strategy in the faculty/school/department is aimed at promoting the development of professional knowledge, education and practice.
7. Physical and learning resources support teaching and learning activities in all settings for the achievement of educational programme outcomes.
8. Practice experience provides learning opportunities which enable the achievement of the stated learning outcomes.
9. Lecturers are involved in the development of practice and professional and academic knowledge.
10. Nursing/midwifery/health visiting lectures and service staff are involved in the selection of students and ensure that the stated entry requirements for specific educational programmes are met.
11. Curriculum design and development reflect contemporary educational approaches and health care practice.
12. The assessment strategy incorporates the requirements of Statutory Instruments, EC Directives, the UKCC's and the Board's standards and the assessment regulations of the higher education institution.
13. The assessment of learning of theory and practice is a continuous process, culminating in a judgement of achievement.
14. Assessors measure student achievement against the performance criteria for the programme.
15. External examiners monitor the assessment process to ensure that professional and academic standards are maintained.
16. Students are supported in the achievement of the learning outcomes of the educational programmes.
17. Programme management ensures that educational opportunities are provided for students to enable them to meet the intended learning outcomes.
18. Educational provision leads to the achievement of fitness for purpose, practice and award.

Table 12.11

The 18 ENB standard statements (ENB, 1997)

overall capacity and capability to deliver education leading to an award in nursing and midwifery' (page 7).
2. Programme approval (indefinite period of approval). Approval of the educational programme is a process which will 'ensure that the curriculum submission complies with professional and academic criteria for a specific award and to ensure that the resources, human physical and financial, will be able to support the programme at the appropriate academic standard' (page 7).

Process
1. Student learning experience

Outcomes
1. Fitness for purpose, practice and award. Separation of fitness for purpose, practice and award is inappropriate for professional education. It is the board's view that professional practice is underpinned by professional knowledge in which academic theory and professional practice are an integral part of the whole learning experience (page 5).

2. Annual monitoring and review of programmes. Annual monitoring and review is defined as *'a process of formative assessment which culminates in a summative judgement of performance at the programme level'* (page 8).
3. Quinquennial review and re-approval of institutions. Quinquennial review is the major summative assessment of total institutional performance, using evidence gained through the annual monitoring and review process measured against the board's standards and institutional goals. This culminates in an overall judgement of an institution's capacity and capability to continue as a board approved institution (page 9).

QUALITY IMPROVEMENT MODELS

Quality improvement (QI) is defined by Peterson *et al.* (1997) as follows:

> *'The term "quality improvement" is used to describe any structured and intentional approach to institutional change that derive from re-workings of industrial or commercial models of quality management, such as continuous quality improvement (CQI) and total quality management (TQM).'*

Total quality management

The most familiar quality improvement model in the literature of higher education is total quality management (TQM), although it is a concept that seemingly evades capture by a single definition.

Lundquist (1998), for example, identifies three key elements of TQM:

1. focus on customer needs;
2. process orientation;
3. continuous improvements.

Sallis (1993) offers a useful insight into the concept of TQM:

> *'TQM is a practical but strategic approach to running an organization which focuses on the needs of its customers and clients. It aims to reject any outcomes other than excellence. TQM is not a set of slogans, but a deliberate and systematic approach to achieving appropriate levels of quality in a consistent fashion which meet or exceed the needs and wants of customers. It can be thought of as a philosophy of never-ending improvement only achievable by, and through, people'* (page 36).

Sallis emphasises the need for a permanent shift in the culture of an organization, from short-term expediency to long-term quality improvement.

Boaden (1997) offers a helpful list of the elements of TQM, distilled from a range of surveys in the literature:

- customer focus, with emphasis on the customer-supplier relationship, internally and externally;
- the commitment of everyone to quality improvement, especially managers;
- training and education are considered an investment;
- the involvement of everyone within the organization in quality improvement;
- a focus on processes;
- the use of teams and teamwork;
- the use of appropriate tools and techniques, reviewed regularly;
- goal-setting, measurement and feedback for all aspects of the business;
- continuous improvement as a philosophy;
- a change in the culture of the organization, i.e. the way people think and behave;
- the inclusion of quality principles into product and service design.

INVESTORS IN PEOPLE STANDARD

In February 1998, the Government published a green paper, The Learning Age: A Renaissance for a new Britain (DFEE, 1998a). The green paper highlights the variable spread and quality of training in the workplace and the need for workplaces to become centres of learning. This will be encouraged by a legislative framework, and Investors in People (IiP) will become the standard for staff development in both public and private sectors.

Investors in People is a national standard for the training and development of people in organizations, and consists of the following elements:

- commitment of top managers;
- written institutional strategy;
- regular review of staff development;
- lifelong learning activities;
- evaluation of effectiveness.

The four principles of IiP

Investors in People is based upon four principles derived from the experience of organizations whose investment in their people has led to improvement in the organization's performance (TQMI, 1996):

1. Commitment. 'The Investor in People makes a commitment from the top to develop all employees to achieve its business objectives.'
2. Planning. 'An Investor in People regularly reviews the needs and plans the training and development of all employees.'
3. Action. 'An Investor in People takes action to train and develop individuals on recruitment and throughout their employment.'
4. Evaluation. 'An Investor in People evaluates the investment in

training and development to assess achievement and improve future effectiveness.'

Each of these principles is further elaborated by a series of statements, and examples are given of the ways in which the standard can be demonstrated. One of the statements under the 'Planning' principle is as follows:

> 2.4: *'A written plan identifies the resources that will be used to meet training and development needs.'*

Examples of resources are given, including money, people, time and facilities.

The process for gaining IiP status

Organizations wishing to gain IiP status must understand the national standard, and undertake an organizational self-evaluation to ascertain the degree to which the organization meets the standard. There must be a strong commitment to the standard throughout the organization, from top management to employees. Evidence of the organization's performance against the standard is gathered and analysed by means of a manager survey and an employee survey, and action is taken to remedy any deficits between the organization's performance and the standard. This evidence is verified by an approved body such as a Training and Enterprise Councils (TEC), and if successful, the organization is awarded IiP status. The organization's performance against the standard is reviewed within three years of approval. The approval process for IiP is overseen by the DfEE.

BS EN ISO 9000 (SERIES)

The British Standards Institute (BSI) published its quality assurance standard as BS5750 in 1979, and developed this as an international standard with ISO in 1984 (Hoyle, 1998). The BS EN ISO 9000 (series) consists of standards for quality assurance and quality management. The quality assurance standards for the design and assessment of quality assurance systems are 9001, 9002, and 9003. This external quality monitoring system, although designed for manufacturing industries, is capable of adaptation to meet the requirements of education and training, and has been adopted by many colleges and universities for their quality assurance systems. It is important to note, however, that it constitutes a standard for an institution's quality system, not its standards for teaching or other activities.

The standard requires commitment by the entire workforce; top management must ensure the effective functioning of the quality system; middle management must ensure that approved policies and objectives are implemented; the workforce must commit itself to adhere to the approved policies. This normally involves a change in the organizational culture, with a commitment to maintaining continuing customer satisfaction. Doherty (1995) describes the implementation of BS EN ISO 9000 at the University of Wolverhampton.

The BS EN ISO 9000 (series) standards

BS EN ISO 9001demonstrates that the organization has the capability to design certain products. BS EN ISO 9002 demonstrates that the organization has the capability to manufacture, install or service certain products, or deliver certain services. BS EN ISO 9003 demonstrates that the organization has the capability to supply products, or perform services, that are verifiable by final inspection or test.

There are 322 requirements to meet Standard 9001, and these require the defining and documenting of procedures relating to the maintenance of quality across all the organization's activities, including auditing of the effectiveness of procedures.

Accreditation for BS EN ISO 9000 (series)

Organizations wishing to register for BS EN ISO 9000 (series) must undergo an external assessment of their quality system by an accredited certification body. The assessment involves sampling the requirements of the standard from a range of activities, personnel, locations, documents, etc. Registration serves as a quality kite-mark for customers and consumers.

QUALITY CIRCLES

Quality Circles are extensively used in Japanese manufacturing, and is a strategy that involves group problem-solving in order to enhance the quality of service. Membership of the group is voluntary, and groups are autonomous in their functioning. They typically consist of between three and twelve people from similar areas of work who meet together for an hour per week during the working day, on an ongoing basis. The group should be trained in problem-solving skills and they focus on problems occurring within their work. Their solutions are implemented directly by them or via management.

Boore (1993) provides an interesting account of the use of quality circles to develop standards for teaching at the University of Ulster. The quality circle groups consisted of academic staff and students drawn from a range of disciplines, and the task of each group was to write standards for a given teaching method. The methods included lectures, seminars, tutorials and placements, and the groups met on two or three occasions only, due to time constraints. The outcomes of the quality circles activity was not limited to the production of standards; the author concludes that staff have gained a greater awareness of the allocated teaching method, and the importance of quality of teaching was highlighted for both staff and students.

REFERENCES

Ashworth, A. and Harvey, R. (1994) *Assessing Quality in Higher Education*, Jessica Kingsley Publishers, London.

Bligh, D. (1998) *What's the Use of Lectures?*, 5th edn, Intellect, Exeter.

Boaden, R.J. (1997) What is total quality management ... and does it matter?, *Total Quality Management*, 8(4), 153–71.

Boore, J. (1993) Teaching standards from quality circles, in *Quality Assurance for University Teaching*, R. Ellis (ed.), Society for Research into Higher Education/Open University Press, Buckingham.

Boyle, P. and Bowden, J.A. (1997) Educational quality assurance in universities: an enhanced model, *Assessment and Evaluation in Higher Education*, 22(2), 111–21.

Cave, M., Hanney, S. and Kogan, M. (1991) *The Use of Performance Indicators in Higher Education*, Jessica Kingsley Publishers, London.

Dearing, R. (1979) *Higher Education in the Learning Society, The Report of the National Committee of Inquiry into Higher Education*, HMSO, Norwich.

DfEE (1997) *National Advisory Group for Continuing Education and Lifelong Learning for the 21st Century*, DfEE document reference:PP62/31326/1197/43, London.

DfEE (1998a) *The Learning Age: Renaissance for a New Britain*, HMSO, London.

DfEE (1998b) *Higher Education for the 21st Century. Response to the Dearing Report*, HMSO, London.

Doherty, G.D. (1995) BS5750 Parts 1 and 2/ISO 9000(series) 1987 and education – do they fit and is it worth it?, *Quality Assurance in Education*, 3(3), 3–9.

Ellis, R. (ed.) (1993) *Quality Assurance for University Teaching*, Society for Research into Higher Education/Open University Press, Buckingham.

English National Board for Nursing, Midwifery and Health Visiting (1993) *Guidelines for Educational Audit*, ENB, London.

English National Board for Nursing, Midwifery and Health Visiting (1997) *Standards for Approval of Higher Education Institutions and Programmes*, ENB, London.

English National Board for Nursing, Midwifery and Health Visiting (1998) *Quality Assurance Manual*, ENB, London.

Flanders, N. (1970) *Analysing Teaching Behaviour*, Addison-Wesley, MA.

Further Education Development Agency (1999) *Standards for Teaching and Supporting Learning in Further Education in England and Wales*, FEDA, London.

Green, D. (ed.) (1994) *What is Quality in Higher Education?*, Society for Research into Higher Education/Open University Press, Buckingham.

Harvey, L. (1999) *Student Satisfaction Manual*, Society for Research into Higher Education/Open University Press, Buckingham.

Higher Education Quality Council (1996) *Guidelines on Quality Assurance*, HEQC, London.

Hoyle, D. (1998) *ISO 9000 Pocket Guide*, Butterworth/Heinemann, Oxford.

Institute for Learning and Teaching (1999) *Consultation Document: The National Framework for Higher Education Teaching*, ILT, York.

Lunquist, R. (1998) Quality improvements of teaching and learning in higher education: a comparison with developments in industrial settings, *Teaching in Higher Education*, 3(1), 51–61.

Perry, P. (1994) Defining and measuring the quality of teaching, in *What is*

Quality in Higher Education?, D. Green (ed.), Society for Research into Higher Education/Open University Press, Buckingham.

Peterson, S.L., Kovel-Jarboe, P. and Schwartz, SA. (1997) Quality improvement in higher education: implications for student retention, *Quality in Higher Education*, 3(2), 131–41.

Quality Assurance Agency for Higher Education (1998) *Quality Assurance: A New Approach*, JEC/98/33, QAA, London.

Sallis, E. (1993) *Total Quality Management in Education*, Kogan Page, London.

Thomas, E. (1993) The first distinguished teaching award in the United Kingdom, in *Quality Assurance for University Teaching*, R. Ellis (ed.), Society for Research into Higher Education/Open University Press, Buckingham.

TQMI (1996) *Investors in People Handbook*, TQM International, Cheshire.

University of Greenwich (1999a) *Academic Quality Assurance Handbook*, University of Greenwich, London.

University of Greenwich (1999b) *Regulations for Taught Awards: September 1999*, University of Greenwich, London.

Winch, C. (1996) *Quality in Education*, Blackwell, Oxford.

PART THREE

TEACHING STRATEGIES

LECTURING

13

It is not surprising that academic personnel in educational institutions are called lecturers, given the predominance of this form of teaching in further and higher education. In lay terms, to lecture someone is to 'go on' at some length about an issue, with the recipient listening either willingly or unwillingly. This is not dissimilar from the educational use of the term lecture, i.e. a particular type of educational encounter in which a teacher transmits information to a number of students, with the teacher doing most of the talking and the students mainly listening or writing.

Lecturing is the most common teaching strategy in adult education (Bligh, 1998), but it does tend to polarize teachers' opinions into those who love it and those who loathe it. The proponents of the lecture method would argue for its use on two main grounds:

1. *A proven track record*. The practice of using lectures to transmit the culture of a civilisation goes back to at least the ancient Greeks, and has therefore stood the test of time. A significant proponent of this viewpoint is the psychologist David Ausubel (Ausubel *et al.*, 1978), who defends the use of lectures for transmission of knowledge. He maintains that it is simply wasteful to ask students to discover everything for themselves, when the transmission mode has been used successfully over generations to transmit the culture of a society. Ausubel's work is described in Chapter 4 (p. 91).

2. *Efficient use of resources*. In an era of significant resource constraints in higher education, lectures make very efficient use of teachers' time, e.g. when giving a lecture to 150 students, the teacher–student ratio is 1:150; this helps to resource small group and laboratory teaching where the ratio may be as low as 1:8. This resource efficiency of lectures is used to good effect in the context of modular programmes. A module is a self-contained unit of learning and modular programmes are now very common in British higher education. Academic awards are made up of numbers of modules at different academic levels, and efficiency gains can accrue by making a given module available to students from a variety of programmes. For example, an introductory module on psychology could be attended by students from a variety of disciplines, such as nursing, social science, and humanities. Hence, a single lecture could address several hundred students at the same time, particularly when used in conjunction with closed-circuit television relays.

The argument about the importance of lectures for the transmission of culture would be disputed by many academics, and is encapsulated in the adage: 'the information from a lecture goes from the lecturer's notes to the students' notes without passing through the brains of either!' Whilst this may be a little overstated, it does raise a serious question about whether lectures actually facilitate students' learning. The argument based upon efficient use of resources would also be challenged by opponents of the lecture method, because it contains the unsupported assumption that lectures actually do make students learn. In fact, the counter-argument is just as powerful, i.e. it might be much more efficient in the long term to use small-group and individual teaching methods, as these may be much more effective in facilitating students' learning.

THE LECTURE METHOD: USES AND SHORTCOMINGS

Evidence from the literature on the educational use of lectures is summarized below:

1. *Purposes*. Lectures are as effective as other methods for conveying information, but less effective for the promotion of thinking skills and the changing of attitudes.
2. *Compulsory attendance*. Students who absent themselves from lectures do less well in examinations and tests.
3. *Time of day*. Morning lectures seem superior to afternoon lectures for the recall of information, but this may not apply to the 'evening-type' of learner, whose maximum physiological alertness occurs between 15.00 hours and midnight.
4. *Length*. Attention declines considerably after some 20 minutes, with a reduction in the amount of information assimilated and noted.
5. *Recall*. Recall on information from lectures is relatively inefficient, falling to something around 20% recall after one week.
6. *Delivery*. Speed of delivery is closely related to the level of difficulty of the material, and evidence suggests that there is a critical level of difficulty and speed, beyond which the material is delivered with a loss of efficiency.

One common criticism of the lecture method is that the information could have been obtained from textbooks just as easily, yet this shows a lack of understanding of the purpose of lectures. Indeed, if they are used only to convey information readily available in other forms such as books, then they are likely to be simplistic or inaccurate due to time constraints. However, used thoughtfully, lectures can complement textbooks by providing:

1. up-to-date research information that has not yet reached the textbooks;
2. a synthesis of viewpoints from a wide variety of sources;

3. clearer explanations of issues and phenomena, with the possibility of demonstration;

4. personal involvement of the students by means of activities during the lecture; and

5. the potential to motivate and inspire students to further study.

However, over-reliance on lectures may lead to dependence on the part of the students, who expect all the information to be handed to them 'on a plate'. All too often lectures are long, tedious and poorly organized, whereas with careful planning and practice they can be an effective vehicle for motivating students.

The advantages and disadvantages of the lecture method are summarized in Table 13.1

Advantages	Disadvantages
Efficiency, i.e. one teacher can communicate with a large number of students	Students' attention may wane
A well-presented lecture may increase student motivation	Students are largely passive
New knowledge may be presented which is not yet in textbooks	Lectures do not cater for individual student's needs
Teachers can integrate the subject matter better than students	Pace of lecture does not suit all students
Good for introducing a new topic	Teacher's bias may be evident
Useful for giving a framework upon which students can build	Students obtain material 'second-hand' rather than from primary sources

Table 13.1

Advantages and disadvantages of the lecture method

LECTURING TECHNIQUES

I firmly believe that lecturing is analogous to acting, each requiring careful scripting, polished presentational skills, and a certain personal charisma for effective performance. This theatrical performance element may not be present in other forms of teaching and can provide a source of stimulation and job satisfaction for those teachers who enjoy the challenge. The requirements of good lecturing are creativity, well-developed verbal-exposition skills, clarity of ideas, an ability to make a subject interesting, enthusiasm and self-confidence. *Verbal exposition* is the term given to the kinds of talking in which the teacher engages during a lecture, or indeed in any other type of teaching, with the exception of individualized instruction. This 'teacher-talk' can be subdivided into a number of modes, the commonest ones being the stating of facts, the defining and classifying of material, asking and answering questions, giving explanations, comparing and contrasting information and evaluating material.

Table 13.2 gives guidelines for planning and delivering lectures, and uses an acrostic arrangement under the headings 'before', 'during' and 'after'. In an acrostic, the initial letters of each of the horizontal statements combine vertically to make another word, and this is a simple way to introduce novelty into teaching. Acrostics can also be used as an

Table 13.2

Guidelines for planning and
delivering lectures

1. **Before the lecture**
    Believe in Yourself
    Explaining
    Focus on Selected Aspects
    Over-learn Your Material
    Rehearse
    Excitement/Anxiety

2. **During the lecture**
    Delivery
    Unusual
    Recap
    Involve Your Audience
    Note-taking
    Get out on Time

3. **After the lecture**
    Average/mean performance
    Focus on Well-done/Less Well-done
    Tape the Lecture and Review
    Experience Other Peoples' Lectures
    Retain a Sense of Proportion

organizing principle for lecturing on a given topic – any topic – provided you have the ingenuity to think up appropriate words, and provided they are not over-used!

COMMENTARY ON THE GUIDELINES FOR PLANNING AND DELIVERING LECTURES

Before the lecture

Believe in yourself
By assuming the role of lecturer, one is, in a sense, claiming to have superior knowledge in comparison to the audience and this may lead to the feeling of vulnerability when facing them. Self-belief is a vital characteristic for successful lecturing; the teacher has an extensive knowledge and experience base which underpins their lectures, and this should provide the confidence to approach the lecture, and the audience, in a positive manner.

Explaining
Explanations are a central activity in most lectures and great care must be taken in their preparation. Explaining is discussed in detail in Chapter 5.

Focus on selected aspects
When planning the lecture it is important to be selective about what to put into it, the temptation being to cram in everything the teacher knows about a topic. Chapter 5 deals with this aspect of planning in more detail.

Over-learn your material

It almost goes without saying that the teacher must know the subject matter of the lecture 'inside-out' if credibility is to be maintained. Students very soon see through any attempts to 'waffle' by a teacher who does not know a particular point or answer. No teacher can know everything about a subject and it can increase stature if a lack of knowledge is admitted. Needless to say, the teacher who constantly has to say, 'I'm sorry, I don't know', has an inadequate background knowledge which requires attention. If the lecture has been prepared some time in advance, or if it has been given previously, the teacher needs to spend time going over the material again to ensure he or she has remembered it.

Rehearse

The analogy with acting emerges again here, with the advice that the teacher should spend time rehearsing various elements of the lecture until he or she is satisfied with the likely impact and timing. A videotape or audiotape recorder is invaluable for providing feedback on these aspects.

Excitement/anxiety

Lecturing to a large audience is often the main anxiety experienced by those new to teaching and it largely stems from the fear of making a fool of oneself by 'drying up' or forgetting what to say. The opening of the lecture is often the most nerve-racking part for the inexperienced teacher, but it is common to find that teachers still experience initial nervousness even after years of teaching. Actors often claim that this initial state of high arousal is beneficial, in that it puts an 'edge' on their performance. However, it is useful to distinguish between arousal and anxiety; arousal applies to the state of wakefulness or alertness of the individual, while anxiety applies to a state of arousal above that required for the optimum level of performance. Anxiety, therefore, reduces the performance effectiveness of an individual. What the lecturer is aiming at is a level of arousal sufficient to bring out the best in the performance without tipping over the edge into anxiety, which would reduce his or her effectiveness.

During the lecture

Delivery

On first entering the lecture room, it is important that the teacher takes a couple of minutes to organize the area, check the overhead projector, etc. Very often the students have been sitting in the room prior to the teacher's entry, having already received a previous lecture and there is a temptation to commence the lecture straight away. So often lecturers begin their session and after a few minutes turn on the overhead projector only to find it is projecting onto the wall or somewhere other than the screen. It is important to spend a moment or two organizing the area, and to let the audience know so they can feel free to talk to their friends until everything is ready. This should ensure that the lecturer feels confident that all is well prior to commencing the lecture.

The introduction to the lecture is very important in gaining the students' interest and attention, so it is well worth attempting to provide a motivating opening. This could involve asking the audience whether anyone has had experience related to the topic, thus making the session relevant to them. It is also good practice to write out on the chalkboard a plan or outline of the sequence of the lecture, so that students may follow each section without losing track of the explanation.

The aim of a lecture is to communicate certain things to the audience and the main medium for this communication is the lecturer's voice. There are three components of the vocal apparatus:

1. *Vocal cords* which vibrate as the breath passes between them;
2. *Resonators* which are the hollow spaces of the mouth, nose and pharynx; and
3. *Speech organs* consisting of the tongue, palate, alveolar ridge, teeth, jaw and lips.

Volume or *loudness* is dependent on the force of the breath striking the vocal cords. Pitch is determined by the length, thickness and tension of the vocal cords, the first two factors being influenced by the size of the larynx. For instance, the small larynx of a child has short vocal cords which give the voice a high pitch. Adult males, on the other hand, possess large larynxes with long cords, producing a low pitch, i.e. a deep voice. Nervous tension will produce a note of higher pitch and this is often detectable in persons who are anxious. Tone is the result of the air vibrating in the resonating spaces.

One of the most important aspects of speech in the lecture setting is *audibility*. This relies particularly on the careful use of consonants, which ensures clarity, and on the ability of the teacher to project his or her voice. It is good technique to stand up straight and speak from the lungs rather than the throat, ensuring that the lungs are well-inflated with each breath. Careful observation of the facial expressions and other non-verbal communication will provide feedback as to whether the rear row of the audience is hearing what is being said.

Expressiveness is another important aspect of speech, as it helps maintain the listeners' interest by providing variety. Variations in intonation are produced by changing the pitch of the voice and also by variations of the volume and rhythm. The use of stress to emphasize important words can make the voice more interesting and the speed of delivery needs to be at a pace suitable for the students to absorb the material and to write notes. Pausing is a strategy that new teachers need to develop; the tendency is to regard any periods of silence as undesirable, although pauses are a necessity during speech, since they provide the punctuation that makes the words meaningful. It can be useful to take a sip of water periodically, as a way of forcing oneself to pause.

One of the major problems that can cause loss of attention during lectures is the *speed of delivery*; this is often difficult to judge when inexperienced and the commonest error is going too fast when nervous. It is helpful for new teachers to keep a card on the desk or lectern with the words 'SLOW DOWN' written on it, which serves to catch their eye from time to time and remind them to think about the speed of delivery.

The aim of any lecture should be to provide an atmosphere of psychological safety in which the students feel free to volunteer comments or questions. If the teacher conveys the impression of warmth and acceptance towards the group, this, combined with a sense of humour, will go a long way towards establishing the rapport that is so essential to learning. Evidence suggests that interest and enthusiasm of the teacher are characteristics that are particularly valued by students, and this can be indicated by emphasis and tone of voice, and also by the use of non-verbal signals.

It is difficult to overstate the fundamental importance of non-verbal communication during lectures. Students emit a variety of non-verbal cues and the teacher can gain valuable feedback on his or her performance by observing their facial expressions, which can convey feelings of surprise, puzzlement or astonishment. The teacher also emits non-verbal signals, so it is important to be aware of the role of such signals.

Gesture can play a useful part in explaining concepts, especially those with spatial relationships, but other gestures may prove distracting, such as fiddling with chalk. Head nodding can be a reinforcer of behaviour and if a learner is talking to the teacher and the teacher nods frequently, this can encourage the learner to continue talking. When lecturing it is also important to engage the students in eye contact periodically, as this indicates interest and confidence. However, it should be noted that the length of time for eye contact should not exceed ten seconds, as this may provoke anxiety. Honesty is a quality which is not often mentioned in connection with verbal exposition and in this context it implies the willingness of the teacher to admit that he or she does not know the answer to something.

Unusual

The inclusion of unusual or novel stimuli can be a powerful strategy for maintaining students' arousal and attention during a lecture. Such stimuli could be pictures, music, poems and activities which have an element of surprise or novelty.

Recap

Recapitulation or repetition should be used frequently, so that the learner is exposed to the information on more than one occasion. Provision could also be made for this at the end of the lecture if time allows, and will help to retain the information for a longer period of time.

Involve your audience

Adult students are never very happy just sitting listening to lectures; what they like to have is some personal involvement in them. There is a wide variety of strategies for involving students in lectures, even when faced with a large number of students. One effective way is to use buzz groups, in which students form groups of four to six by swivelling around to face the ones behind them, without moving their seats. These small buzz groups then spend a couple of minutes discussing some aspect of the topic and then feedback is invited. The use of incomplete handouts is another way of ensuring student participation; the handout contains only key headings or diagrams and the student is required to fill in the details gleaned from the presentation. A quiz or test given at the end of the lecture may also serve to focus students' attention on the material presented!

Note-taking

This is discussed in detail in Chapter 19 (p. 497), but it is helpful to note a few key points here. There are both advantages and disadvantages in taking notes during a unit. Taking notes provides a permanent record of the information which is then available for review at a later date. Another advantage is that the information is actively processed and encoded in their own words. Bligh (1998) summarizes 29 studies showing that note-taking aids memory, and 20 studies showing that note-taking aids revision. On the negative side, notes may be inaccurate, and students may miss important points whilst writing down previous ones. On balance, though, I favour note-taking if it is done effectively, i.e. recording the key points rather than trying to write down everything word-for-word. At degree level, it is more important to note key references given in the unit, so that the original source can be accessed later, avoiding reliance on secondary sources.

Get out on time

It is quite common to find that lectures over-run their allotted time, and I think this is a cardinal offence! Students find it difficult enough to maintain attention during the normal span of a lecture, and over-running simply compounds the problem. There are also knock-on effects on the students' next class or lunch break, and it delays access by other groups to the lecture room. One of the causes of over-running is an over-ambitious lecture plan for the time available. These lecture plans seem to exert a powerful influence over teachers, who slavishly follow them until the bitter end, often regardless of the time or circumstances. From the teacher's perspective, the lecture plan contains important material that must be covered by the end of the lecture, even if this results in running late to do so. On the other hand, the students' perception is quite different, in that the important aspects of their college day are more likely to be the coffee and lunch breaks when they meet with their friends and peers. The teacher should aim to finish five minutes before the official end of the lecture, to give students and themselves a break before starting their next session.

After the lecture

Average/mean performance
Teachers often worry unduly if a lecture does not go as well as they would like, but it is important to see it in the context of their average performance. Some lectures go very well, others we would rather forget; it is not helpful to spend time worrying about a less than satisfying one-off performance. The teacher should aim for a good overall standard of performance, but realize that there will inevitably be minor variations from day to day.

Focus on well-done/less well-done
When evaluating a lecture it is helpful to try to focus on those aspects that were well-done, and those that were less well-done. By adopting this system the teacher will hopefully avoid distorting the evaluation by agonizing over a single unsatisfactory episode.

Tape the lecture and review
Evaluation of a lecture can be much more effective if the teacher can videotape one from time to time. It is a salutary experience to watch yourself performing as a lecturer, but by and large it is an encouraging activity that can boost confidence considerably.

Experience other people's lectures
Giving lectures can be quite an exciting experience for teachers, but it is easy to forget what it is like from the audience's point of view. It is helpful for teachers to attend lectures from time to time just to remind themselves what it feels like to sit in a lecture, especially if it is not particularly interesting or well-presented. Also tips and ideas may well be picked up that can be used in later lectures!

Retain a sense of proportion
The problem with the lecturing/acting analogy is that teachers may feel they have to produce virtuoso performances in every lecture. Clearly, some teachers have a flair for lecturing, while others are merely competent; the important thing is to be yourself. A sense of proportion is a great asset in lecturing; if the teacher attempts to incorporate every good point of style gained from observation of colleagues, then there will be little room left for the most important quality that the teacher possesses, namely individuality.

LECTURING AND STUDENT PARTICIPATION

Lecturing is often thought to be a one-way process, and this would seem to be the case when dealing with large groups of students. However, it is surprising just how much interaction can be generated in a lecture, provided that the teacher and the group have good rapport. The two following examples relate to human biology.

Lecturing by the 'structure and related function' approach

This approach involves an inductive style of lecturing, which draws out the students' existing knowledge and stimulates thinking skills. It has a certain crossword type of appeal and can be used to teach a topic for the first time, or for revision and consolidation prior to examinations.

Table 13.3 shows the basic matrix for this approach, which can be used to study any organ of the body. If the subject is being introduced to a class for the first time, then the teacher may wish to provide the information in a normal lecture manner for the column headed 'Structure'. The related functions can then be elicited from the students using inductive techniques and these functions can often be worked out even though the students have no prior knowledge of them. This has the effect of making the students discover, by reasoning, the related functions of an organ. These are written down in the 'Related function' column, opposite the structure to which they refer. Table 13.4 is an example that shows the matrix being applied to study of the heart. The section on macroscopic structure only has been completed to give the reader an idea of how the matrix works.

Table 13.3

Matrix for 'structure and related function' approach

	Structure	Related function
Organ		
Position and boundaries		
Macroscopic structure		
Microscopic structure		
Blood supply		
Lymphatics		
Nerve supply		
Anatomical relations		

Use of this approach is also beneficial to the teacher, as it quickly reveals any weaknesses in their own knowledge of the subject. It also provides a basis for the students' individual study of an organ. It can be varied by transposing the columns and asking the students to work out how the structure is designed to carry out each function. For example, the following questions might be asked during the study of the heart: 'What properties would you include in a design for the lining of the heart? What materials would you use?'.

	Structure	Related function
Macroscopic	MYOCARDIUM: middle layer of cardiac muscle; contains areas of specialized cardiac muscle	Acts as a syncytium, cells all contract as one; has property of myogenic rhythm
Microscopic	SINU-ATRIAL NODE: in right atrium, called pacemaker ATRIO-VENTRICULAR NODE: in right atrium; very small diameter fibres	Has fastest rate of self-excitation; initiates impulse. Delays passage of impulse down bundle until atria have contracted

Table 13.4

Section of completed matrix for heart

This will hopefully elicit such things as smoothness, anticoagulant properties and simple squamous epithelium.

Lecturing by the 'inductive build-up' approach

This is quite a useful approach, particularly for revision purposes, and is almost entirely done by inducing from the students their knowledge, except when the teacher has to clarify or correct a statement. This approach works quite well with the respiratory system to illustrate the sequence of events during respiration. The technique is similar, in that the students are invited to contribute their ideas about the sequence, commencing with the cells of the respiratory centre in the medulla responding to the level of carbonic acid in the blood perfusing them. Figure 13.1 shows this sequence as it might appear at the end of such a

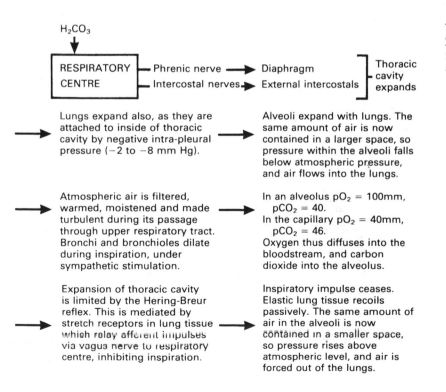

Figure 13.1

Sequence for 'inductive build-up approach' as applied to respiration session, on the chalkboard or flipchart. Again, I find that the fine detail helps to clarify any mistaken ideas. The fact that the bronchi and bronchioles dilate during inspiration and constrict during expiration provides the explanation as to why the patient with bronchial asthma has more difficulty breathing out than breathing in. The normal constriction during expiration is accentuated by the triad of spasm, oedema and secretion.

VARIANTS OF THE LECTURE

The standard format for the lecture is capable of many adaptations to suit the purposes of the teacher and three such variants will be discussed: demonstrations, team teaching and dialogue.

The demonstration

A demonstration can be defined as a visualized explanation of facts, concepts and procedures. The purposes of demonstration can be broadly classified into:

1. those designed to show the learner how to perform certain psycho-motor skills; and
2. those designed to show the learner why certain things occur.

In the former, the learner must reproduce exactly the behaviour that is demonstrated, whilst in the latter the behaviour is intended only as a strategy to aid the learner's understanding of a concept or principle. Each of these is now examined in turn.

Demonstrating a psycho-motor skill

In Chapter 4, the theory of skills acquisition was discussed, so we will bear these principles in mind when planning a demonstration. Table 13.5 gives a checklist for giving a demonstration.

Commentary on Table 13.5

It is good practice actually to put the sub-skills on the chalkboard in the correct sequence, so this can serve as a guide when the learner is prac-tising the skill. Whatever the purpose of the demonstration, it is impera-tive that each learner can see what is going on, and this implies very careful arrangement of the room and the lighting. Provision of seating is often considered unnecessary when giving a demonstration, but the students should be comfortable, so that they can give maximum concen-tration to the demonstration.

If closed-circuit television is available, it can provide a valuable addition to the demonstration, in that the camera can be placed so that it 'shoots' over the shoulder of the teacher, giving a 'demonstrator's-eye view' of the skill.

A full-speed total demonstration of the skill, at the commencement of the demonstration, gives the learner an overall 'Gestalt' of the form of the total skill. If the teacher has not demonstrated the skill in class

Table 13.5

Checklist for giving a demonstration

Before the demonstration
1. Formulate the learning outcomes
2. Perform a skills analysis and determine the sequence
3. Assess entry behaviours of students, and determine prerequisites
4. Formulate the teaching plan, with particular reference to:
   (a) ensuring optimum visibility, and
   (b) preparation of all materials

During the demonstration
5. State the learning outcomes to the students
6. Motivate them by explaining why the skill is important
7. Demonstrate the total skill at normal speed
8. Write the sequence of part-skills on the chalkboard or overhead projector, as a checklist for the step-by-step demonstration
9. Demonstrate each part-skill slowly, in the correct sequence
10. Obtain feedback by questioning and observation of non-verbal behaviour
11. Avoid the use of negative examples and variations in technique

After the demonstration
12. Provide immediate supervised practice, with adequate time allowance
13. Provide verbal, rather than physical, guidance
14. Make the environment psychologically safe by providing a friendly atmosphere and constructive criticism
15. Remember that initial interest may wane, so provide motivation and encouragement
16. Remember that students will acquire the skill at different rates, so individualize the planning to cater for the fast and slow learner

before, or not for some time perhaps, then he or she is well-advised to practise the skill a day or so before the class is due. This will have benefits not only from the point of view of the skill itself, but also from the timing. Some teachers like to teach a skill using examples of how not to do it, and others like to include one or two variations of the technique. A common example of this is aseptic technique, which has permissible variations within a framework of principles. However, when teaching a new skill, most authorities would agree that learning is facilitated by teaching only one method of performing the skill and omitting any negative examples. This will minimize the effects of psychological interference that would otherwise arise due to the similarity between the original material and the variations or negative examples. Of course, once the learner has become proficient in the skill, then interference from other techniques is unimportant.

It is crucial to formulate the objectives and prerequisites before commencing the lesson plan, just as in preparing any kind of lesson. As is seen in Chapter 16, the skills analysis will provide a detailed breakdown of the types of behaviour that constitute the total skill and these must then be set out in the correct sequence. This is a very important step, as it is not always appreciated that the learner must not only remember the techniques for each sub-skill, but also the correct sequence of these.

The single most important aspect of the demonstration of a psychomotor skill is the provision of immediate practice for the students. A demonstration can only provide information about the cognitive and affective aspects and the psychomotor components must be learned through the students' own muscles, by practice. It is often tempting, when teaching a skill in a clinical setting, to take over from the student in order to 'show' how to do it. Of course, this is quite valid if the student is unsure of the correct technique, but generally speaking, he or she must be allowed to learn the skill by doing it themselves. It is thus that students receive the proprioceptive feedback from their own muscles and joints, which in turn modify their performance. No amount of 'showing' by the teacher will provide the necessary kinaesthetic feedback, without which no skill can be learned. Learning a skill can be frustrating and tiring, so it is essential that the atmosphere is friendly and relaxed. Testiness on the part of the teacher will only lead to tension in the students and this in turn will lead to poor performance and increase in errors. This is why it is so important to allow sufficient time for practice and to bear in mind that not all students will master a skill at the same rate. In this kind of situation, competition between students can be quite counter-productive, so the teacher needs to emphasize that individuals differ in their rates of learning and that it does not matter if some people acquire a particular skill more quickly than others. What is important is that every student actually acquires the skill, not the speed of acquisition.

Demonstrating a principle or concept

Let us take as an example the concept of osmosis, a fundamental concept in medical science, which is readily demonstrated by a simple experiment using two glass beakers, each containing a piece of raw potato. The first jar is filled with plain water and the second with water containing a tablespoonful of salt. After several hours, the potato in the beaker of salt water is seen to be shrivelled and dried up, whilst the potato in the first one remains much the same. If teaching the concept of osmosis in a deductive fashion, then the teacher would first explain and define the term and give examples from human physiology. The demonstration could then follow, as a further example. In the inductive method, however, the demonstration would be presented first and the students put into groups to decide how the findings could be explained. Hopefully, they would arrive at a definition of the phenomenon of osmosis having explored the possibilities.

Team teaching

A classic definition of team teaching is that of Shaplin and Olds (1964):

> *'an instructional organization in which two or more teachers are given responsibility, working together, for all or a significant part of the instruction of the same group of students'.*

There is often a measure of confusion with regard to the exact meaning of the term and many people claim to be using team teaching when the nurse teachers simply work in one or two teams within a department. However, within these teams, the individual teacher plans and delivers the teaching of a particular area, such as orthopaedic nursing, whilst another does likewise for paediatric nursing and so on. There is not necessarily a sharing of planning or of delivery, each one doing the preparation and teaching of his or her own area. In team teaching, on the other hand, the team actually plans each session together and also does the teaching together for a particular group of students. The methods of teaching are decided by the team and the lecture method can be employed to good effect here.

Organization of team teaching

For team teaching to be a viable proposition, there are some necessary prerequisites. At least two teachers who share a common interest in trying out new ideas are required. They should be people who do not feel threatened by a close working relationship with their colleagues and should be prepared to have their ideas criticized or questioned. It is probably wise to introduce team teaching into just one area of a given module initially, taking care to evaluate the effectiveness before enlarging the use of it. The key to successful team teaching lies in two areas, the interpersonal relationships of the team members and the quality of the planning. If these two aspects are good, then the presentation of the lessons will be very effective. There is considerable planning required for team teaching and this in turn makes large demands on the time of the teachers involved. Each lesson in the team-teaching situation must be planned by every member of the team, as each will normally be involved in its presentation. Without this careful, co-operative planning, the sessions will lack polish and convey an impression of disorganization to the students. During the planning stage such issues as the learning outcomes, teaching methods and evaluation are aired within the team and each member may question and argue the merits of a particular approach. It may not be necessary to have a leader in a teaching team, as then each member is free to be as creative as he or she wants to be. The actual lecture plan is best done in the form of a script to ensure that each team member knows exactly which area and at what time their contribution occurs, although experienced team teachers learn to 'freewheel' very much with each other.

Implementing team teaching

Team teaching can be a very exciting experience for students, provided that the team can create the right level of relaxation and confidence with each other. During ordinary lectures, some students soon lose their concentration and attention wanders; team teaching can provide the necessary change of stimulus that will maintain their interest, particularly if the interchange between teachers is relatively frequent. When it works well, team teaching can provide much more stimulation and variety than an ordinary lecture, because each teacher can act as critic or evaluator of the other's points of view. Obviously, this needs great psychological safety if threat is to be avoided, but here again, the quality of interpersonal relationships between team members is the crucial factor for success.

Team teaching does, of course, increase the resource requirements, since there are two or more teachers occupied in doing what one teacher might normally undertake. This extra resource demand needs to be carefully evaluated, but not dismissed out of hand as being impractical; the use of team teaching may make more effective use of time, thereby reducing the total amount of teaching time required in a particular course component. In addition, team teaching can also act as valuable staff development, in that teachers are in a position to work together and evaluate their teaching in a way that cannot happen in the ordinary course of events. It still seems rare for teachers to sit-in on other colleagues' lectures, so it might be that team teaching has hidden extras that help to compensate for the additional resource demands.

Dialogue

This variant of the lecture is not common in higher education. The principle of dialogue is that two teachers or colleagues either in nursing, or with health-related interests, sit together in a lecture-type situation with an audience. The two participants agree in advance what the topic for discussion will be and they then spend the time in the lecture engaging in a dialogue about the issues in question. This type of activity is very familiar to television audiences, since it is a common technique for raising people's awareness of particular issues. Two leading personalities from some walk of life engage in dialogue about an issue and there may or may not be a chairperson.

This technique of dialogue can be very useful for value-laden issues and can involve such personnel as a chaplain, a service manager and indeed, any two persons with views on a particular issue. The audience is not normally involved in the dialogue, but are privy to the thinking and argument of the two participants. Since lectures are not very useful for generating changes in attitude or for dealing with issues involving the affective domain, it would seem that dialogue could be a useful way of raising students' awareness and feelings about issues in nursing and health care.

REFERENCES

Ausubel, D., Novak, I. and Hanesian, H. (1978) *Educational Psychology; A Cognitive View*, Holt, Rinehart and Winston, New York.
Bligh, D. (1998) *What's The Use of Lectures?*, 5th edn, Intellect, Exeter.
Shaplin, J. and Olds, H. (1964) *Team Teaching*, Harper and Row, New York.

SMALL GROUP TEACHING AND EXPERIENTIAL LEARNING

14

The juxtaposition of small group teaching and experiential learning within this chapter is no coincidence. These two educational strategies are very much inter-related and inter-dependent, but it is useful to identify the characteristics of each before going on to explore them in more detail.

SMALL GROUP TEACHING

The term *small group* is difficult to define. Brown (1996) emphasizes the importance of context in defining what constitutes a small group, i.e. the term can apply equally to three or four students working on a project, or the subdividing of a large lecture group into small groups of twenty or more.

Group size

Clearly, the size of the group will have an effect on the processes occurring within it, particularly with regard to the amount of face-to-face interaction with other group members. With numbers greater than about 25, this becomes impossible and subgroups have to be formed in order to allow for it.

Group size has another important bearing on learning: the larger the group, the less time each individual member will have available for contribution. Let us take a typical one-hour group session; if there are 30 students, each will have a maximum possible contribution time of two minutes: with a group of only ten students, the individual contribution time becomes six minutes. If we assume that not all students contribute to the same extent, it becomes quite probable that certain students will gain at the expense of others; it is interesting to note that none of the above timings include any input from the teacher and the more the teacher becomes involved, the less time there is for student participation.

Purpose of small groups

The concept of a small group is not defined solely by the numbers of students involved; it also includes the purpose of the group. Broadly speaking, the function of an educational small group is to put the student at the centre of things; to allow opportunities for face-to-face interaction with other group members in order to exchange ideas and feelings; to be challenged by other people's viewpoints – in short, to expand the student's universe of awareness. Brown (1996) suggests that working in small groups can help students to develop interactive and collaborative skills that are necessary for employment and research.

For many teachers, small group teaching is the essence of education, providing them with the opportunity for more intimate and rewarding engagements with students than is possible in lectures. The term small group teaching covers a very wide range of strategies and techniques and is one of the main ways in which students learn from and through experience.

EXPERIENTIAL LEARNING

Although experiential learning is not confined to a single teaching or learning method, small group strategies do provide a major vehicle for many aspects of it. Hence the inclusion of both strategies in this chapter.

David Kolb's theory of experiential learning was discussed in Chapter 3 (p. 62), so the present chapter will focus on more practical aspects of experiential learning. At its simplest, experiential learning is learning that results from experience, but since almost everything in life constitutes experience, this becomes an impossibly global notion. Essentially, experiential learning is learning by doing, rather than by listening to other people or reading about it. This active involvement of the student is one of the key characteristics of this form of learning, together with student-centredness, a degree of interaction, some measure of autonomy and flexibility and a high degree of relevance.

Kolb (1984) identifies the characteristics of experiential learning:

1. Learning is best conceived as a process, not in terms of outcomes.
2. Learning is a continuous process grounded in experience.
3. The process of learning requires the resolution of conflicts between dialectically opposed modes of adaptation to the world.
4. Learning is an holistic process of adaptation to the world.
5. Learning involves transactions between the person and the environment.
6. Learning is the process of creating knowledge.

From these key characteristics, Kolb offers a working definition of learning:

'Learning is the process whereby knowledge is created through the transformation of experience' (Kolb 1984, p. 38).

The term *experiential learning* is used in a number of ways in education; some apply it specifically to the learning of 'interpersonal skills', whilst others see it as pertaining to 'field placements' away from the educational institution. It is useful to distinguish between learning *from* experience and learning *through* experience (Burnard, 1990). The former involves utilizing past experiences to gain new insights, whereas the latter consists of deliberately planned experiences to facilitate learning. In other words, both 'there and then' and 'here and now' experiences can be useful learning stimuli.

Burnard (1991) describes a study in which nurse teachers were interviewed about their perceptions of experiential learning and experiential learning methods. The range of definitions given by respondents was quite wide-ranging, and included:

- tautological definitions (experiential learning is learning from experience);
- all-encompassing definitions (any activity could be experiential);
- time-related definitions (learning from the past and the present);
- practical definitions (learning from clinical placements);
- personally focused definitions (gaining awareness); and
- contrast-with-tradition definitions (less cognitive input).

Although the study used a very small sample, the results graphically illustrate the wide range of perceptions that these nurse teachers have about the concept.

Experiential learning as therapy

In Burnard's study, one of the respondents suggested that for him experiential learning was more like doing therapy, and this view is supported by Rogers (1983) and Heron (1986). It is important, however, that nurse teachers are fully aware of the problems associated with the blending of teaching and therapy. The primary objective of an educational group is the learning of particular aspects of the curriculum, whereas the purpose of a therapeutic group is helping group members to 'heal' themselves in a therapeutic setting. Although it is important for students to understand the working of therapeutic groups, the teacher must be careful to avoid running educational groups as therapeutic groups, since there are ethical and moral implications such as informed consent of students.

Experiential learning: cross-references to other chapters

Experiential learning is a very pervasive strategy in education, and is addressed in some detail in Chapter 16, Teaching in Clinical and Community Settings, and Chapter 18, Teaching Interpersonal Communication Skills.

GROUP DYNAMICS

Whatever the nature of the group, there are a number of fundamental processes that are identifiable and a knowledge of these will help the nurse teacher to understand the dynamics of a given group.

Social roles

In any given group, there are many social positions called social roles; the family has roles called 'father' and 'mother', nurse education has roles called 'teacher' and 'student' and the individual 'in his time plays many parts'. A number of roles are played concurrently, as with a post-registration student who is also a ward manager; others are played sequentially as with the roles of child, adolescent, adult and elderly person.

Types of role

It is useful to differentiate between *ascribed* roles and *achieved* roles in society; the former are roles that cannot be altered without difficulty, such as sex roles and social class and the latter are roles that are achieved by the individual's own volition, such as the roles of husband, engineer and so on. Primary roles are those that are always played, i.e. sex roles and social class; *secondary roles* are linked to economic awareness and employment and *tertiary roles* are occasional ones such as 'captain of the local netball team'.

Group norms

Group norms are defined as required or expected behaviours and beliefs of group members, which may be covert or overt. *Covert* or *implicit* norms are usually typified by the phrase 'it just isn't done', whereas *overt* norms are usually formulated as explicit rules of behaviour. In nursing, there are explicit rules about the way in which uniform is worn, but in clinical settings, there may be implicit norms such as, 'The ward manager likes it done this way'. It could be argued that norms are simply roles that are applied to all group members rather than to different concepts.

Both roles and norms may be considered as either imposed or emergent. *Imposed* roles are those that arise from outside the group, such as the appointment of a new head of department; *emergent* roles are those arising from within a group, such as the election of a chair-person. Norms may also arise from outside the group as when a nurse teacher lays down the rules for conduct in a small group session. Alternatively, the group may itself develop norms for behaviour and these are often termed *group rules*.

Group conformity and decision making

The notion of group conformity has attracted considerable attention by researchers over the years and there are a number of classic experiments in this area of social psychology.

Sherif's work

Sherif (1935) used an optical illusion known as the 'autokinetic effect' to study conformity in groups; this effect occurs when a stationary point of light is viewed against a dark background and appears to move. Subjects were asked to judge the amount of movement of the point of light in two experimental conditions; one group made individual estimates and then came together as a group and the other group did this in the opposite way by making a group decision first and then making individual estimates. In both conditions, subject's individual judgements were influenced by the group norm for the amount of movement.

Asch's work

Asch (1956) studied conformity by using experiments that required subjects to judge the lengths of lines in comparison to a line of standard length. Subjects were seated in front of a screen and shown the standard line alongside three comparison lines and they had to say out loud which line was equal to the standard one. In reality, only one of the subjects was genuine, the remainder being confederates of the experimenter and these confederates all gave responses that were obviously wrong. About one-third of the genuine subjects gave judgements that were wrong, despite the evidence of their own eyes.

These two studies show that group pressure is a powerful agent for conformity, although one could argue that the Asch study shows that two-thirds of the subjects did not conform to group norms. It could also be said that the Asch experiment dealt with physical judgements, whereas normal social interaction is concerned very much more with social judgements, where there is no objective criteria for judgement.

It is useful to ask why subjects conform to a majority judgement; the prevailing notion has been that subjects fear rejection by the group if they deviate from the group norms, whereas conformity leads to rewards. This notion has been criticized as being too simplistic by Eiser (1980). He cites several studies that indicate that a consistent minority can influence the majority of a group to alter its position. Eiser argues that individuals may want to differentiate themselves in a group and that in certain circumstances, such innovation may be valued by the group if it leads to useful new directions.

Risky shift phenomenon

Another phenomenon of group decision making is that known as the 'risky shift'; groups who have to make decisions that involve risks tend to take riskier decisions as a group than when making individual decisions (Wallach and Kogan, 1965). This is explained by the notion of diffusion of responsibility, where individual responsibility for failure is diffused throughout the group, resulting in a feeling of less personal responsibility.

Diffusion of responsibility

Diffusion of responsibility was investigated by Latane and Darley (1968) who studied bystander intervention. Subjects were given questions to fill in purporting to be a consumer survey and were seated in a room either alone or with someone else. A simulated emergency was enacted in an adjoining room and the time subjects took to respond to this was measured. There were four experimental conditions in this study, the subject being either alone, with a friend, with a stranger or with a confederate of the experimenter. Results showed that subjects were much more likely to respond when alone than when with someone else, particularly a stranger. Again, responsibility for intervention is said to be diffused between two people and this has the effect of inhibiting social behaviour. Diffusion of responsibility may also explain the phenomenon called 'social loafing', where the output of individuals may reduce when he or she is part of a group, particularly if the individual contributions cannot be easily measured, as in clapping or pushing a car.

Social facilitation and inhibition

The presence of others can be either inhibiting or facilitating, depending upon the nature of the task. *Audience effects* is the term given to the effects on an individual's performance of having other people observing it, whereas *coaction effects* are those that result from other people actually performing alongside the individual in question. Coaction effects are very much in evidence in athletics, where pacemakers help athletes to increase their performance.

Bond and Titus (1983), reviewing a large number of studies on social facilitation, consider that task complexity is the main determinant of social facilitation. The presence of others has a facilitating effect on both speed and accuracy of performance with simple tasks, but decreases them when the task is complex.

Tajfel (1978) suggests that an individual's commitment to a group depends upon the contribution it makes to his or her sense of *positive social identity*. If it fails to provide this, the individual has several options:

1. He or she may leave the group, but this may not be possible if there are pressing reasons for remaining, such as employment or important values associated with membership.
2. He or she may remain as a group member but try to improve the status of the group by some means or other.
3. He or she may attempt to justify the undesirable features of the group to make them acceptable.

An example might be useful here to help in understanding Tajfel's notion. Let us take a trained nurse who entered nursing some years ago because he or she always wanted to be a nurse. Lately, this nurse may have felt that nursing had lost a lot of its standing as a desirable social role in comparison with other professions such as teaching or social work. According to Tajfel's proposal, the nurse would have three options. Option 1 would be to leave nursing, but in the present climate of unemployment this may not be wise. Option 2 could lead the nurse to become an advocate for evidence-based practice, which emphasizes the scientific nature of nursing practice, and hence raise its perceived status. Option 3 could lead the nurse to attempt to justify the fall in status by attributing it to the growth of materialism in society and the lack of personal commitment to caring in young people nowadays.

Communication and interaction in groups

The study of communication and interaction in groups has tended to fall into two distinct types of approach: those in which the pattern of communication is under the control of the experimenter, and those in which the natural pattern occurring during group interaction is observed.

Experimenter-controlled communication

These studies involve small numbers of subjects who work on a task, each of whom has an item of information necessary for successful completion of the task in question. Hence, subjects must pool their information and these experimental studies seek to explain which patterns of communication facilitate completion of the task (Bavelas, 1948; Leavitt, 1951; Mulder, 1960). Subjects were organized into four different patterns of communication as shown in Figure 14.1 and could only communicate directly with those subjects with whom they were connected.

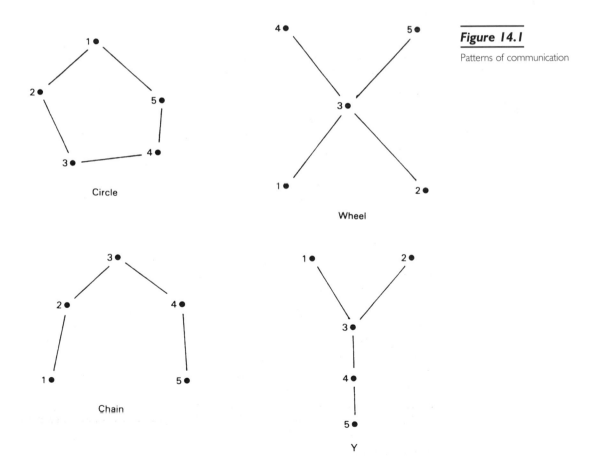

Figure 14.1

Patterns of communication

It can be seen that in each pattern there are differences in the number of other people that any particular subject has to go through in order to communicate with other members. In the chain, for example, subject number one has to relay their message through three people if he or she wishes to communicate with subject number five. In the circle, subject number one can communicate directly with both number five and number two; in the 'Y' pattern and the wheel, subject number three occupies a key position, which is often identified as leader. The speed of problem solving was faster in the 'Y' pattern and the wheel, but as the really interesting role was performed largely by subject number three, peripheral members experienced less enjoyment than subjects in the circle.

Communication in natural group settings

A number of researchers have investigated groups interacting in a natural group setting, the best-known example being that of Bales (1950). He observed groups working in committees and classified the contributions of individual members into twelve main categories, as shown in Table 14.1.

Table 14.1

Bales' interaction process analysis

Reactions	Task area		Problems
Attempted answers	4.	Gives suggestions, direction, implying autonomy for others	Control, evaluation, orientation
	5.	Gives opinion, evaluation, analysis, expresses feeling, wish	
	6.	Gives orientation, information, repetition, confirmation	
Questions	7.	Asks for orientation, information, repetition, confirmation	Orientation, evaluation, control
	8.	Asks for opinion, evaluation, analysis, expression of feeling	
	9.	Asks for suggestion, direction, possible ways of action	
	Social-emotional area		
Positive	1.	Shows solidarity, raises others' status, gives help, reward	Reintegration, tension-management, decision
	2.	Shows tension release, jokes, laughs, shows satisfaction	
	3.	Agrees, shows passive acceptance, understands, concurs, complies	
Negative	10.	Disagrees, shows passive rejection, formality, withholds help	Decision, tension-reduction, reintegration
	11.	Shows tension, asks for help, withdraws out of field	
	12.	Shows antagonism, deflates others' status, defends or asserts self	

These contributions are divided into two major areas, those concerned with the task in question and those termed social-emotional reactions, the latter being either positive or negative. Bales' system provides a method for analysing the working of a group in a systematic way.

Lawrence (1986) suggests that small groups develop through the following processes:

- forming;
- storming;
- norming;
- performing;
- informing.

The first stage refers to individual commitments to the group, whilst storming refers to the stage of conflict and hostility within the group. This is followed by the stage of norming, in which the emphasis is on interaction and harmonious relationships. The performing stage is concerned with pursuance of the goals of the group and this is followed by informing, which involves the development of systems for communicating with other groups.

Sociometry

Sociometry, as the name implies, is concerned with the measurement of social relationships within groups and its principal tool is the sociogram. Each group member is asked a question about which other group members they would like to work with in a given situation, or which members they would not wish to work with. The members' choices are plotted in the form of a sociogram, as illustrated in Figure 14.2.

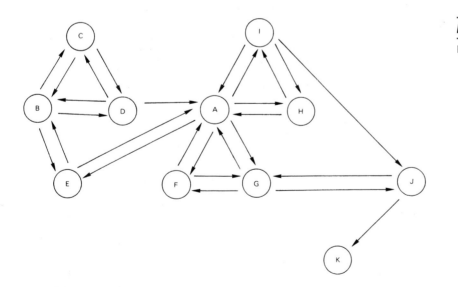

Figure 14.2

Example of a sociogram

Each student is represented by a letter (A–K) and the arrows drawn joining the letters indicate the direction of choice for each of the eleven students.

Structures

There are a number of typical structures revealed by a sociogram: the most popular student (A) – who receives six out of the eleven choices – is called the 'star'; other typical structures shown are 'mutual pairs', 'triangles' and 'chains'. It may also be possible to identify an 'isolate', who is not chosen by anyone, or who decides not to make choices.

Target sociogram

An alternative way of plotting a sociogram is to use a target sociogram, as shown in Figure 14.3. The most popular students are placed in the innermost circles and the least popular in the outermost ones, giving a clear indication of choices. Sociometry has a number of advantages:

1. sociograms show relationships from the group members' point of view;
2. choices are uninfluenced by the teacher/experimenter;
3. sociograms can show subgroupings in classes; and
4. sociograms are easy to collect, either in writing or verbally.

Figure 14.3

Target sociogram

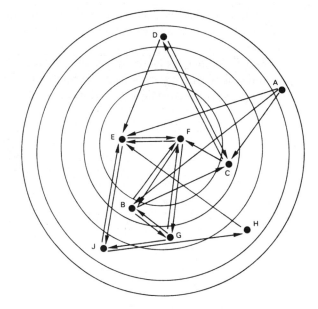

There are some disadvantages, however, that need to be borne in mind; many teachers may find the notion ethically unacceptable to use with students, particularly if 'social engineering' is used on the basis of data from sociometry. Intermediate relationships are not indicated, giving a rather 'black-and-white' picture of the relationships in the group. The actual design of the sociogram depends as much on artistic talent as on rational rules, so that two sociograms from the same data may give quite different impressions. Also, for groups of more than about 15, sociograms become impossibly complex.

Another way in which sociometric data can be analysed is by use of sociometric indices, and these can be of use when comparing the same individual in a variety of groups. Sociometric indices reduce the great amount of visual detail in a sociogram into relatively simple numerical values that allow comparison. The following are examples of indices.

1. Individual's choice status (CSi):

   CSi = (Number of persons choosing i) / N–1

2. Individual's rejection status (RSi):

   RSi = (Number of persons rejecting i) / N–1

3. Group cohesion (CO):

   CO = (Number of mutual pairs) / (Possible number of mutual pairs)

The use of indices may give the impression that sociometry is an 'exact science', whereas the reliability of positive choices leaves much to be desired (Harper, 1968). The validity is also questionable, in that choices may reflect the day-to-day changes rather than deep group structure. Perhaps the old maxim about 'analysing data with a microscope that was gathered with a rake' needs to be borne in mind when considering sociometric indices!

Area	Examples
Intellectual	Trying out ideas for size Clearing up misunderstandings Clarifying issues Follow-up of key lectures Development of critical, logical thinking Solving problems Examining evidence and assumptions Applying theory to practice
Affective	Self-evaluation Personal development and confidence Tolerance of ambiguity Motivation Attitude change
Social	Awareness of other people's strengths and weaknesses Sensitivity to others Identification with a group Group cohesion Ability to listen to others Tolerance of opposing viewpoints Independence Closer teacher–student relationships
Expressive	Developing power of expression Developing public-speaking skills Ability to formulate an argument Ability to engage in debate
Experiential	Participating in experiential activities Reflecting upon experiences Analysing the implications of the experience

Table 14.2

Aims and purposes of educational small groups

AIMS AND PURPOSES OF EDUCATIONAL SMALL GROUPS

There are many aims or purposes of small group teaching in education; the main ones are outlined in Table 14.2.

It can be seen that the use of small group teaching has benefits not only in terms of academic learning, but in the development of social skills and confidence in the presence of other people. In nursing, these social skills are vital to the proper functioning of the practitioner and the expressive skills that small group work generates can make a significant contribution to the political dimension of the profession by ensuring that nurses can argue effectively from their unique perspective.

REFLECTION IN SMALL GROUP AND EXPERIENTIAL LEARNING

One of the most useful strategies for learning in small groups or experiential learning is reflection, and the teacher can assist the student in this process by using a model devised to promote reflection (Boud *et al.*, 1985). The model consists of a series of stages through which the student nurse should progress, having completed an experience. For example, the student may have completed the admission of a patient for surgery, and some time later takes time to reflect on this using the following stages.

1. *Returning to the experience.* During this first stage the student is encouraged to simply 'replay' the whole experience over again, describing what happened but not judging it.
2. *Attending to feelings.* The aim of this stage is to put students in touch with their own feelings about the experience. They should try to utilize any positive feelings they may have about it, such as the pleasure felt by making the patient feel welcomed and reassured. Some feelings can actually form barriers to learning, so these need to be removed by such means as laughing about an embarrassing question inadvertently asked during the admission, or by expressing feelings to another person. This removal of obstructing feelings is vital if learning is to take place.
3. *Re-evaluating the experience.* This final stage consists of a number of substages, which in essence involve the students in associating the experience with their existing ideas and feelings about admission, and in testing for consistency between them.

This model of reflection needs to be practised until the students feels comfortable with each stage and this is best accomplished by sharing the reflections with other students.

PLANNING AND IMPLEMENTING SMALL GROUP AND EXPERIENTIAL LEARNING

Small group teaching and experiential learning is more challenging than many teachers realize, so it is essential to plan carefully for its implementation.

The experiential taxonomy

A helpful framework for planning and implementing small group and experiential learning is that of Steinaker and Bell (1979). They describe an experiential taxonomy that can be used as the basis for writing learning outcomes for all kinds of small group teaching and learning. The taxonomy can be used for a single lesson or for a complete curriculum course. The taxonomy is shown in Table 14.3, and Table 14.4 shows two applications to nursing for each of the main categories.

Taxonomic level	Description
1.0 Exposure	Consciousness of an experience
2.0 Participation	Deciding to become part of an experience
3.0 Identification	Union of the learner with what is to be learned
4.0 Internalization	Experience continues to influence lifestyle
5.0 Dissemination	Attempt to influence others

Table 14.3

The experiential taxonomy (Steinaker and Bell, 1979)

Taxonomic level		Nursing applications
1.0 Exposure	(i)	I see an injection given
	(ii)	I hear about Orem's self-care model
2.0 Participation	(i)	I administer an injection
	(ii)	I attempt to use Orem's self-care model
3.0 Identification	(i)	I become competent in giving injections
	(ii)	I become adept at using Orem's self-care model
4.0 Internalization	(i)	Giving injections is now part of my life
	(ii)	Orem's self-care model is now part of my life
5.0 Dissemination	(i)	I teach other students to give injections
	(ii)	I show other students how to use Orem's self-care model

Table 14.4

Nursing applications of experiential taxonomy

The physical environment

As with all learning settings, the physical environment should be as pleasant and comfortable as the facilities allow. It is useful if particular rooms are designated as discussion rooms so that students associate them with democratic participation and equality. The main aspect of the physical environment, though, is the arrangement of seating (and desks if used). Some people feel that small group methods are best when students are seated without desks, as this lends an air of informality to the group. Certain students, however, prefer to have a surface upon which they can jot down key thoughts, especially when the group is working on a specific task that requires writing.

A good rule of thumb is to ensure that whether desks are used or not, every group member has the same facility, including the teacher. It is common to see a group of students sitting in a circle without desks, with a teacher firmly ensconced behind one; this inequality may serve to

Figure 14.4

Seating patterns for small group teaching

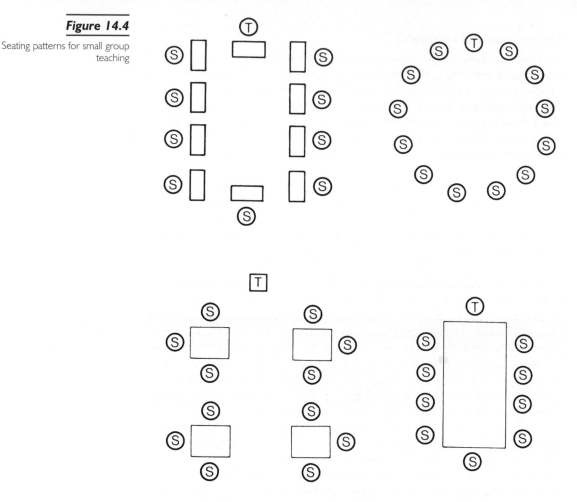

highlight the differences in status between teacher and students to the detriment of group effectiveness. There is a variety of arrangements for seating during group work, some of the common ones being illustrated in Figure 14.4:

1. The 'U' arrangement is useful for teacher-led discussion, as each member can be seen clearly and, equally, the students can see any material the teacher may want to show to them.
2. The circle, with or without desks conveys a sense of equality amongst all members of the group; it is particularly intimate when chairs alone are used and even a group of 15 can create a feeling of close personal contact.
3. The idea of a number of 'horseshoes', each consisting of a table around which three students are seated, can provide a very effective way of breaking larger groups into subgroups. The seating arrangement ensures that each student can see the teacher during plenary periods, but each 'horseshoe' can work independently with its members on some aspect of a topic or problem.

This arrangement can also capitalize on shortage of space, where a large circle is not feasible.

4. The 'committee' arrangement is a useful one for small groupwork that has more formal purposes, providing a large surface, in the form of a central table, around which each member is seated. Although each member can engage in eye contact with the rest of the group, the shape of the table can make a big difference to the pattern of interaction. A rectangular table has a natural 'head' at either end, and students occupying these may be seen as the leader or chairperson, whereas a round table has no such natural positions of power. A rectangular table has corners and students occupying these seats tend to make the least contribution to discussions; people generally interact most with those sitting diametrically opposite, again this being more obvious in a rectangle than a circle.

Re-arranging seating

One of the common errors that inexperienced teachers make is to rearrange seating in the classroom without adequate explanation to the group. Students of all ages tend to be quite sensitive about their personal seat and usually sit in the same place for all sessions. If they suddenly find that the seating arrangements have been altered they may become resentful; indeed, many an unwitting student teacher has entered a classroom only to find that their carefully planned seating arrangement has been returned to its normal state by the students.

The emotive nature of seating positions is such that the teacher must ensure full and adequate explanation as to why he or she is wishing to rearrange it. A few minutes spent in explaining one's philosophy of teaching and the importance of the students' contributions can save a great deal of trouble later on by giving students rational, sincere reasons for such a rearrangement. Students are usually tolerant of such innovations, provided they have been consulted before it is implemented. If a group is particularly resistant to rearrangement, it may be wise to leave the seating as it is, but to use a small group activity early in the lesson that requires students to interact with others. This will encourage natural pairing and movement, which can be capitalized on for the remainder of the session.

Psychological environment

The ideal environment for small group and experiential learning is that which is termed a 'learning community'. This is characterized by a climate of acceptance, support and trust, where each member of the team acknowledges that he or she is still learning and where the needs of students are recognized. This notion of a learning community can apply to both the higher education institution and the clinical or community area, and contains an implicit value judgement that students are equal to trained staff in all respects other than those of age and experience. In a learning-community approach, opportunities for learning are made available and professional growth is encouraged by graded responsibility. A large element of negotiation is typical of this approach, where students can determine what they want to learn and the means by which this will be achieved and evaluated.

Establishing trust

The establishment of trust among group members is fundamental to successful small group and experiential learning. The length of time the small group is likely to be together is an important factor. For example, small group techniques may be used on a study day, and in this short timescale it would be impossible to develop group identity. On a programme of study, on the other hand, small groups may well remain together for months or years, and it is therefore crucial that the group is given the time and opportunity to foster interpersonal relationships and trust. This means that the teacher must avoid the temptation of setting the group tasks and issues too early. Taking time to facilitate group cohesion will pay dividends later on when the group is able to work effectively without interpersonal conflict and competition.

TECHNIQUES FOR FOSTERING RELATIONSHIPS IN SMALL GROUPS

There are a great many ways in which small groups can be made aware of individual members.

Pairs exercises

One technique is a pairs exercise which aims for maximum interaction. Group members are asked to form pairs, choosing someone they do not know. Each member spends two minutes introducing himself to the other. After this, group members are asked to find another partner whom they do not know, and spend two minutes each on explaining what they hope to gain from the group membership. This pairing continues until all the group has met each other, using topics such as 'My feelings about small group work', 'Problems in my current job', etc.

In another example, group members are asked to form pairs, and each member must choose a character from literature, theatre, films or television whom they would most like to be. They must explain the reason for their choice, taking up to two minutes to do this.

Developing trust

When members of a small group trust each other, they are able to contribute without fear of being ridiculed if their suggestion seems wrong; indeed, such suggestions may be seen as creative rather than stupid and may lead the group into a new direction. Students need to be able to try out their ideas, and this can only be encouraged in an atmosphere of psychological safety. Where there is trust in a group, each student is free to concentrate his or her energies on learning, rather than wasting them on building up defensive barriers against attacks from other group members. Trust may be developed using techniques which involve the group members in such activities as being led around the room blindfold. Other examples are given in Chapter 18. Yet another important way in which trust can be developed is the use of group evaluation at the end of each session. The group is asked to allow five minutes at the end for some spontaneous evaluation of the group's performance.

Participation of the teacher

There are many roles that the teacher can adopt in small group work; he or she may function as the leader, taking the major responsibility for the conduct of the group, or alternatively, adopt varying degrees of involvement, such as facilitator, resource person and group trainer.

The presence of the teacher is more likely to influence a very small group, but be less obtrusive in a larger group. Indeed, the teacher may decide to leave the group entirely on their own during group work, but being available close by, but out of sight, should the group feel they need assistance. If the teacher decides to be involved in the group, there is always the danger that they will see the teacher as the leader, even if the position has been made clear that the teacher's function is as facilitator only.

Establishing the right climate

The teacher's role is invested with authority and it is difficult for students to overcome this barrier. Compare the interaction of a group of student nurses talking in the local pub and their contributions in a small group learning session. It is obvious that lack of knowledge or interest is not the main factor for the poor response so commonly found in group work; rather, it is the climate of the situation that determines how well students involve themselves in discussions. Presumably, in the local pub there is no danger of humiliation from other people, since it is generally accepted that individuals have the right to express their opinions, however unusual these might be. In addition, the group in the pub are usually friends and a degree of trust is present, which adds to the climate of psychological safety. If this atmosphere can be captured during group work in the college of nursing, then there would be fewer problems of participation. Very often it is the teacher's own anxiety that stifles the spontaneous flow of ideas and opinions; the teacher must learn to trust the group to control their own discussion to a large extent, even if he or she is acting as their leader. If the teacher leads the group, then it is vital that he or she avoids evaluating the members, since they may become hesitant about giving their own opinions.

Importance of organization

Many of the dissatisfactions that are experienced with the use of small groups stem from the fact that they have not been properly organized. Because a small group is informal does not mean that it can be conducted in an off-the-cuff manner, and it is sensible to indicate to the students the goals to be achieved and the roles they must assume during the discussion. Each member must be prepared to contribute something to the group, and the importance of this should be explained at the first meeting. The teacher must be aware of attempts to participate by members and, if these are unsuccessful, should assist. A careful watch of non-verbal communication will provide good feedback as to how the students are feeling, and will also reveal such non-productive behaviour as opting out, dominating and seeking sympathy.

Styles of small group teaching

It is possible to identify four styles that the teacher might adopt during small group teaching (Royal College of General Practitioners, 1986):

1. *The authoritarian style.* This style is one in which the teacher is seen as the authority – telling the students what is important and asking questions, largely to clarify whether they understand. There is no place for dissent or argument; the teacher's view is the correct one.

2. *The Socratic style.* This ancient style relies on a question-and-answer technique, with the teacher asking questions and the student answering them. The teacher's questions are not random, but are used to elicit what the student knows, with each answer acting as a stimulus for the next question. The teacher only supplies information when it is apparent that the student does not know the answer. This technique is really intended for individual students, but it is a style that many teachers adopt during small group work, with the answers being supplied by the group as a whole rather than by a single individual.

3. *The heuristic style.* This style acknowledges that both teacher and students have areas of shared knowledge and ignorance and that both parties also have areas of knowledge that the other lacks. This style puts the student in a position of responsibility for finding out information.

4. *The counselling style.* This focuses on the student's feelings about the material to be learned and about their interaction with the teacher. The goal is for the students to understand their own behaviour and this is accomplished by the use of reflective questions and other counselling techniques.

In the experiential taxonomy referred to earlier, the role of the teacher changes as the student ascends the hierarchy of levels, as shown in Table 14.5.

Table 14.5

Role of the teacher in experiential learning

Taxonomic level	Role of teacher
1.0 Exposure	Motivator
2.0 Participation	Catalyst
3.0 Identification	Moderator
4.0 Internalization	Sustainer
5.0 Dissemination	Critic and evaluator

BASIC CLASSIFICATION OF SMALL GROUP TEACHING

The classification of small group teaching presents a major conceptual problem, in that there is a bewildering array of possible types. It is useful to distinguish between these basic types of small group and the various techniques that might be used with each. For example, role-playing is really a technique that can be used in many types of small group, so it is not included here as a basic type of group. On the other hand, 'syndicate work' seems to have a very specific function and is structured in a particular way, and is thus seen as a basic type of group. The following section explores a number of basic types of small groups in education, and the various techniques that might be used as part of these basic types of group.

Seminar groups

In higher education, a seminar group is mainly concerned with academic matters rather than with individual students and commonly involves the reading of an essay or paper by one group member, followed by a discussion by the total group on the topic. The teacher may decide to be the leader, or may delegate leadership to the group. It can be a motivating strategy in nursing, where a student presents a paper on some aspect of nursing and then participates in a discussion with the group. The presentation of a seminar by the student can be counted as an assignment for continuous assessment purposes and this may serve as a motivating factor in ensuring a good quality seminar.

Tutorial groups

Tutorial groups can take many different forms, and the term is often used synonymously with 'seminar'. It can also mean a one-to-one encounter with a student, an encounter with three or four students and a teacher, or can be synonymous with a controlled discussion. Clearly, the purpose of the tutorial group will largely determine its organization; a one-to-one tutorial is usually related to individual student progress and comments upon specific aspects of the student's work. The same kind of function can be achieved with three or four students together, although this may inhibit some individuals from speaking as freely as they might if they were alone.

The term *tutorial group* is often used for convenience to describe the collection of personal tutees for whom a teacher has responsibility, and this is discussed in detail in Chapter 15 (p. 344)

Controlled-discussion groups

In this form of discussion group, the teacher assumes leadership and the purpose is to clarify points raised during a lecture and to develop the ideas that it contained. Thus it can provide feedback to the teacher on the level of understanding achieved in a lecture and gives an opportunity for further explanation if the students have any difficulties with regard to the subject matter.

Free-discussion groups

In contrast to the controlled discussion, this type of discussion is under the control of the group members and the teacher acts merely as an observer and resource person. The topics and direction are decided by the group. This can be a useful method in nursing for developing autonomy in the students, by giving them responsibility for their own learning. In addition, the fact that the topic has been chosen by the students may increase the motivation of the group.

Issue-centred or subject-centred groups

An issue-centred group has as its focus an issue that has no right or wrong answer, and which is usually controversial or provocative. Topics such as 'Is nursing really a profession?' or 'Should resuscitation be carried out on the terminally ill?' provide an opportunity for students' opinions to be questioned and attitudes to be changed. It also provides a forum for public presentation of an individual student's own beliefs and values and gives practice in the efficient presentation of arguments.

Step-by-step discussion groups

This involves a prepared sequence of material designed by the teacher and consisting of key questions or issues that are to be used to draw out the students' own knowledge about the topic. It utilizes inductive technique rather than didactic presentation.

Problem-solving groups

In this form of small group discussion, the students are given a problem to solve and are usually provided with certain sources of information from which to draw their solutions. The problem may be something that requires a single correct answer, or may involve a number of correct answers, the students being required to decide which one is most appropriate to the situation.

Brown and Atkins (1988) identify four main stages in problem solving that equate to the following questions:

1. *What is the nub of the problem?* This question gets at the core of the problem, and may identify sub-problems, conflicts and contradictions.
2. *Have I met a similar problem before?* By recalling similar problems from past experience, the student may discover that the solution arrived at then will apply to the current problem.
3. *What approaches can I use?* Students may have to resort to trial-and-error experimentation if the solutions in Stage 2 above are not successful.
4. *How should I check the solution?* This stage involves checking whether the solution feels right, and also reflection upon the strategies used to solve the problem, as part of the development of students' problem-solving skills.

The main purpose of problem-solving groups is to encourage critical thinking by the students and this method has had considerable success in the teaching of medicine at McMaster University in Canada. The nursing faculty there has also developed a problem-solving approach to nurse education, using real and simulated patients. A common strategy for problem-solving groups is to present a detailed case history of a patient and then to ask specific questions related to nursing or medical science. The students are required to define the problems and to devise nursing measures that will help to overcome.

Learning-through-discussion groups

Learning-through-discussion (LTD) groups were described originally by Fawcett-Hill in 1969 and are similar in some respects to the free group discussion outlined above. However, in an LTD group, the topic is decided by the teacher rather than the students. The teacher's role in LTD is that of resource person and group trainer only; they do not take part as a group member. The roles normally taken by a teacher or chairperson are seen to be the responsibility of each and every group member. Fawcett-Hill maintains that students have little preparation for involvement in small-group work and so need to have a plan by which to proceed (Fawcett-Hill, 1969). The purpose of this method is to enhance learning of course material by utilizing the skill of each group member.

There are three parts to the LTD method, the group cognitive map, group roles and skills and criteria for an effective group.

Group cognitive map

The group cognitive map is a plan that gives a rational sequence of steps for the group to follow, thus minimizing the possibility of aimless discussion. An example is given in Table 14.6.

The group will have been given some assignment to read prior to the meeting and the cognitive map is designed to guide the group through their discussion of it. Steps 1 to 3 of the cognitive map are concerned with:

1. defining the terms and concepts of the assignment;
2. stating the main message; and
3. identifying the major themes and sub-themes.

Step 5 allows discussion of the main themes and sub-themes, from the author's point of view, while Step 6 attempts to integrate the material with the student's past learning thus applying it to real life situations. Step 8 involves the personal opinions and feelings of the group members. Obviously, this method can be applied to discussion of a lecture, not just of reading.

Group roles and member skills

In order for the group to be successful, each member must assume the following roles when appropriate: initiating the discussion, volunteering

Table 14.6

Example of a group cognitive map for anxiety in hospital patients

---

Step 1   Definition
Anxiety, fear, phobia, stress, tension, psychoanalytic, id. ego, super-ego, learning theory, limbic system, reticular activating system, coping mechanisms

Step 2   General statement of message
'Nurses can help prevent anxiety in patients by the use of thoughtful nursing care and interaction.'

Step 3   Identification of major themes and sub-themes
1.   Psychology of anxiety
    (a)   Definition of terms
    (b)   Theories of anxiety
    (c)   Effects of anxiety
            physiological
            psychological
    (d)   Measurement of anxiety

2.   Nursing the patient in situations of anxiety
    (e)   Admission to hospital
    (f)   Prior to surgery
    (g)   Dying

Step 4   Allocation of time
    Step   Time
    5   5 min
    6   5 min
    7   15 min
    8   20 min
    9   5 min

Step 5   Discussion of major themes and sub-themes

Integration of material
    e.g. relate to patients whom you have nursed with anxiety.

Step 7   Application of material
    e.g. to next ward allocation, when dealing with pre-operative patients.

Step 8   Evaluation of author's/lecturer's standpoint

Step 9   Evaluation of the group's performance

---

and requesting information and reactions, rephrasing and exemplifying points, confronting other members' contributions, clarifying and summarizing, timekeeping, spreading the participation by inviting members to comment, encouraging others to contribute by giving praise, etc., relieving tension by joking, evaluating and setting standards for the group's work.

It often takes some time for these roles to be internalized in each group member, but once this has occurred the group will become truly efficient. There are a number of non-productive roles that Fawcett-Hill identifies, which must not be allowed to happen in the group. Behaviours such as aggression, withdrawing, fooling around, status-seeking, dominating, seeking sympathy, pushing a special interest and competing are all counter-productive to the aims of a group and each member is responsible for watching for these.

Criteria for an effective group
Fawcett-Hill outlines the main criteria which must be present for a successful group.

1. The climate must be warm, non-threatening and psychologically safe.
2. Learning is approached as a co-operative venture.
3. Learning is seen as the main reason for the group. Everyone participates and interacts.
4. Leadership is distributed throughout the group.
5. The sessions are enjoyable.
6. Material is covered adequately and efficiently.
7. Evaluation is an integral part of the function of the group.
8. Members come prepared and attend regularly.

The LTD method can be a very powerful tool for small group discussion, and the time spent training the students will be amply rewarded by the learning achieved. This kind of group work has implications far beyond the learning task being considered. The member roles and skills provide sound training for future committee work and stimulate the development of responsibility for one's own learning. An LTD group can function without the teacher even being present. It is better not to try to teach every small group session by this method, as the constant use of any method will lead to boredom on the part of the student. My own experience of this method has convinced me that it provides an interesting form of learning for group members, and also encourages strong interpersonal relationships between them. Any teacher attempting this method for the first time should be aware that the group will feel initial frustration until the method has been internalized and should thus provide considerable support and encouragement in the early part of the group training.

Syndicate groups

This type of group is valuable for putting students in a position for discovery learning. The total class is given a major topic and then divided into small groups of about six members. Each of these small groups selects one aspect of the major topic and studies this over a period of two weeks or so. Contact with the teacher is maintained intermittently to report progress. When the work has been completed, each group reports its findings to the total group, after which the findings are assessed and interpreted by the teacher and a grade awarded.

Project groups

The project method can be defined as a unit of purposeful experience in which the educational needs and interests of the student determine the aims and objectives of the activity and guide its process to a conclusion.

Characteristics

The main characteristics of the method are that the students are very much involved in the formulation of the aims and objectives of the project and that they are actively participating in the learning experience. Projects may be done by individuals, but more commonly they are undertaken by a small group of about six members. The main topics can be suggested by the teacher, or left completely to the student's imagination, but in both cases it is crucial for the teacher to ensure that the aims of the project are clarified, so that the students are in no doubt as to the purpose of such an exercise. The kinds of aims that a group project can foster are the ability to work co-operatively in groups, collection of information, development of confidence in decision-making and many others.

Motivation and projects

For the project method to be successful, it is necessary to have motivated students and this in turn requires subject-matter areas that are seen to be interesting and to contain scope for individuality and imagination. It is common for students to be required to undertake community-based projects, such as a neighbourhood study, and this allows the students scope to be imaginative.

For example, when doing a neighbourhood study, one of my small groups decided to focus their project on access to local facilities by individuals confined to a wheelchair. One of the students sat in a borrowed wheelchair and two other students accompanied him to the local shopping centre. This was an example of experiential learning for the students, as it soon became apparent that it was extremely difficult to withdraw money from a cashpoint due to the position of the dispenser on the wall of the bank. Similarly, the students tried to gain access to a well-known tourist attraction, but found that it was impossible to do so in a wheelchair. The findings of the students were reported back to the rest of the group, and provided very thought-provoking discussion about life in a wheelchair.

History of the project method

The project method itself is not a new development, having its origins in the 1920s. The method was first described by John Dewey of Columbia University and further developed by his colleague W.H. Kilpatrick. Dewey's philosophy was that the process of educational thought was more important than the results of such thought, and he believed that a child would undergo mental growth if he actively participated in solving a problem that he saw as real. Use of the project method declined in the 1950s, but with the advent of the Nuffield Foundation Science Teaching Project and the personal topic in the Certificate of Secondary Education, interest in the method has revived.

A number of advantages are claimed for the use of the project method, including greater interest for the student, development of resourcefulness and independence in learning and the opportunity for the student to use important skills such as the identification and analysis of problems and the exploration of solutions. On the other hand, this method has its critics, and the main disadvantages are the time-consuming nature of project work and the difficulty in evaluating the student's achievement.

Planning for project work

When planning to use the project method for the first time, the teacher of nursing should ensure that the exercise is carefully organized. Groups may be allocated by the teacher, or selected by the students according to personal preference. The latter has the advantage of allowing them to work with friends, which may increase motivation and spur their efforts to succeed. As indicated earlier, it is important for the teacher to clarify the purpose of the project so that the enthusiasm and co-operation of the groups are obtained and it is equally necessary to allocate sufficient time for the work to be accomplished.

When the groups have chosen, or have been allocated, a specific subject area then they decide amongst themselves which objectives and methods of inquiry they will use. The teacher must not control the direction of approach, as this would stifle independence and enthusiasm. The progress of each group's project should be monitored by the teacher, but only to ensure that difficulties are being overcome and that the most efficient techniques of data collection are being used.

The channels for obtaining information from personnel in the hospital or community must be clearly understood by the group. It is important to check that personnel who are likely to be approached by students are willing to spend time talking to them. The form of presentation of the projects should be decided before the students commence their work. All projects should be written up regardless of the form of presentation and the teacher can negotiate with the group as to whether the projects are presented to the total group, or simply submitted to the teacher in written form. My own preference is for a presentation to the total group, as this is seen as the culmination of the students' work and reinforces their feelings of accomplishment and success. Assessment of project work is discussed in Chapter 8 (p. 222)

Small group projects then give students the opportunity for more intensive study of a topic, challenging them to seek more widely for resources and giving experience in the skills of problem solving and decision making, all of which are important for the changing role of the nurse.

Experiential learning groups

These groups are characterized by the use of experiential techniques to develop greater expertise in a variety of fields, for example, teaching in clinical and community settings (discussed in Chapter 16) and interpersonal communication skills (discussed in Chapter 18).

Focus groups

This is a qualitative research technique that is frequently used in nursing and health research. Focus groups are discussed in Chapter 20 (p. 520).

Synergogy groups

Synergogy utilizes the notion of synergy, i.e. that the sum of the work of a group of individuals is greater than that of any individual alone.

The central concept is teamwork, and the synergogy system involves the use of peer-teaching and teamwork for the achievement of specific outcomes. The system is described in detail in Chapter 5 (p. 123)

TECHNIQUES FOR TEACHING SMALL GROUPS AND EXPERIENTIAL LEARNING

So far we have identified a number of types of educational small group, each having fairly specific purposes or functions. Within any one of these basic types, there are a number of techniques that might be employed to help group members to achieve the purpose of the small group. Again, it is useful to categorize them according to their main purpose, although some techniques have a wide range of application. Table 14.7 identifies the categories.

Table 14.7

Categories of techniques for small group teaching

Category	Techniques
1. Techniques to maximize group members' interaction with each other	Snowball groups; square-root or crossover groups; buzz groups
2. Techniques to generate creative solutions	Brainstorming; synectics
3. Techniques to generate data	Carousel exercise
4 Techniques to develop group members' self-awareness and empathy	Role-play; simulation; gaming; case-study
5. Techniques to develop group members' presentational ability	Debate; seminar; peer-tutoring; microteaching; square-root technique
6. Techniques for applying knowledge and skills to real-life	Role-play; simulation; case-study; brainstorming
7. Techniques to develop group members' awareness of group processes	Fishbowl technique; peer review; group-interaction analysis

Snowball groups

As the name implies, this technique involves group members in subgroups of ever-increasing size until the total group is involved together. It begins with each individual group member working on a problem and then sharing this information in pairs. Each pair then joins with another pair for further work on the problem and then these tetrads join with each other to form groups of eight. Work continues in this fashion until the entire group comes together to share its ideas in a plenary session. The work can become progressively more detailed as the 'snowball' grows and this technique is useful for getting every member of the group involved in participation.

Square-root or crossover groups

This technique is extremely useful in a number of ways, the starting point being the number of students in the total group. The teacher takes this total number and forms a series of horseshoe-shaped groups, each containing the number of students that equals the square root of the total group. Thus, if there are 16 students, each horseshoe group will contain four students; if there are 25 students, each horseshoe group will contain five students.

Each student is then given a card with a letter and a number on it, which determines the group in which each student starts, as shown in Table 14.8, for a group of 16. After an appropriate amount of time spent in discussion of an issue or problem, the groups disband and reform according to their numbers, i.e. all the number ones form a group, as do all the number twos, number threes and number fours. This means that each contains only one member of the original group, thus giving the maximum exchange of ideas. At the commencement of the new groups, each member is required to give a summary of what their previous group's findings were and this also helps to break the ice in the new group.

Group A	Group B	Group C	Group D
A1	B1	C1	D1
A2	B2	C2	D2
A3	B3	C3	D3
A4	B4	C4	D4

Table 14.8

Square-root technique for a total group of 16 members

Buzz groups

Buzz groups consist of from two to six members and are most frequently used to provide student involvement during a lecture or other teacher-centred session. For example, during a lecture on post-operative nursing care, the large class can be asked to form buzz groups to discuss the complications of surgery for three or four minutes. The group leaders then feed back their contributions to the total group. It is often a good idea simply to ask the first row to turn and face the second and the third to turn and face the fourth and so on. These rows can then be segmented into groups of six students and this system minimizes the reorganization of the room. Buzz groups can be used more than once in any given lecture, and provide the students with social activity and involvement, helping to maintain their level of arousal during the lecture. It is often a useful way to begin a session to ask them to form buzz groups and write down everything they know about a subject, for example, the structure of the heart. This can be fed into the main group and forms the basis of the lecture.

Brainstorming

This is another effective method of obtaining creative solutions to a problem (Osborne, 1962). The idea is for each member to generate as many ideas as they can about the problem in question. The emphasis is on free expression of ideas, and no criticism is permitted, however unlikely the suggestions. De Bono (1986) suggest that there are three main features of a brainstorming session: 'cross-stimulation', 'suspended judgement' and a 'formal setting'. Cross-stimulation refers to the effects of other people's ideas on an individual and the fact that these ideas may interact with existing ones to produce creative solutions. As the name implies, suspended judgement means that no criticism of suggestions is allowed, however silly the ideas may seem. It is important that the leader or chairperson be on the lookout for any evaluative comments and stop them immediately. It is not vital to produce entirely new or novel ideas; indeed, it may be that an old idea is the best solution to a difficulty in certain situations.

A formal setting is important so that participants can feel that there is something special about the group and thus be less inhibited about saying things that might seem ridiculous. The organization of a brainstorming group involves a leader or chairperson and someone to make notes of the ideas as they arise; it is helpful to use audiotape recording to ensure that no ideas are lost. The brainstorming activity can take any amount of time up to a maximum of about 30–40 minutes, and frequently lasts only some 5–10 minutes.

The activity itself is only a means to an end, so there has to be an evaluation session in order to see what the next steps should be. This evaluation should take place some little time after the brainstorming session itself, and involves the sifting out of all the useful ideas into three categories: those ideas that are of immediate use; those that need further exploration; and those that represent new approaches.

Synectics

Synectics is a system of problem solving that aims to produce creative solutions by making people view problems in new ways. Creative ideas are seen as involving the making of new connections between ideas, and one way of facilitating this is the use of the 'SES box steps' method (SES Associates, 1986). This method is based on the assumption that all problems contain a paradox or contradiction that can only be solved if new connections can be made. It uses the notions of analogy and metaphor to create these new connections and there are four distinct steps in the process:

1. identify the paradox, which is the essence of the problem;
2. develop an analogy or metaphor to provide a creative, different viewpoint;
3. identify the unique activity associated with the metaphor or analogy; and
4. apply equivalent thinking, in which the unique activity is transferred to the current problem, resulting in a new idea for its solution.

An example will be useful to help understanding of this series of stages. Consider the following problems. A health visitor wishes to put on health promotion sessions on the topic of safety in the home, for mothers of young children. Despite local advertising, however, there is a very poor turnout.

1. *Paradox*: Health promotion sessions may be perceived by mothers as less attractive than other forms of social interaction, such as visiting friends or attending coffee mornings with other mothers and young children.
2. *Analogy*: Sales parties are a well-established strategy for selling all sorts of goods, such as clothes, perfume, and gifts. The salesperson brings her wares to someone's home, and a number of friends, relatives and their children are invited over by the person hosting the party.
3. *Unique activity*: The salesperson combines business with a social setting, including company and refreshments.
4. *Equivalent thinking*: The health visitor must combine the health promotion message with an opportunity for social interaction. This means she must organize her classes as social events, e.g. by providing refreshments, and creating an opportunity for social interaction in an atmosphere of informality.

The carousel exercise

This is an excellent and novel way of generating data from a group of students and also for the development of interviewing skills. The first step is for the teacher to identify a series of topics or sub-topics that will be the focus of the session. The group is then divided into two, half of

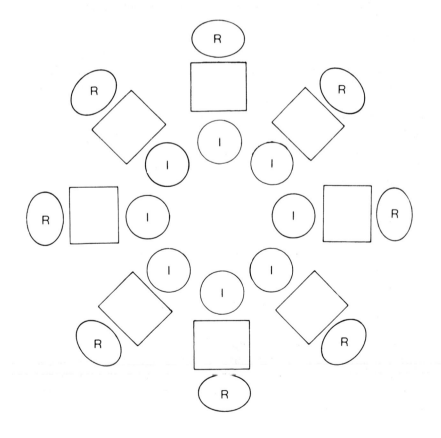

Figure 14.5

Carousel exercise – arrangement of seating

whom will be interviewers and the other half who will be respondents. Each interviewer is given a sheet of paper that is blank apart from a question that is written across the top of the page. The desks are arranged in a circle, with the interviewers seated on the inside facing out and the respondents seated on the outside facing in, as shown in Figure 14.5.

This arrangement ensures that there is a pair of students sitting opposite one another and separated by a desk. At a given signal from the teacher, each interviewer proceeds to ask their respondent to answer the question at the top of their sheet of paper and to answer it as fully as possible. Each interviewer has a different question and five minutes is allowed for each interview, after which time the teacher signals 'all change' and the outer circle of interviewees moves round to the next seat on each person's right. The inner circle of interviewers remain in the same position throughout the exercise and every five minutes, a new respondent arrives opposite each of them. They proceed to ask their question to each respondent as they appear, recording the various answers on the same sheet of paper.

Eventually, all the outer circle will have been interviewed by each of the interviewers and the latter will have a sheet of different responses to their question. This data can then be analysed to reveal the opinions of those group members who were in the outer circle. It is desirable to then exchange the roles, so that the outer group become the interviewers and vice versa, thus generating twice as much data for analysis.

Simulations

A simulation is an imitation of some facet of life, usually in a simplified form. It aims to put students in a position where they can experience some aspect of real life by becoming involved in activities that are closely related to it. Airline pilots spend time working in flight simulators, which are identical to the flight deck of an aircraft and in which the pilots can gain simulated experience of handling emergencies that cannot (for safety and/or expense reasons) be gained in any other way. For example, they are able to practise emergency procedures for such things as sudden depressurization, failure of engines, etc., and this experience should transfer to the real-life setting, if it is ever required. The notion of 'transfer of learning' underpins all aspects of simulation, the aim being to use the simulated experience to help the student to learn how to cope with the real thing.

Using simulation in nurse education

In nurse education, a commonly used simulation is that of the cardiac-arrest procedure or 'crash-call'. The teacher organizes the simulation by providing an authentic environment that simulates a ward setting, with a 'patient' in a bed, a locker, charts, etc. Certain staff or students are designated roles such as anaesthetist, sister, relatives and nurses and the whole scenario of what happens when a patient has a cardiac arrest is enacted. The scenario can be used to give student nurses an insight into how the procedure operates and in this instance, would serve as a demonstration. Alternatively, students can be asked to take the part of the student who discovers a patient with a cardiac arrest and to imitate the procedures required following such detection. By this means it is possible to give the student experience of a situation, without the associated anxiety of learning it initially in the real-life setting.

Transfer of learning

It is always debatable whether or not there is 'transfer of learning' to the real-life setting, but at the very least, the student will have had an opportunity to internalize the sequence of procedures required and to appreciate the urgency of the whole situation. One of the important hallmarks of a simulation is that the students are not required to act out any kind of script; they are expected to behave and react in any way they feel is appropriate. In other words, a simulation involves the students in being themselves, and dealing with situations using their normal, everyday behaviour. Whatever the scenario of the simulation may be, the students are expected to be themselves and to deal with the situations presented.

Simulations in first aid

One of the most valuable areas in which simulation can be used is that of first aid. Although this topic has some theoretical basis, the main emphasis is on practical techniques, so it is important to teach first aid in a way that helps students to cope with real-life situations. I prefer to use the first part of each session introducing the concepts in question and then demonstrating the techniques required. I then invite volunteers to join in with a simulation, in which they are required to give first-aid treatment to a 'casualty', and the simulation should be as realistic as possible within the limitations of the college setting. With a little imagination and dramatic flair, it is quite possible to create a scenario that simulates to a reasonable extent a first-aid emergency such as a head injury, a fracture, poisoning and the like. The aim is to create a simulation that is as near as possible to the real-life situation that the student will encounter, so that the established behaviours and procedures can be transferred easily to the new setting.

Simulations and role-play

The term *simulation* is closely related to the concepts of role-play and gaming; indeed, many simulations will involve an element of role-playing by other people, even though the students in question remain themselves. For example, a teacher may wish to do a simulation involving the admission of a mentally disturbed patient to the admission ward. A student is first identified who will be the admitting nurse, whilst another student or teacher will undertake the role of the disturbed patient. In this scenario, one nurse will be acting out the role of a disturbed patient, i.e. he or she will indulge in role-play; the other nurse, however, will simply behave and react in the way they feel appropriate in order to carry out the admission, i.e. they remains themselves throughout the simulation.

When carrying out simulations, it is important that the teacher should give full briefing beforehand and allow sufficient time for an adequate debriefing at the end. These aspects are discussed in the next section on role-play.

Role-play

Role-play is derived largely from the work of Moreno on psychodrama, and utilizes acting and imagination to create insights into the student's own behaviour, beliefs and values and those of other people. Students are required to take on someone else's identity and to act as they think that person would behave. Although some scripting is essential to delineate the role, this should be kept to a minimum so that the student can act out the role in their own way.

Counter-attitudinal role-play

Role-play can be an excellent way of creating empathy with other people's points of view, particularly if the student is given a role that is opposite to the position or viewpoint currently held. This counter-attitudinal role-play forces the students to consider issues and feelings from the other person's point of view and can help them to gain insight into why that person's behaviour is occurring. One of the important points about role-play is that the student, after some initial self-consciousness about the role in question, then quickly settles down to project their own character and values into the role. It is this identification with the role that forms the basis for subsequent debriefing and experiential learning. Role-play can be used for almost any social situation and is the

Table 14.9

Examples of role-play scripts in nursing

Role-Play Number 1

Nurse
You are a post-graduate nurse working in the Burns Unit.
 You are nursing a young woman who has had severe burns to the face; she is called Sally and is aged 17. She asks to talk to you. You go over to her bed.

Sally
You are a 17-year-old and have experienced severe facial burns. Although the pain is now much easier, you are desperately worried about the long-term effects on your appearance. You don't have a steady boyfriend, but do enjoy going out with boys. You decide to talk to the staff nurse.

Role-Play Number Two

Nurse
You are a post-graduate student nurse working in the plastic surgery children's ward.
 A toddler has been admitted for repair of hare-lip and cleft palate, accompanied by his mother. The child is called Gary Turner and has a severe deformity. His mothers asks to speak to you after the admission formalities are completed.

Mother of Gary
You have arrived at the hospital with your toddler son Gary, who is being admitted for repair of hare-lip and cleft palate. The deformity is quite severe and you are wondering how successful the operation will be. You decide to ask the staff nurse about the operation after she has finished the admission.

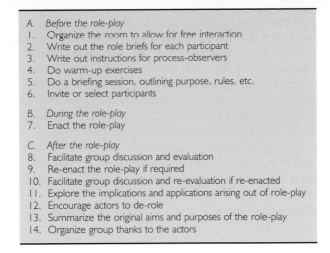

A.	*Before the role-play*
1.	Organize the room to allow for free interaction
2.	Write out the role briefs for each participant
3.	Write out instructions for process-observers
4.	Do warm-up exercises
5.	Do a briefing session, outlining purpose, rules, etc.
6.	Invite or select participants
B.	*During the role-play*
7.	Enact the role-play
C.	*After the role-play*
8.	Facilitate group discussion and evaluation
9.	Re-enact the role-play if required
10.	Facilitate group discussion and re-evaluation if re-enacted
11.	Explore the implications and applications arising out of role-play
12.	Encourage actors to de-role
13.	Summarize the original aims and purposes of the role-play
14.	Organize group thanks to the actors

Table 14.10

Checklist for organizing role-play

method *par excellence* for exploring interpersonal communication skills. Some examples of brief role scripts are given in Table 14.9 and a checklist for organizing role-play is given in Table 14.10.

Briefing for role-play

As mentioned earlier, a vital part of the process of role-playing is that of briefing and debriefing of participants. Briefing is an important preliminary process prior to many kinds of small group activity and is particularly pertinent to role-playing situations. Briefing involves giving prior guidelines about rules, intentions and goals, and is designed to ensure that participants benefit from the subsequent activities. It is not necessary to declare the outcomes beforehand, particularly if this might 'give the game away'; many role-play activities are designed to allow students to discover things for themselves, so it is important not to pre-empt this.

One of the essential rules of role-play is that no member of the group should be allowed to be a passive observer; any students who are not directly engaged in one of the acting roles should be given the job of 'process observers'. This implies that they are actively observing the role-play, including the verbal and non-verbal signals emitted by the actors. Such process observation is a crucial part of the feedback and debriefing session that follows the role-play.

Debriefing

Debriefing occurs after the activities have been concluded and can be seen as having three stages:

1. a description of what occurred;
2. sharing of participants' feelings about the activity; and
3. the examination of the implications of the activity for future work.

The first stage simply asks participants and observers to describe what occurred during the role-play; this is followed by a sharing of group members' feelings about the activity and it is important to have an atmosphere of mutual trust for this stage. The final stage involves the application of what has been discussed to the real world of nursing and where the insights gained can be shared with other students. The actors may receive much useful feedback from the observers about their personal skills of communication and the group as a whole can benefit from the range of ideas and values generated by the role-play. Since a great deal of emotion can be generated during role-play, it is important that the participants are encouraged to de-role at the end, so as to establish contact with reality again. This can be done by simply having students say out loud that they are out of role and that they are their normal selves again.

Gaming

Gaming is the third of these closely related concepts of simulation and role-play; gaming differs from simulation by the fact that it has very precise sets of rules and is usually competitive in nature. Unlike simulation, games have no scenario, being complete in themselves and participants behave as their normal selves. Educational games are simply extensions of recreational games, such as board-games, card-games and quizzes, and the aim is to create a method of learning that is both enjoyable and beneficial.

Case studies

Case studies are textual descriptions of specific situations that may either be genuine or fictional and that provide a trigger for the discussion of issues and the examination of real-life events. Case studies differ from simulations in that they offer the student a cognitive view of the event rather than an experiential one. However, it is possible to use a case study as the basis for a simulation or role-play, with students taking the parts of the characters involved.

Case studies usually entail making decisions about particular courses of action or, alternatively, making judgements about decisions contained within the case study. Case studies can be used to very good effect in bringing theoretical issues closer to the real world of nursing; for example, students may be given a case study of the nursing care of a patient and asked to evaluate the care given in the light of their own knowledge and skills. In some instances, it is useful to use fictional studies to abstract the typical features of issues or problems, but generally speaking, it is better to use real-life examples, since these are based on actual nursing practice.

Writing a case study

Writing a good case-study is time-consuming and difficult and Davis (1985) suggests three basic questions that need to be addressed when planning a case-study:

1. *What is the major issue or problem?* This needs to be clearly stated along with any subordinate problems related to it.
2. *What facts does the student need?* It is important to include all relevant data required to deal with the problem or issue, but not to overload the case-study with superfluous material.
3. *How should the material be presented?* This involves deciding on the sequence of the material, such as background to the case, significant facts, use of the past or present tense and inclusion of statistics. The writer must avoid putting in personal opinions, keeping only to factual material.

One of the great uses of case studies is to integrate information from a wide range of topics in nursing; in order to solve a nursing-care problem in a case study the students will need to integrate their knowledge of biological and behavioural science, nursing science and other areas. When using the case study method the teacher must be very familiar with every detail of the case, so that he or she can be of greatest use to the group during the discussion. The teacher needs to be particularly careful that the group does not skim over the case study too quickly, thereby missing many of the important aspects. It is very useful to jot down an evaluation of how the session went, so that this is available for reference when the same case study is used again.

The fishbowl technique

This technique is very useful for process observation of group behaviour. The total group is divided into two and one of these subgroups arranges itself into a circle for discussion and interaction. The other subgroup arranges itself outside the first circle concentrically and can then observe the inner group as though it were in a fishbowl. After the inner group has completed its interaction, the outer group can give feedback and evaluation about the group processes.

Debate

Although commonly thought of as a large-group technique, debate can be used to good effect in small group teaching. Debate is a formal way of examining issues that can be very exciting to the participants as well as the audience and it has the added advantage of not only raising the students' awareness of issues and values, but also giving them the opportunity to formulate an argument and present it in a public arena.

Debate is quite easy to set up; the teacher can choose a number of issues, or the group may come up with its own list. Four students are required to present their view, two speaking for the motion and two against it. Following the presentations, the issue is opened up to the audience to contribute and then a vote is taken on whether the motion is carried or defeated. Debate is particularly useful for topical, emotive issues and can serve to make students examine their beliefs and values about such issues.

Microteaching

Microteaching is a small group activity that has many uses in nurse education. Essentially, microteaching consists of a cycle of events as those outlined in Figure 14.6. It can be seen that the cycle consists of the performance of some microskill, i.e. some aspect of a social or psycho-motor skill such as asking questions, which is recorded on videotape. This recording is then played back to the small group; the performer firstly evaluates their own performance and then the group members contribute their evaluation. The performer then replans the performance using the feedback gained during the analysis. The performance is then repeated, incorporating the changes suggested in the analysis and this is also videotaped. The video is then replayed, further analysis takes place and the cycle is repeated as often as is required until the performance is satisfactory. Microteaching can be a very potent tool for the acquisition of skills, but it does need a fair amount of time in order to allow students the chance to teach and re-teach several times.

Figure 14.6

The micro-teaching cycle

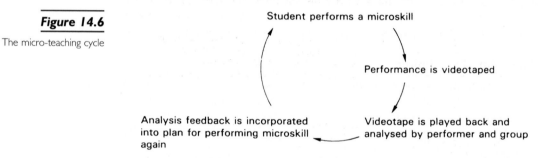

Student performs a microskill

Performance is videotaped

Videotape is played back and analysed by performer and group

Analysis feedback is incorporated into plan for performing microskill again

Field visits

A well-established technique in nurse education, field visits can provide insight when extending students' experience of nursing. Visits can be clinical (to a hospice or specialist centre) or non-clinical (to museums or public utilities). Within programmes for initial registration, it is common to find that students are required to undertake field visits as part of a neighbourhood study, e.g. to the local government offices, sports centres, supermarkets, etc. Briefing and debriefing are important if the maximum learning value is to be gained from the visit. Figure 14.7 gives an algorithm for planning such a visit.

Exercises

Exercises are particularly common in experiential learning, and consist of structured sequences in which students are actively involved, often containing written instructions. Exercises consist of dyadic, triadic or small group activities, usually ending in a discussion of participants' feelings about the exercise.

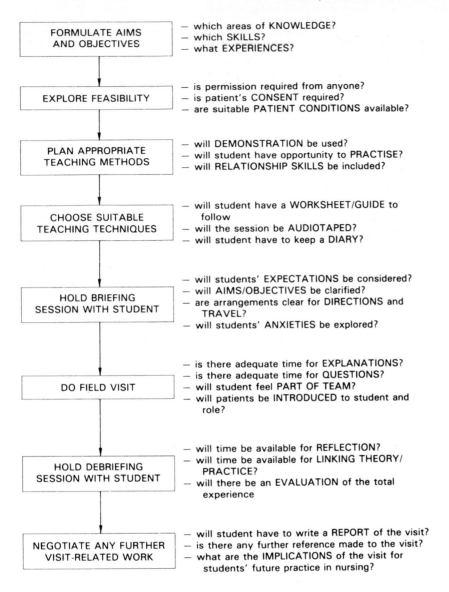

FORMULATE AIMS AND OBJECTIVES	— which areas of KNOWLEDGE? — which SKILLS? — what EXPERIENCES?
EXPLORE FEASIBILITY	— is permission required from anyone? — is patient's CONSENT required? — are suitable PATIENT CONDITIONS available?
PLAN APPROPRIATE TEACHING METHODS	— will DEMONSTRATION be used? — will student have opportunity to PRACTISE? — will RELATIONSHIP SKILLS be included?
CHOOSE SUITABLE TEACHING TECHNIQUES	— will student have a WORKSHEET/GUIDE to follow — will the session be AUDIOTAPED? — will student have to keep a DIARY?
HOLD BRIEFING SESSION WITH STUDENT	— will students' EXPECTATIONS be considered? — will AIMS/OBJECTIVES be clarified? — are arrangements clear for DIRECTIONS and TRAVEL? — will students' ANXIETIES be explored?
DO FIELD VISIT	— is there adequate time for EXPLANATIONS? — is there adequate time for QUESTIONS? — will student feel PART OF TEAM? — will patients be INTRODUCED to student and role?
HOLD DEBRIEFING SESSION WITH STUDENT	— will time be available for REFLECTION? — will time be available for LINKING THEORY/PRACTICE? — will there be an EVALUATION of the total experience
NEGOTIATE ANY FURTHER VISIT-RELATED WORK	— will student have to write a REPORT of the visit? — is there any further reference made to the visit? — what are the IMPLICATIONS of the visit for students' future practice in nursing?

Figure 14.7

Algorithm for planning field visits

Body movements

Also extensively used in experiential learning, physical contact may or may not be involved in this kind of experience, but is common in the various forms of 'warm-up' exercises prior to interpersonal skills sessions. Relaxation also comes under this heading .

Guided imagery and meditation

Guided imagery is being increasingly used in clinical practice, particularly in pain management. For example, a patient might be asked to imagine s/he has flown to a peaceful island, far away from the pain. In nurse education, these experiential techniques are useful for gaining greater self-awareness. The student sits comfortably relaxed, with eyes closed and with the verbal help of the teacher, imagines she is back in a pleasant place of her choosing. She is prompted to involve all her senses in this re-creation.

Meditation is also carried out in a relaxed environment with eyes closed and there are many techniques for this. One of them consists of simply attending to one's thoughts as they pass through the mind.

Instrumentation

A variety of instruments are used to facilitate activities, the commonest being questionnaires and inventories that direct the student to self-exploration.

COMMON DIFFICULTIES IN SMALL GROUP AND EXPERIENTIAL LEARNING

The teacher may find that difficulties arise from time to time in a small group and these require sensitive handling. It is usually better to deal with them as they arise, but occasionally it may be necessary to have a private word with a group member after the session has finished.

Multi-speak

A common problem in small group discussion is that of all the members talking at once (multi-speak), which leads to a chaotic situation where no progress is made. The teacher should exert firm, friendly control to bring the session to order and a sense of humour is invaluable in keeping the atmosphere informal, while at the same time maintaining order. Very often there is a vocal member of a group who tends to monopolize the session and it is important not to 'squash' them, as motivation can easily be lost. Ignoring the contributions may lead to extinction of the response, but it usually makes the student feel hurt and resentful. Possibly the best solution is to remind them gently that other group members need a chance to air their views also.

Hogging the limelight

A similar problem is that of the student who attempts to engage the teacher in a dialogue, to the exclusion of the rest of the group. This often arises when a student wishes to show that he or she has a particular piece of knowledge or expertise that the other students do not. Again, sensitive handling is required and a particularly useful strategy is to deliberately open out the dialogue to the rest of the group by using such statements as, 'You are raising some interesting points here, would anyone else like to comment or react to any of them?'

Conflict

Group discussions can become very heated, especially when debating an issue that is emotionally charged, such as abortion. However, conflict is not always undesirable, as productive conflict can be an effective aid to learning. It is useful to reassure the group that disagreement is quite in order, but that it should be the opinion of another group member that is questioned and not that person as an individual. Each group member is respected, but his or her opinions are open to challenge and disagreement.

Emotional outbursts

Occasionally, the teacher may be confronted with an emotional outburst by a group member and one of the most dramatic of all gestures is that of a student walking out of the group. It is always difficult to know how best to handle such a situation. Resisting the temptation to follow the individual, the teacher should stay with the group and attempt to help them to realize that such behaviour (flight, rather than fight) is one way that people have of coping with anxiety or anger; it is important to convey to the group that this is not a major disaster. However, it is extremely important for the welfare of the group as a whole that the teacher make contact with the distressed student before the next group meeting to discuss the incident with a view to deciding how best to raise it with the group.

Whilst every student has the right to behave in this way when under stress, the teacher cannot ignore the effects of such behaviour on the rest of the group. It might be that at the next meeting the student concerned with the incident should be invited to make a statement to the group about their feelings at the time and thus use the incident as a positive learning experience for all concerned.

Unwillingness to participate

Another common problem in small groups is that of the student who is unwilling to participate. Arguably, every individual has the 'right to remain silent' but this obviates the whole purpose of an educational small group. However, the teacher must acknowledge that students will differ in the degree of confidence they possess for making public contributions and this may be due to a variety of factors including basic personality, lack of knowledge, feelings of lack of personal worth or inadequate preparation. On the other hand, it may be the teacher's own style that is inhibiting a student; if the climate of the group is not conducive to psychological safety, then it is unlikely that students will risk contributing to discussion, lest they be humiliated or made to feel inadequate in some way.

The previous background and experience of students will also influence their desire to contribute to group discussions; in certain cultures, the teacher is seen very much as an expert who is not to be questioned and this may be difficult to overcome. Childhood experience of college teachers who humiliated students may have left scars that ensure that the student is never again put in such a position. Some of these factors may be impossible to change, although the teacher can do a great deal to ensure that the group members are valued and respected. Students can be invited into the discussion by gentle questioning, particularly in areas that rely upon student opinion rather than hard fact, since there is no likelihood of giving an incorrect answer.

It may well be that such reticent students require more specific help in the building up of confidence in public, by a systematic programme of interaction that begins in pairs and gradually builds up to larger numbers, but such provision has obvious resource implications for the institution.

REFERENCES

Asch, S. (1956) Studies in independence and conformity: a minority of one against a unanimous majority, *Psychological Monographs*, **70**(9), 416.

Bales, R. (1950) *Interaction Process Analysis: A Method for the Study of Small Groups*, Addison-Wesley, Cambridge, MA.

Bavelas, A. (1948) A mathematical model for group structures, *Applied Anthropology*, 7, 16–3.

Bond, C. and Titus, L. (1983) Social facilitation: a meta-analysis of 241 studies, *Psychological Bulletin*, **94**, 265–92.

Boud, D., Keogh, R. and Walker, D. (1985) *Reflection: Turning Experience into Learning*, Kogan Page, London.

Brown, G. and Atkins, M. (1988) *Effective Teaching in Higher Education*, Methuen, London.

Brown, S. (1996) The art of teaching small groups, *New Academic*, Autumn 1996, Spring 1997.

Burnard, P. (1990) *Learning Human Skills*, 2nd edn, Heinemann, London.

Burnard, P. (1991) Defining experiential learning: nurse teachers' perceptions, *Nurse Education Today*, **12**, 29–36.

Davis, R. (1985) Some suggestions for writing a business case, in *Teach Thinking by Discussion*, D. Bligh (ed.), SRHE/NFER-Nelson, Guildford.

De Bono, E. (1986) Brainstorming, in *Teach Thinking by Discussion*, D. Bligh (ed.), SRHE/NFER-Nelson, Guildford.

Eiser, J. (1980) *Cognitive Social Psychology*, McGraw Hill, London.

Fawcett-Hill, W. (1969) *Learning Thru Discussion*, Sage, CA.

Harper, D. (1968) The reliability of measures of sociometric acceptance and reflection, *Sociometry*, **31**, 210–27.

Heron, J. (1986) *Six Category Intervention Analysis*, Human Potential Research Project, University of Surrey.

Kolb, D.A. (1984) *Experiential Learning: Experience as the Source of Learning and Development*, Prentice Hall, New York.

Latane, B. and Darley, J. (1968) Group inhibition of bystander intervention in emergencies, *Journal of Personality and Social Psychology*, **10**, 215–21.

Lawrence, G. (1986) Social procedures of task-orientated groups, in *Teach Thinking by Discussion*, D. Bligh (ed.), SRHE/NFER-Nelson, Guildford.

Leavitt, H. (1951) Some effects of certain communication patterns on group performance, *Journal of Abnormal Social Psychology*, **46**, 38–50.

Mulder, M. (1960) Communication structure, decision structure and group performance, *Sociometry*, **23**, 1–14.

Osborne, A. (1962) *Applied Imagination*, Scribner, New York.

Rogers, C. (1983) *Freedom to Learn for the 80s*, Merrill, OH.

Royal College of General Practitioners (1986) Tutorial Styles, in *Teaching Thinking by Discussion*, D. Bligh (ed.), SRHE/NFER-Nelson, Guildford.

SES Associates (1986) The SES box method for creative problem-solving, in

Teaching Thinking by Discussion, D. Bligh (ed.), *SRHE/NFER-Nelson, Guildford.*

Sherif, M. (1935) *The Psychology of Social Norms*, Harper, New York.

Steinaker, N. and Bell, M. (1979) *The Experiential Taxonomy: A New Approach to Teaching and Learning*, Academic Press, New York.

Tajfel, H. (1978) *Differentiation between Social Groups: Studies in the Social Psychology of Intergroup Relations*, Academic Press, London.

Wallach, M. and Kogan, N. (1965) The role of information, discussion and consensus in group risk taking, *Journal of Experimental Social Psychology*, **1**, 1–19.

15 Tutoring and counselling skills

Within higher education, it is usual to differentiate between the terms *teaching* and *tutoring*. The latter can be defined as a relationship between a tutor and a student that includes a range of functions, other than formal teaching and assessment, that support students in their progression through a programme of study. Some institutions make the distinction between academic tutors and personal tutors, whereas others combine these two aspects in a single tutorial role. A closely-related term that is used in clinical and community settings is *mentoring*, which applies to a member of staff in the placement setting who carries out a range of roles not dissimilar from that of a tutor. Mentoring is discussed in detail in Chapter 16 (p. 426).

THE CONTEXT OF TUTORING

Tutoring is acknowledged as an important aspect of a student's educational experience, and this is underlined by *The Charter for Higher Education* (DfEE, 1993). The Charter explains the standards of service that students, employers, and the general public can expect from universities and colleges and other bodies involved in higher education in England, and refers specifically to tutoring: 'You should receive well-informed guidance from your tutors and careers staff and appropriate access to counsellors'. However, the expansion of student numbers, combined with a diminishing resource base, has had an adverse impact on the personal tutoring system in some institutions. The importance of personal tutoring is nicely captured in the following quote:

> *'The purpose of having a personal tutoring system is primarily to provide an anchor on which the support system of the university rests. The personal tutor is needed by all students, including those who enjoy a relatively straightforward passage through university' (Wheeler and Birtle, 1993).*

Approaches to tutoring

Tutoring can take place in three main ways:

1. as a face-to-face meeting between tutor and student, on a one-to-one basis;
2. as a face-to-face, small group activity;
3. at a distance, via remote links.

Many would claim that the most effective form of tutoring is the face-to-face meeting between a tutor and a single student, as this focuses solely upon that student's needs, and also ensures confidentiality. However, it is much more resource-efficient, in terms of tutor-time, to have small group tutorials, and students may benefit from the views of other group members. A combination of both approaches is probably best from the students' point of view, as they get the advantages of both.

Students on open and distance learning programmes may only attend an institution once or twice in a given semester, so the option of frequent face-to-face tutorials, or small group tutorials, is not available. In this case, tutoring occurs via remote communications such as terrestrial mail, telephone, fax, and email. Whilst these one-to-one tutorials offer the advantages of a sole focus on students' needs, and confidentiality, the absence of face-to-face communication is felt by many to be a disadvantage. Tutoring on open and distance learning programmes is addressed in Chapter 11 (p. 289).

Models of tutoring

There are three models of tutoring in common use in higher education, each of which has advantages and disadvantages.

Model 1. The student is allocated a personal tutor for the entire programme of study, whose role includes academic and pastoral support. The tutor is responsible for the marking of all the student's assessment work.

Model 2. The student is allocated a personal tutor for the entire programme of study, whose role is to provide general academic support and pastoral support. In this model, the student's assessment work is marked by the appropriate course (module) co-ordinator rather than by the personal tutor.

Model 3. The student does not have a personal tutor as such. Students are tutored by the course co-ordinator(s) of the course(s) they are currently studying, who are also responsible for marking their assessment work.

Model 1 has the advantage that continuity of tutoring is maintained throughout the student's programme of study, fostering the development of a strong tutorial relationship. However, that is fine, provided that the tutor/student relationship is a good one. If not, the student is saddled with that tutor for the rest of the programme, unless mechanisms exist for transfer to another tutor. A further disadvantage is that the tutor is responsible for marking all the students' assessment work, and since no teacher is expert in all aspects of a given curriculum, there is the danger of a lowering of academic standards.

Model 2 is designed to overcome the disadvantages of Model 1; marking of students' assessment work is done by the course co-ordinator, an expert with respect to a given course, so standards are maintained. However, the marking workload for course co-ordinators may be excessive, and contradictory advice about assessment requirements may be given by the personal tutor and the course co-ordinator.

Model 3 offers the protection of academic standards, but the personal and pastoral aspects of tutoring may be diminished or lost, depending on the degree of commitment of a given tutor.

THE TUTORING ROLE

Within higher education, it is not customary for students' attendance at tutorials to be compulsory, but they need to be aware that failure to take the opportunity may disadvantage them in their progression through a programme. For example, failure to attend tutorials may well be cited as evidence if the student should appeal against a decision of the Board of Examiners. The venue for tutorial meetings is normally the tutor's room, but if the room has shared occupancy with other staff, it is better to find an alternative room with more privacy. Tutees can be contacted by letter or by a message on the notice-board, but either way it is important to make contact as early as possible in the programme. During the induction period, I prefer to make out a list with times when I am available, and invite tutees to fill-in their names against a time slot. Once tutees have chosen a slot, it remains theirs for the duration of the programme, making it less likely they will forget their tutorial time. New students may feel uncomfortable having a one-to-one tutorial as their very first; it is therefore advisable to hold a group tutorial for the first meeting, so that the purpose and process of tutorials can be clarified.

The tutorial role commonly includes teaching and assessment, but the role also comprises a wide range of other elements including:

- encouraging and supporting;
- informing and advising;
- liaising and representing;
- monitoring;
- coaching;
- negotiating;
- profiling;
- counselling.

These elements are illustrated in Figure 15.1, and discussed in the following section.

Encouraging and supporting

It is invaluable for the student to have a personal tutor who can provide the necessary encouragement when things become difficult, as well as a friendly, sympathetic person to whom the student can unburden themselves. This element is no less important for mature post-registration students, since they often have difficulties with course-work and assessment if they have not been engaged in formal study for some considerable time. The relationship between the tutor and course member is paramount. The course member needs to be able to express views, opinions, and feelings in an atmosphere of psychological safety. However, the tutor should also expect to be challenged about

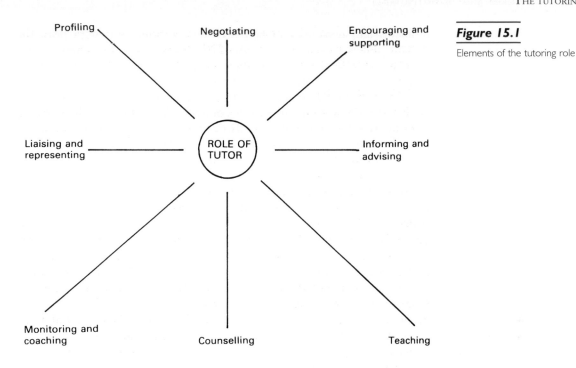

Profiling Negotiating Encouraging and supporting

Liaising and representing ROLE OF TUTOR Informing and advising

Monitoring and coaching Counselling Teaching

Figure 15.1

Elements of the tutoring role

his or her views and beliefs as the tutees grow in knowledge and confidence.

Informing and advising

The personal tutor is a valuable learning resource for tutees, particularly in relation to coursework and assessment. The tutor should ascribe to the course member appropriate independence and autonomy as a learner, so that critical thinking and enquiry is encouraged. Advising is one step beyond information-giving, in that the personal tutor is making suggestions or recommendations to the tutee believed to be in the tutee's best interests. One of the pitfalls of giving advice is that it removes the individual's autonomy to some extent. On the other hand, it is quite appropriate as a form of helping, provided that it is used thoughtfully. The sheer weight of experience often enables the tutor to see things more clearly than the tutee, although this is no guarantee of infallibility.

Student services

Tutors should be aware of the kind of service provided by the institution's student services, such as guidance and careers advice, welfare and financial advice, medical services, nurseries and child care, and sport and recreation.

Liaising and representing

It is good practice for tutors to undertake liaison visits to discuss their students' progress with practice-placement staff. This can often forestall problems and tensions and help to foster relationships with both the student and with placement staff. Liaison with other teachers is also necessary to ascertain how the tutee is functioning in his or her various groups. Tutors are often called upon to furnish reports of students' progress to funding bodies, and to support students' claims for study leave and funding for courses. It is sometimes necessary for the personal tutor to attend examination boards to provide information about factors affecting a student's performance.

Monitoring and coaching

Monitoring of student progress is a key responsibility of the tutor that can be achieved in a number of ways. Academic work can be monitored by noting the grades given for assignments, and clinical practice by direct observation, ward reports and informal feedback from both trained staff and student. Here again, self-assessment is an important tool to foster, so that the student can compare his or her own internal monitoring with that of the tutor and placement staff. Coaching is the term given to the remedial assistance provided by the tutor to help overcome specific learning difficulties. It is also used to refer to tutorial sessions for assessment examination revision and the marking of specimen examination answers.

Negotiation

One of the basic tenets of adult education is that students should be actively involved in the educational process, including any decisions about the curriculum that affect them. In the past it was common for educationalists to prescribe the goals, methods of learning, and evaluation without involving the student in these decisions. The principles of adult education include negotiation of curriculum elements. By definition, to negotiate implies reaching mutual agreement or compromise, so the negotiation needs to be more than simply a token involvement of the student.

Learning contracts

One of the more effective ways of using negotiation is by drawing up a contract for learning which is then signed by both parties. The theoretical basis of learning contracts is discussed in Chapter 3 (p. 59).

A learning contract is not a substitute method of learning, its sole purpose is to give the student a degree of control over the goals, content, methods and evaluation of some aspects of the curriculum. The balance between the relative proportion of teacher-prescribed activities and negotiated ones will depend upon the nature of the student's programme and the ethos of the institution.

The experience of negotiating a contract puts the student in an active role with regard to learning, in marked contrast to the passive acquiescence in an entirely imposed curriculum. The autonomy conferred by contract learning tends to be a potent motivating force, and the negotiated work is perceived as being the student's own, rather than that imposed by the teacher. It puts the responsibility for learning squarely with the student, an important factor for lifelong learning.

Contracts can vary greatly in the amount of work required and in the time available for completion. They can be used effectively for just one day of a study module, for example, where students are told that a particular day is unprogrammed to allow them to negotiate what they would like to do. Obviously, the contract for this kind of experience will be relatively limited, given that the students have only a short time to spend on their chosen activities. However, this exercise can be a good way of introducing the notion of contract learning to a group before more ambitious use in the programme.

Figure 15.2 shows a pro-forma for a learning contract; the headings will normally be prescribed by the institution. Each component of the contract is negotiated with the tutor and then signed by both parties.

Learning outcomes	Learning resources and strategies	Evidence of accomplishment	Validation of evidence

Figure 15.2

Example of a pro-forma for a learning contract

Negotiating a contract requires the student to have effective planning skills and good time-management skills. Although it is quite feasible to negotiate for the grade, it is relatively uncommon to find this facility in higher education. The system of grading assessments seems to imply that all students are capable of achieving the highest grade in all areas, and anything less is seen as an indication of weakness. This takes no account of the interests of the student, nor of the fact that few individuals are good at everything. It seems sensible to allow a student to negotiate for a C grade in some parts of the course, and for B or A grades in others. Obviously, a pass grade would be the minimum acceptable grade, but the choice of negotiating for a grade allows the student to concentrate efforts into his or her areas of interest.

The criteria for contracts at different grades need to be standardized to ensure fairness in assessment. It is quite in order for the tutor to state some non-negotiable aspects of the contract such as an emphasis on health rather than disease and in this case the students would have to focus on this aspect, whilst allowing freedom in the choice of the other elements of the contract.

Student profiling

The keeping of records is a key aspect of the role of personal tutor and has many serious implications. Accurate records are a necessary requirement for assessing student progress throughout a course and serve as legal documents in the event of disciplinary action. Profiling has arisen out of the move towards more involvement of students in their education, coupled with a desire to convey the widest possible picture of the student's abilities and interests.

Profiles are not methods of assessment, but rather a means of recording a wide range of assessments such as skills, attitudes, attainments and personal qualities (Hitchcock, 1990). Hence, profiles take a holistic view of the individual rather than the narrow view obtained only from examination results. Few people are good at everything; individuals have areas of greater and lesser expertise whatever their seniority, although professionals must always be judged as competent within their field. Thus, nurse teachers, whilst being basically competent in all areas of teaching, will naturally be better at some things than others. Many teachers are most at home in the lecture setting, while others prefer the small group setting. If we accept this, then the idea of a single overall grade becomes meaningless.

To state that a student maintained an average grade of B over a course means that the areas of greater or lesser expertise are being lost in the notion of average performance. It is surely better for all concerned to be able to read an account of the student's abilities and interests that bring out this range of achievement.

Purposes of profiling

Hitchcock (1990) gives several advantages of profiling which, although focused on the school sector, have relevance for nurse education.

1. *Greater student motivation.* This is largely due to the ethos of profiling, which emphasizes co-operation and recognition of achievement. Students should have the opportunity to participate in their formulation, as in the case of self-assessment of progress.
2. *Improved relationships and communication.* Profiling requires one-to-one communication and encourages development of personal relationships between tutor and tutee. The student is asked to consider her progress over the last module, and to bring written comments to the meeting with the personal tutor, where both parties then discuss the student's progress from their respective points of view.
3. *Facilitation of guidance and counselling.* The process of profiling involves close interaction between tutor and tutee, and this can facilitate pastoral care where appropriate.
4. *Improve diagnosis of learning needs.* Profiling can lead to better diagnosis of learning needs when this is built in as part of the formal profiling process.

5. *Improved selection information for employers.* Profiles are intended for public consumption and act as references for prospective employers and other interested parties.

Types of profiles

Hitchcock (1990) gives five categories of profiles:

1. *Student recording.* These contain such things as personal achievements and self-assessments.
2. *Student/teacher negotiated records.* These are compiled jointly by student and teacher.
3. *Criterion checklists.* Student achievements are matched against pre-determined criteria.
4. *Comment banks.* Statements relevant to the student are selected from a prepared computer bank and structured in prose form.
5. *Grid-style profiles.* A series of hierarchical statements are given, and the most appropriate one ticked to indicate the student's level of achievement.

Data Protection Act

When dealing with profiles, tutors need to be aware of the Data Protection Act, which applies only to computer-stored data; tutors must adhere to the main principles:

1. personal data shall be obtained and processed fairly and lawfully;
2. personal data shall be held for specified lawful purposes only;
3. personal data held for any purpose shall not be used in any manner incompatible with that purpose;
4. personal data shall be adequate, relevant and not excessive for the purpose for which it is held;
5. personal data shall not be kept longer than is necessary for the purpose;
6. an individual shall be entitled
   (a) to be informed of any data held by user,
   (b) to have access to such data, and
   (c) where appropriate, to have data corrected or erased; and
7. users must take appropriate security measures against unauthorized access/disclosure/alteration/accident, etc.

CHARACTERISTICS OF EFFECTIVE TUTORS

The quality of a tutorial relationship is very much contingent upon the interpersonal communication skills of the tutor; some individuals seem to possess these skills naturally, others need to be trained. Nurse teachers come from a culture of caring that is inherent in the role of the professional nurse, and this is carried forward to their tutoring role. Experience suggests that the personal characteristics shown in Table 15.1 are helpful in facilitating tutor/student relationships.

Table 15.1

Characteristics of effective tutors

1. *Self-awareness*
   This refers to the degree of self-knowledge tutors have about themselves, and is considered a fundamental requirement for helping others. Self-awareness of their strengths and weaknesses allows tutors to be more insightful when dealing with students.

2. *Trust*
   Effective tutor/student relationships require a climate mutual trust and can be engendered by appropriate self-disclosure by both parties, and a warm, open, honest approach toward each other.

3. *Acceptance and respect for the student*
   The tutor should demonstrate acceptance of the student as a person in his or her own right, and must convey respect for the student's worth by treating him or her as an equal. It is also useful to remember that nursing is only a part of the student's life; there are many other competing activities involved, each of which is perceived as important by the student.

4. *Retaining individuality*
   In personal tutoring, it is important to be one's natural self; Carl Rogers calls this 'Genuineness', i.e. the tutor should come across as a real person rather than as some kind of ideal model.

5. *Empathic understanding*
   This is another Carl Rogers term, which refers to a tutor's ability to put themselves in the students' shoes in order to see and understand things from their students' perspective.

6. *Credibility*
   Personal credibility is important as a basis for mutual respect, so the tutor needs to be seen as a good teacher as well as a sympathetic tutor.

USING COUNSELLING SKILLS IN TUTORING

In Figure 15.1, counselling was identified as one of the roles of the tutor, but it would be more correct to state that the tutor uses *counselling skills* when tutoring. This distinction is important; counselling itself is generally considered to be a specialist endeavour for which practitioners require high-level education and training. It is therefore not the province of amateurs, be they nurses or higher education teachers. As well as requiring a qualified expert, the counselling relationship should be a conscious contract between two individuals, i.e. the client should decide whether or not he or she wishes to enter into such a relationship, having been informed about the nature of it. There is no justification for tutors attempting to undertake amateur counselling of a student without the latter being aware of it. However, it is helpful for teachers to have an understanding of the distinction between professional counselling, and the use of counselling skills by other professionals.

The nature of counselling

The term *counselling* is used in three senses (Nelson-Jones, 1993):

1. *To describe a helping relationship*. This refers to the core qualities of the counsellor, and includes emphatic understanding, respect for the client, and genuineness.
2. *As a set of activities and methods*. These activities and methods include the empathic relationship with clients, and theoretical approaches such as psychoanalytical, behavioural, and rational-emotive.

3. *As a special area for providing services*. The difference between psychological therapies and counselling lies in the type of clients. In counselling, the focus is on clients in non-medical settings who are less disturbed than those receiving psychological therapy in hospitals.

The British Association for Counselling (BAC) suggests that the task of counselling is to give the client the opportunity to explore, discover and clarify ways of living more resourcefully and towards greater well-being. Hence, counselling can be seen as a helping relationship that assists the client to become self-directing. It differs from the other forms of helping referred to earlier, since they rely on the expertise of the tutor; counselling assumes that the client has the necessary resources to deal with the problem. Woolfe (1996) makes an interesting point about the lack of evaluation by counsellors:

> '*Counselling psychology can be seen as reaction to the somewhat mechanistic view of human beings inherent in more traditional psychological paradigms based upon a conventional model of the nature of science and the technique of scientific investigation. It would be unfortunate, however, if counselling psychology came to be seen as anti-science, nor is this the case. Indeed, its development as a discipline derives in part from the failure by counsellors to evaluate their practice, which remains as much an art as a science'* (p. 9).

Approaches to counselling

There is a variety of theoretical approaches to counselling, including humanistic, behavioural, psychodynamic, and cognitive, each reflecting the particular theoretical stance of the practitioners.

Humanistic or person-centred approach

The foundation of this approach lies in the work of Carl Rogers, who believed that each individual has within themselves a capacity for self-actualization, i.e. to fulfil their potential. However, in some situations, such as loss, or major life changes, the individual's capacity to cope is weakened, and s/he may require the services of a counsellor or skilled helper. According to Rogers, the qualities required of a facilitator are genuineness, trust and acceptance, and empathic understanding. The work of Carl Rogers is discussed in detail in Chapter 3 (p. 53).

Behavioural approach

The basis of this approach is behaviourist psychology, and its main tenets:

- the importance of observable behaviour;
- the effect of environmental stimuli on an individual's behavioural response;
- the importance of reinforcement in the learning of behaviours.

Hence, behavioural approaches focus on the counsellor's role in observing clients' behaviour and actions, and the influence of events in the external world upon these. Goals are established in the form of objectives to be achieved, include the means by which they will be achieved, and the criteria for assessing that achievement.

The work of key behaviourists such as Watson, Thorndike and Skinner is discussed in detail in Chapter 5 (p. 111).

Psychodynamic approach

This approach is based upon the work of Sigmund Freud and his followers, and emphasizes the importance of the unconscious motivation, i.e. things that we are unaware of, in determining behaviour. Another important psychodynamic concept is that of defence mechanisms such as repression or reaction-formation. The role of the counsellor in this approach is to help clients to bring these unconscious factors into their consciousness, and thereby understand what is causing their problems.

Psychodynamic theory is discussed in detail in Chapter 2 (p. 22).

Cognitive approach

Cognitive approaches are concerned with the way that clients think, and aim to deal with distortions and unreal thinking. There are two main approaches in this category: reality therapy, and rational-emotive therapy. The former focuses on the importance of getting the client to recognize reality, and this can be done by the counsellor challenging clients' perceptions of reality, and helping them to re-orientate themselves. Rational-emotive therapy concerns an individual's processing of life events and the link between her/his beliefs and feelings; a client's belief system may cause him to draw invalid inferences from problem situations in his life, and the result is often unhappiness or distress. The role of the counsellor in this approach is to identify any irrational beliefs the client may hold, and helping him to adopt more rational ones.

The counselling process

There are different ways of approaching the counselling process; the following model is a well-established one.

The 'skilled helper' model (Egan, 1981)

This is a developmental model that is firmly based in the person-centred approach of Carl Rogers. It serves as a map to guide the helper through the helping process, and identifies the skills he will need at each stage. There are three stages in the model, but the counsellor may need to traffic back and forth between the stages during the interview.

1. *Exploration.* In this first stage the role of the helper is to establish a warm, trusting, non-threatening relationship with the client to enable him to explore the problem from his own frame of

reference, and to focus on specific concerns. It is important to communicate acceptance of the client for what he is, and also to convey attention. *Active listening* is more than simply listening to what the client is saying; it involves paraphrasing the client's words, reflecting back to the client what the counsellor thinks he is feeling, and making a summary of what the client has said in order to clarify understanding by both parties. The counsellor should help the client to focus on specific, concrete concerns using open and closed questions, and also on the client's strengths as well as weaknesses.

2. *New understanding*. During this stage the counsellor helps the client to see himself and his concerns from alternative perspectives and to focus on ways in which the client might cope more effectively using his own strengths and resources. In addition to the stage I skills the counsellor will use *advanced empathy*, which involves sharing hunches about the client in order to reveal hidden meanings and feelings. The client is helped to use alternative frames of reference for viewing his situation and concerns, and in this stage the use of confrontation by the counsellor helps the client to explore discrepancies and distortions in his perspective. *Immediacy* is used to bring what is happening between the client and the counsellor into the 'here-and-now'. Self-disclosure by the counsellor of her feelings or experiences should only be used if it will help the client to progress, otherwise it will remove the client-focus of the interview.

3. *Action*. In this stage the counsellor's role is to help the client to consider the action he wants to take, in the form of concrete attainable goals, and the resources and skills he may require. The client may need to be helped with decision-making and problem-solving skills, and will require support and encouragement. Brainstorming may be helpful as a way of encouraging creative thinking, and role-play can help the client to practice new behaviours or skills.

Miller's five-stage model for the first session with a new client

Miller (1999) describes a five-stage model for the first session with a new client, which nicely illustrates the counselling approach.

1. *Pre-interview considerations*. This takes place before the actual counselling interview, and consists of pre-planning of the interview and making the initial contact with the client. Pre-planning the interview involves thinking about the client' issues and problems, and this information is gained from the referring person's perceptions. Planning the initial contact involves such aspects as the date, time and venue for the appointment; the counsellor's contact details; and the type of communication used to make the appointment, i.e. telephone or letter.

2. *Meeting and engaging the client*. The venue needs to offer privacy

and confidentiality, and the seating should be positioned to facilitate discussion. The opening of the interview should involve the exchange of names and greetings, and clarification of the counsellor's role. The purpose of the meeting should be articulated, and the time allocation for the interview made explicit. Reference should be made to the need to take notes during the interview. Rapport is built up between counsellor and client by the former taking the lead initially, and using questioning to encourage the client to talk. Careful listening and observation of the client's responses is important, and it is helpful to set small, achievable goals to keep the interview focused. In order to maximize the time available for the interview, it is important to identify the main concerns of the client early in the interview and to prioritize these in terms of their importance to the client. Care must be taken to be precise in the use of words so as to avoid misunderstanding.

3. *Gathering information and making an assessment.* It is helpful for the counsellor to gather more information about the problem in a variety of ways, e.g. third-party information; critical incidents or precipitating factors; the impact upon relationships, etc. The counsellor should use careful questioning to identify the client's beliefs about the problem, and offer appropriate relevant information affecting the problem. One of the more difficult aspects of this stage is helping the client to manage her/his concerns, and one useful strategy is to re-frame the problem to provide an alternative perspective for the client's consideration, and to identify any resources that the client has used in the past. Near the end of the interview, the counsellor should make an assessment of the client on the basis of information gained in the interview.

4. *Decision-making and ending the session.* In this stage, the counsellor must make decisions on a number of aspects, such as whether or not to continue with the counselling; the frequency of sessions and the interval between them, etc. Miller emphasizes the importance of maintaining a neutral, professional relationship, and avoiding giving advice or interpretations at this stage. Time should be made available for the client to ask any questions or comments, but this should not involve a lengthy review of the entire session. It is useful to obtain some feedback from the client about her/his perceptions of the session, and it is also helpful to summarize before closing the session in a appropriate way.

5. *Post-session tasks and reflection.* In this final stage following the end of the session, the counsellor needs to make a careful record of the key points of the interview, bearing in mind that the client is entitled to see her/his records. The information gleaned during the interview is used to review the counsellor's pre-interview hypothesis, and consideration needs to be given to how the referring person will be given feedback. Miller also highlights the importance of consultation and supervision for the counsellor as a support mechanism.

Using counselling skills in tutoring

Earlier in this section, a distinction was drawn between tutors acting as counsellors to students, and tutors using counselling skills in their tutorial relationships. It was emphasized that the former was inappropriate for a number of reasons, but that the latter were helpful in facilitating the tutor/student relationship.

The British Association for Counselling sums up the latter nicely:

'Within another role the counselling skills user may help someone to recognize feelings, thoughts and behaviours and, when appropriate, to explore them in greater depth' (BAC, 1999).

The difference between nursing skills and counselling skills is nicely pointed out by Pratt (1994):

'Janet was a district nurse who opted to take a six-day course entitled "An Introduction to Counselling Skills". Before the course Jan believed she already knew what "counselling" was, and although in practice she sometimes found the going a bit tough and had suspicions that there were aspects of counselling she needed to know more about, she was basically attending the course to brush up her skills and to confirm that she was on the right track. In the initial workshop and discussion, it became clear that giving advice and information were, at best, very low priorities when using counselling skills. Also, and contrary to Jan's actual experience hitherto, finding "answers" or even ways forward in the troublesome situation she and her patient were discussing were seen to be much more the responsibility of the patient than herself' (p. 1).

Pratt also draws a distinction between the locations in which counselling and counselling skills are used; the former normally takes place in a consulting room or other appropriate venue designated for counselling. Counselling skills, on the other hand, are used in largely impromptu settings such as corridors, classrooms, treatment rooms or community nurses' cars.

Basic counselling skills

Table 15.3 identifies a range of basic counselling skills that can be used by tutors. These are generic skills common to interpersonal communication, and Chapter 18 discussed a range of these skills including verbal and non-verbal communication (p. 462), self-awareness (p. 464), effective listening skills (p. 473), and effective questioning skills (p. 474).

BAC code of ethics and practice guidelines

The British Association for Counselling have developed a *Code of Ethics and Practice Guidelines for Those Using Counselling Skills in Their Work* (BAC, 1999), and they state that counselling skills are being used:

1. when there is intentional use of specific interpersonal skills which reflect the value of counselling;

Table 15.2

Basic counselling skills

Skill	Description
Attending	Shows complete attention to client by non-verbal signals, i.e. eye-contact; relaxed open posture, leaning forward; sitting opposite client; close proximity without invading client's personal space
Observing	Watching client's non-verbal behaviour for signs of stress or incongruity with what is being said
Active listening	Concentrated listening, not only to the message, but also to the prosodic, paralinguistic and indexical features of speech
Summarizing	Making a summary of what client has said helps to clarify understanding for both parties
Reflecting	Paraphrasing client's words, or saying what counsellor thinks client is feeling
Questioning	Need to avoid interrogation; use open questions rather than closed, to allow expansion by client
Silence	Effective use of silence can encourage client to talk. Counsellor needs to control own anxiety about lengthy periods of silence
Independence	Giving client responsibility for solving their own problem by appropriate questions
'Concreting'	Assisting client to give concrete examples of how he or she is behaving or feeling

2. when the practitioner's primary role (e.g. nurse, tutor, line manager, social worker, personnel officer, helper) is enhanced without being changed;
3. when the client perceives the practitioner as acting within their primary professional or caring role which is *not* that of being a counsellor.

It is clear from this statement that the difference between counselling, and the use of counselling skills in tutoring, lies in the fact that the tutor retains her primary role of tutor throughout the tutorial relationship.

Focus of the BAC code of ethics

The BAC code of ethics and practice guidelines should be followed by tutors who use counselling skills as part of their tutoring role. These focus on the following areas:

1. *Values.* Tutors should embrace the values of integrity, impartiality, and respect for the student; counselling skills must be used in a non-exploitative way.
2. *Confidentiality.* Tutors should reach agreement with the student at the outset about the extent of confidentiality, and be careful not to inadvertently disclose information given in confidence.
3. *Competence.* Tutors should consider the appropriateness of using counselling skills within a tutorial relationship, and consider whether they are adequately prepared for the use of such skills. They should recognize the limits of their competence, and also need to consider whether the student is aware of the purpose of

using counselling skills in the tutorial relationship. They should also recognize when it is appropriate to refer the student elsewhere.

4. *Supervision.* It is recommended that tutors who use counselling skills should undergo regular, non-managerial supervision to monitor the tutor's counselling skills work. The supervisor should be experienced in the use of counselling skills.

MAKING STUDENT REFERRALS

Tutors need to be aware of their own limitations, and be prepared to accept the need to refer the student elsewhere for further help. Examples of such referral might be a medical practitioner, a professional counsellor, or a legal advisor. Referral should not be seen as a failure on the part of the tutor; rather, it is an indicator of the competence of the tutor in recognizing that alternative help is required for the student. It is better if the student makes the arrangements for referral, as he is more likely to keep an appointment made by himself. As part of the overall student services, all institutions of higher education have a counselling and advisory service, and it is to this service that students should be referred, with the student's agreement, for further counselling.

PITFALLS OF TUTORING AND COUNSELLING

Although the benefits of tutoring are well acknowledged within higher education, there are also pitfalls of which both tutors and students need to be aware.

Inappropriate tutor–student relationships

One of the hallmarks of successful tutoring is the development of a supportive and trusting relationship between the tutor and the student, but herein lies a potential danger. Tutors and students need to be aware that, if the student's learning and development are to be facilitated, there must be boundaries to the tutorial relationship.

Given the unequal distribution of power between tutor and student, there is the possibility that a tutor could abuse the tutorial relationship for reasons of personal gain, e.g. romantic, sexual or financial gain. Students correctly perceive their tutor as having considerable influence over their progression through their programme; s/he is often the person who comments on assessment drafts, grades their coursework, and produces reports and references. This puts the tutor in a position of considerable power in relation to the student, and it is very much to the latter's advantage to keep their tutor 'sweet'.

It is important to state at this point that there is nothing illegal about a relationship between a tutor and a student, because in higher education the students are adults, and can make such decisions for themselves. Nevertheless, universities frown upon inappropriate relationships between tutors and students when the tutor is involved in teaching or assessing the student in question.

Most institutions of higher education will have a policy on relationships between staff and students, which advises members of staff to consult in confidence with their head of department if a relationship has existed, or does exist, between themselves and one of their students. This enables alternative teaching, tutoring and assessment arrangements to be made for that student.

Amateur psychoanalysis

A good tutor/student relationship is based on trust and confidence, so it is not surprising that students may wish to bring personal problems to the attention of their tutor. In attempting to explore the problem, tutors may engage in a degree of analysis that is beyond their sphere of competence. Because nurse teachers, and particularly mental health teachers, have a good grounding in psychology, there is the temptation to stray into areas that can only be described as 'amateur psychoanalysis'. Tutors are not psychotherapists, nor are they qualified or employed as such. They should therefore recognize these limitations, and if they feel that a student may be in need of psychotherapy, then they should use the referral system to address this issue.

REFERENCES

British Association for Counselling (1999) *Code of Ethics and Practice Guidelines for Those Using Counselling Skills in Their Work*, BAC, London.

DfEE (1993) *Higher Quality and Choice: The Charter for Higher Education*, HMSO, London.

Egan, G. (1981) *The Skilled Helper: A Model for Systematic Helping and Interpersonal Relating*, Brooks/Cole, Monterey.

Hitchcock, B. (1990) *Profiles and Profiling: A Practical Introduction*, Longman, Harlow.

Miller, R. (1999) The first session with a new client: five stages, in *The Trainee Handbook: A Guide for Counselling and Psychotherapy Trainees*, R. Bor and M. Watts (eds), Sage, London.

Nelson-Jones, R. (1993) *The Theory and Practice of Counselling Psychology*, Cassell, London.

Pratt, J. (1994) *Counselling Skills for Professional Helpers*, Central Book Publishers, London.

Wheeler, S. and Birtle, J. (1993) *A Handbook for Personal Tutors*, SRHE/Open University Press, Buckingham.

Woolfe, R. (1996) The nature of counselling psychology, in *Handbook of Counselling Psychology*, R. Woolfe and W. Dryden (eds), Sage, London.

PART FOUR

SPECIFIC TEACHING TOPICS AND CONTEXTS

16

Nursing, midwifery and health visiting practice is carried out in a range of workplace settings, including hospital wards and departments, community health centres, GP surgeries, schools, nurseries, day centres, residential homes, and industry. It is therefore self-evident that these settings constitute important learning environments; indeed, experiential learning is based on the premise that learning gained through experience is more meaningful and relevant than that acquired in classrooms.

Some people prefer to use the term *learners* to describe individuals who are pursuing an education or training programme in the workplace, but given that everyone is now meant to be a 'lifelong learner', the term student seems a more appropriate distinction. Within a given workplace setting, there is a variety of individuals who can be classed as 'students' at one time or another:

1. *Pre-registration students*. These are students undertaking an educational programme in a higher education institution leading to an academic award and registration as a nurse or midwife. Their presence in the workplace is on the basis of a placement, i.e. they spend a given amount of time in a range of workplace settings, but are not part of the workforce of those settings.
2. *Post-registration students*. These are qualified registered nurses or midwives who are undertaking either:
   (a) an educational programme in a higher education institution leading to an additional academic and/or professional award; or
   (b) an in-house programme of professional development.

Most of these are in-service students, i.e. they are undertaking their studies on a part-time or flexible basis, whilst maintaining their responsibilities as members of the workforce in a given workplace setting. However, some post-registration programmes, such as health visiting, lead to a further professional registration and are therefore classified as being both pre-and post-registration! These programmes require full-time attendance, and the students undertake placements in a range of community workplace settings.

3. *National Vocational Qualification (NVQ) students*. These are normally health care assistants who are undertaking an NVQ programme at a college of further education leading to an NVQ award. These are part-time in-service programmes with an emphasis on workplace learning and assessment.

From the foregoing discussion, it can be seen that workplace settings in nursing, midwifery and health visiting provide the learning environment for a whole range of personnel, including those undertaking formal programmes, and those receiving informal, and often spontaneous, teaching as part of their day-to-day practice. Hence, this environment for learning becomes a crucial factor in the success or otherwise of the personnel involved, so it behoves nurse teachers to appreciate the social dynamics of the workplace. Chapter 14 (p. 355) contains a detailed discussion of group dynamics, but selected aspects relating to the workplace are included below.

GROUP DYNAMICS AND THE WORKPLACE

The workplace does not simply provide an environment for learning the knowledge and skills required for practice, it also serves as a vehicle for pre-registration students' socialization into the profession of nursing or midwifery.

Socialization

From early infancy, individuals learn the values, knowledge and patterns of behaviour that make them a member of their particular society; the process by which an individual undergoes induction into these expected behaviours or roles is termed *socialization*, and is a lifelong process involving transmission of culture.

Primary socialization

This begins in infancy and is mediated through the immediate family; sex roles, social class morals and manners are all part of this early socialization process.

Secondary socialization

This begins once the child commences school, and this is influenced not only by teachers but by peers; the latter exert a powerful effect as the child moves into adolescence, when peer-group pressure may result in behaviour at variance with the child's family or society.

Occupational socialization

This is a particular kind of secondary socialization, which involves the induction into specific occupational roles after leaving school. Nursing culture has a powerful influence on new members, socializing them into the role of nurse, with all its attendant values and behaviours. In the past, there was great emphasis on conformity and obedience to superiors and a very rigid code of personal and professional behaviour.

Socialization may begin in anticipation of future rules and this anticipatory socialization is important in facilitating the eventual uptake of such roles. Many girls are socialized into nursing from an early age by means of play, especially that associated with hospitals and caring. The mass media is a powerful influence on such socialization and may well be responsible for sex-role stereotyping and racism. Television, newspapers and even children's books may portray nursing as being the exclusive preserve of women; indeed, women are commonly portrayed in occupations such as nursing, teaching, domestic work and catering, rather than in engineering or medicine.

The public nature of work-based teaching

One of the major differences between classroom teaching and workplace-based teaching is that the latter is a much more public endeavour. In the classroom, the teacher is normally alone with the students; in contrast, the workplace is populated by a wide range of people including:

- nursing and medical staff;
- practitioners from the professions allied to medicine, e.g. physiotherapist, occupational therapist, medical laboratory technicians, etc.;
- support workers and administrators;
- patients, clients, relatives and friends;
- counsellors, ministers of religion.

It is very likely that much of the teaching will take place in this public arena, so it may be helpful to explore the effects of an audience on human performance. The mere presence of an audience may facilitate or hinder behaviour, the so-called 'audience effect'. For example, many actors and athletes feel that they need an audience in order to perform to their fullest ability, and this effect is supported by studies.

The effect of having someone actually performing a task with another person (i.e. co-acting) has also been studied extensively; the classic study by Allport (1924) concluded that the presence of a co-worker enhances the speed and quality of work on simple tasks. On the other hand, the presence of others can exert an inhibitory effect on behaviour and this has been demonstrated in a number of interesting studies.

Latane and Darley (1968) showed the effect of the presence of other people on an individual's reaction to emergency situations. They conclude that people are less likely to intervene in an emergency if other people are present and this can be explained by diffusion of responsibility. If a person is alone when he or she encounters an emergency, then that person is solely responsible for his or her actions. If, however, other people are present, each individual may feel that their own responsibility is reduced and this makes them less likely to become involved.

Roles and norms

Within the workplace setting, roles and norms exert a significant influence. Roles are actions within a given status, such as the leadership role of the ward manager. Norms are standards or values of behaviour, which may be formal or informal. Formal norms in a workplace setting are imposed by the organization, such as a requirement for practice to be evidence-based. Informal norms develop from within the group as a result of interaction; for example, one ward may have a norm involving a particular way of organizing the daily workload. Individuals tend to conform to the prevailing norms of the workplace, and there is evidence that norms may develop over a short period. In a classic study on group norms, Sherif (1936) demonstrated the rapid convergence to a group norm of individuals' opinions regarding the extent of apparent movement of a spot of light in a darkened room. Hence, individuals who join a workplace setting will be expected to adhere to the norms, or risk alienation or ostracism.

Labelling theory and expectancy effect

Another aspect of group dynamics that has significance for workplace settings is that of labelling and expectancy effect. In sociological terms, labelling is the assigning of an individual to a category as a means of classifying his behaviour or state. Hence, 'ill' is a label used to distinguish people who are not healthy; 'vandal' is a label that distinguishes people who exhibit antisocial behaviour involving damage to property.

Labelling, then, involves classifying people who deviate from what is considered to be normal; the term *deviance*, however, is used to indicate a negative social evaluation.

Primary deviance

This is the assigning of a label to particular behaviours or states judged by society as deviant; these behaviours are socially defined and will vary between different cultures. The behaviours that a society considers deviant may change over the course of time; in the UK, it used to be considered deviant to attempt suicide, or to live as a couple without being married, whereas nowadays these behaviours are seen in quite a different light.

Secondary deviance

Once society has assigned a label to an individual, certain consequences may occur and these are termed. When a person is labelled 'deviant' he or she becomes stigmatized or disgraced in the eyes of society; depending upon the nature of the deviance, the individual may be shunned or worse – this is particularly true for labels such as 'rapist'. Many diseases, however, can stigmatize the sufferer, especially mental illness, epilepsy, AIDS and even such problems as deafness or blindness. Indeed, it can be argued that the diagnosis of such conditions in itself constitutes labelling of primary deviance, setting in train a series of predictable social consequences.

The 'self-fulfilling prophecy'

A second major effect of labelling is that of changes in the individual's self-concept; as a result of social reactions to the original label, the affected person begins to respond in a way that is compatible with that label. In other words, he comes to believe that he is what the label says he is and produces stereotyped behaviour that accords with it. This phenomenon has been termed the 'self-fulfilling prophecy' – a prophecy that comes true solely because it has been made. For example, a ward manager labels a student nurse as 'lazy' and people begin to react to him according to his label; eventually the nurse begins to accept the label and his behaviour becomes lazy. Obviously, there must have been an initial episode that led to the label, but it may have been a 'one-off' incident entirely untypical of the individual.

The notion of self-fulfilling prophecy has been explored in education, where it is known as 'teacher-expectancy effect'. There is a good deal of evidence about the effect of people's expectations on certain outcomes; experimenters have to be cautious when interpreting results because such results may be due to the 'Hawthorne effect' – a variation in subjects simply due to the fact they are being observed. The presence of an observer may have either positive or negative effects on the performance of students that are totally unrelated to the style of teaching given.

In a classic study (Rosenthal and Jacobson, 1968), carried out in an American school, teachers were given false information about some of the children in their classes; these children were purported to have unusual academic potential and were called 'spurters', but in reality they were randomly selected from the total class. The children were given tests of non-verbal intelligence at the start of the experiment and again at four months and eight months and results showed that the 'spurters' had gained significantly more in terms of IQ than the other children. This was ascribed to the fact that teachers' expectations of the 'spurters' had acted as a self-fulfilling prophecy, which made them achieve more. The study has been criticized on methodological grounds, but there is some support from other studies that teacher-expectancy can influence learning.

THE WORKPLACE LEARNING ENVIRONMENT

The qualified staff are a key factor influencing the learning environment in hospital placements, the role of ward manager being particularly influential. Not only do they have control of the management of the area, but also serve as role-models for nursing practice. The leadership style and personality of the ward manager are important determinants of an effective learning environment, as demonstrated in a series of classic surveys in the 1980s (Orton, 1981; Fretwell, 1983; Ogier, 1982, 1986; Pembrey, 1980).

Characteristics of a workplace environment conducive to learning

The following summarizes the main perceptions of students in these research studies with regard to the characteristics of a good clinical learning environment.

A humanistic approach to students

Qualified staff should ensure that pre-registration students are treated with kindness and understanding and should try to show interest in them as people. They should be approachable and helpful to students, providing support as necessary, and try to foster the students' self-esteem. In the case of colleagues undertaking post-registration programmes, qualified staff need to be sensitive to their study needs, a point easily overlooked when a colleague has been working in the clinical area for some time as a full-time practitioner.

Team spirit

Qualified staff should work as a team and strive to make the student feel a part of that team. They should create a good atmosphere by their relationships within the team.

Management style

This should be efficient and yet flexible in order to produce good quality care. Teaching should have its place in the overall organization and students should be given responsibility and encouraged to use initiative. Nursing practice should be consistent with that taught in the university.

Teaching and learning support

Qualified staff should be encouraged to act as supervisors, mentors, preceptors, and assessors as appropriate. Opportunities should be given for students to ask questions, attend medical staff rounds, observe new procedures and have access to patients/clients records. Non-nursing professionals such as doctors, physiotherapists, dieticians and chaplains can also contribute to the learning environment provided they are made to feel part of the total team. It is important for the ward manager to spend a little time with new non-nursing colleagues in order to explain the ethos of the ward or department in relation to learning, thus encouraging them to see themselves as a resource for student learning.

It is not always appreciated that students themselves are very much a part of the learning environment and not merely the passive recipients of its influences. An effective environment will encourage the students to take responsibility for their own learning and to actively seek out opportunities for this. Critical thinking and judgement are fostered in an atmosphere where the student can question and dissent without feeling guilty or disloyal.

An important part of the learning process is experimentation, in which the student can try to apply concepts and principles in different ways; this implies that the student will need to adopt different approaches to patients and to be innovative. There may be other students in a clinical area and this peer support can be invaluable. By planning for two students to work together, there can be substantial benefits for both, provided they take time to discuss approaches and decisions and their underlying rationale.

The learning environment in community nursing

So far we have discussed learning environments with reference to hospital settings, but the environment is equally important when students are in community placements. Prior preparation in advance of a student placement is vital to ensure that the student gains the most from it. It is good practice to establish empathy with the student many weeks before the actual placement, for example, by the mentor giving the student his or her work and home telephone numbers in order to discuss expectations, and also 'housekeeping' issues such as transport arrangements, etc.

The physical environment is clearly very different from that of a hospital, particularly when it involves domiciliary visits to patients in their own homes. Nursing staff are guests in this situation, with no right of entry and consequently, much of the teaching will occur by observation, with discussion following later after leaving the patient's home. Much of this discussion takes place in the practitioner's car in a one-to-one setting, calling for very good interpersonal skills on the part of the teacher. The practitioner needs to put the student at ease and treat him or her as an equal. The effects of a strained relationship are much more difficult to cope with when there are only two people involved.

Clinics and post-natal groups provide another community learning environment for students. When running a well-baby clinic the mentor can combine tutorials for both student and parent, since the information is common to both. In community placements, media resources tend to be less readily available than in hospital settings, and hence the mentor places greater reliance on discussion and role modelling strategies.

Stress and the workplace learning environment

The concept of work-related stress has become a major issue for employers and employees, evidenced by the increasing numbers of claims for compensation arising out of work-induced, stress-related illness. Indeed, the term has now become a normal part of our everyday experience of living, exemplified in the expression, 'I'm really stressed-out'.

There can be few work settings that have more potential for stress than hospitals or community health settings; the very nature of the work involves staff in close contact with patients who are themselves often distressed and traumatized.

The nature of stress

Stress is a difficult concept to pin down, but it is generally thought of as consisting of two components:

1. *Stressors.* These are events in our lives that threaten our physical or mental well being.
2. *Stress responses.* These are our reactions to the stressors we encounter.

The reaction of the individual to stressors occurs in three well-defined stages termed 'the general adaptation syndrome' (Selye, 1956):

1. *The alarm reaction.* This is a short-term reaction characterized by changes in physiology such as increased heart rate, respiration, endocrine activity and sympathetic-nervous-system activity. This combination is commonly referred to as the 'fight or flight' reaction.
2. *Resistance to stress.* In this stage the body processes return to normal and the individual adapts to the stress.
3. *Exhaustion.* This rarely occurs in psychological stress, although it is common in extreme physical conditions such as severe exposure. Here, the individual has used up all the resources for coping, and death may occur.

This adaptation syndrome is non-specific, in that it occurs when the person encounters any form of stress, of whatever severity.

One approach to stress is called 'person-environment fit theory' (Caplan, 1983), in which stress is defined as either:

- demands that exceed the individual's capability to fulfil, i.e. s/he is overwhelmed;
- an individual's capability exceeds the demands upon her/him, i.e. s/he is underwhelmed. This is typified by the case of an individual whose work does not sufficiently 'stretch' her/his capabilities.

Effects of stress upon the individual
The impact of stress can be classified into two main categories: the effects of stress on students' performance in the workplace, and the effects of stress on the health of students and staff in the workplace.

Effects of stress on students' performance in the workplace
An individual's level of emotional arousal has a significant effect on her/his subsequent performance, including cognitive as well as physical performance (Hebb, 1972). Each individual has an optimal level of arousal at which they perform at their best; under-arousal or over-arousal results in a deterioration in performance of learning tasks, particularly complex ones. Figure 16.1 shows the Yerkes–Dodson law on the relationship between emotional arousal level and performance.

It can be seen that arousal beyond the optimal level for a particular individual will cause a deterioration in performance. This effect is commonly observed in life-threatening situations, where individuals' behaviour often becomes disorganized and irrational, i.e. the phenomenon called panic. It is important to note that well-learned behaviours are much less likely to be disrupted by hyper-arousal than complex activities that require the integration of information, as the latter require more information-processing by the brain. So it is likely that a member of staff who is suffering from stress may be able to continue to perform many of the more routine, well-learned skills, but will be less

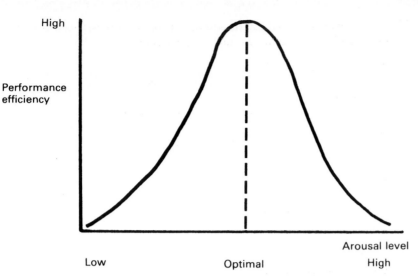

Figure 16.1

Yerkes–Dodson law: emotional
arousal level and performance

able to cope with more complex and demanding situations in nursing practice.

Stress can also affect an individual's ability to concentrate on tasks and to retrieve information from memory, due to the intrusion of distracting thoughts about the possibility of failure. In the context of examinations, this has been termed *test anxiety*. Another aspect of stress-related behaviour is the tendency for the individual to stick to inappropriate patterns of behaviour because they are unable to consider alternatives. Atkinson *et al.* (1993) cite as an example the behaviour of some people trapped in a burning building; they died because they continued to push at doors that were designed to open inwards.

The effects of stress on the health of students and staff in the workplace
The reaction to stress will vary from individual to individual, with some experiencing feelings of anger and aggression, and others apathy and depression. Relationships can be affected, and some individuals make find solace in alcohol. Anxiety is another common symptom of stress, and there is evidence that it can impair the response of the immune system, leading to illness. There is also evidence of a link between stress and heart disease, especially in relation to the 'Type A personality', which is discussed in Chapter 2 (p. 31).

Sources of stress in the workplace
The categorization of sources of stress in organizations by Cooper and Marshall (1976) is adapted below to provide a framework for thinking about sources of stress in the clinical and community workplace.

1. Job-related stressors:
   - too much work to get through in the time available;
   - insufficient staff to support practitioners;

- inadequate availability of equipment or resources;
- little opportunity to use higher level skills.
2. Role-related stressors:
   - role ambiguity, e.g. lack of clarity about boundaries of role;
   - role-conflict, e.g. between role as practitioner and manager;
   - inadequate staff development for role;
   - role-conflict between work and family.
3. Relationship-related stressors:
   - conflict with superiors;
   - conflict with subordinates;
   - difficulties with colleagues from other health disciplines.
4. Career-related stressors:
   - pressures of continuing professional development;
   - expectations of promotion;
   - fear of redundancy.
5. Organization-related stressors:
   - inadequate communication;
   - internal politics;
   - secrecy and lack of trust.

Cooper (1999) gives a list of stressors that are specific to nurses working in outpatients departments:

- volume of patients;
- aggressive patients;
- unpredictable workloads;
- always in the public eye;
- new technology;
- lack of managerial supervision;
- fluctuating shift times;
- lack of time for training.

Coping with stress in the workplace

Many of the stressors encountered in the workplace will be beyond the individual practitioner's power to change. The organization carries a responsibility for the health and safety of its employees, and the increasing incidence of litigation on the grounds of stress-induced illness is forcing organizations to look more seriously at workplace stressors.

One of the most important elements of coping is being able to recognize the signs of stress in oneself, and to attempt to identify the main stressors involved. This enables coping strategies to be mobilized at a relatively early stage before the stress gets to a more serious level. The following coping strategies are commonly identified in the literature:

- Avoid taking on more work than you can cope with, by developing your assertive ability to say no to requests.
- Delegate jobs to other colleagues where possible.
- Always ensure that breaks are taken outside of the workplace area,

e.g. go to the staff dining room for coffee, and go outside to the shops at lunch time.

- Undertake relaxation techniques at appropriate times, such as physical-relaxation techniques and meditation.
- Suggest to management that stress reduction programmes should be made available for staff.
- Try setting up a stress support group in the workplace, where colleagues can share their experiences.
- Use the individual performance review/appraisal system to bring to the attention of management the workplace stressors you have identified, e.g. lack of staff development for your role; inadequate resources, etc. This will ensure that they are formally recorded with the organization, an important point if evidence is needed at a later date.
- Report to your GP if your symptoms of stress are severe. Not only may treatment be provided, but a formal record is made which may be important evidence if needed at a later date.

Managing emotion in the workplace

Clinical and community settings are, by their very nature, places of intense emotions. These encompass positive emotions, such as excitement, joy, elation, and also negative emotions, such as anger, frustration and fear. It is interesting to note that both positive and negative emotions can equally disrupt normal functioning in an individual, including their relationships with others, and their ability to make judgements and take decisions. It may be necessary for nurses, midwives and health visitors to manage other people's disruptive emotions in the workplace, be it those of colleagues, patients or clients, and a number of principles of good practice for managing other's emotions are suggested by Ostell *et al.* (1999):

1. *Deal with the emotional reaction before attempting to resolve the problem.* The individual's disruptive level of emotion needs to be reduced so that they can begin to consider their problem rationally, and the authors' suggest two approaches to this. Apologising to the individual can be helpful if there is a justifiable grievance of some kind, e.g. a patient having to wait in the accident and emergency department for a long time, or if the recipient of the outburst is responsible in some way for the circumstances provoking the outburst. An alternative approach is to use reflective statements such as 'I can see that you are unhappy about....', which may help defuse the emotion, but they may well have the opposite effect if perceived as stating the obvious.

2. *Avoid behaviour that heightens adverse emotional reactions.* When responding to disruptive emotional outbursts it is self-evident that one should avoid any behaviours that might exacerbate the other person's emotional state. Hence, any form of confrontation should be avoided, and it is important not to become angry when

dealing with an angry person, as this will simply fuel their emotional reaction.

3. *Employ behaviours likely to dissipate adverse emotional reactions.* It seems normal to offer sympathy to individuals' who demonstrate disruptive emotional reactions, but this can often reinforce the adverse emotional reaction by seeming to agree with their view of the circumstances. It is preferable to use empathy to show that the person's circumstances are understood, and this can be done by reflecting their views back to them, and by non-judgemental questioning.

4. *Recognize differences between emotions.* The authors' point out that all emotional reactions should not be treated in the same way, because different emotions tend to be stimulated by different patterns of thinking, e.g. anger commonly arises when an individual's demands have been denied; anxiety when individual's anticipate unpleasant consequences that they perceive to be beyond their control.

5. *Where appropriate, attempt to find a solution to the underlying problem.* Finding a solution to the underlying problem can only occur once the disruptive emotional reaction has subsided. It is important to find a solution in order to prevent similar outbursts when the circumstances are encountered again. A counselling approach can be useful here, but advice and instructions are also helpful in some cases.

6. *Learn to 'actively accept' reality.* There are some problems causing adverse emotional reactions that are not capable of solution, e.g. bereavement, redundancy; in such cases, the individual must learn to accept reality by letting go of these unattainable desires. However, this may take considerable time, and the help of a professional counsellor may be required.

Auditing the workplace learning environment

In order to be considered as an appropriate placement for pre-registration students, a workplace must meet the standard laid down by the relevant National Board for Nursing, Midwifery and Health Visiting. The ENB standard for practice experience is shown in Table 16.1.

Guidelines on educational audit have been produced by the English National Board for Nursing, Midwifery and Health Visiting (ENB, 1993a).

Practice placement audit focuses on six categories:

1. *Student learning experience/evaluation.* This includes provision for orientation, appropriate and accessible learning opportunities, adequate length of placement, ethos, appropriate care model, staff commitment, and mentorship system.

2. *Academic staff perspective.* This includes commitment to relationships with placement staff, maintenance of clinical competence,

Practice experience provides learning opportunities which enable the achievement of the stated learning outcomes.

Criteria
1. There is a strategy for the selection and monitoring of practice experience for the provision of learning opportunities which enable achievement of the learning outcomes of the programme
2. Practice provision reflects respect for the rights of health service users and their carers
3. The provision of care reflects respect for privacy, dignity and religious and cultural beliefs and practices
4. Care provision is based on relevant research-based and evidence-based findings
5. Pre-registration nursing and midwifery students' experience includes the 24-hour cycle of patient/client care
6. Plans for practice experience demonstrate equity of opportunity for individual students' learning experiences
7. The number and skill mix of clinical staff and the experience available support the achievement of the learning outcomes of the educational programme
8. A named person who holds effective first level registration on the Professional Register and other professional and academic qualifications and experience commensurate with the context of care delivery supervises and assesses students in health care settings
9. A named person who holds professional and academic qualifications and experience commensurate with the context of care delivery supervises and assesses students in non-health care settings
10. In non-health care settings a first level registered nurse/midwife/health visitor liaises with and supports the named person and student

Table 16.1

The ENB standard for practice experience (ENB, 1997)

integration of theory and practice, monitoring of placement evaluation, and staff development of unit staff.

3. *Service provider unit staff perspective.* This includes a commitment to individualized care, team approach, multidisciplinary teamwork, communication with the college, commitment to the PREP standards by service managers, and appraisal system.
4. *Purchaser requirements.* This includes identifiable and agreed standards, and quality assurance mechanisms.
5. *Environment.* This includes adequate physical environment to deliver quality care, to facilitate development of competencies, to provide teaching and learning opportunities, space and equipment, and health and safety requirements.
6. *Quality assurance mechanisms.* This includes congruence of curriculum and placement, unit staff preparation, monitoring and annual review mechanisms, system for ensuring clinical knowledge base of academic staff, and adequate supervision of students.

PLACEMENT SUPPORT SYSTEMS FOR STUDENTS AND STAFF

Supervision

The term *supervisor* is used in a general sense to indicate someone who oversees the work of another, and this meaning is captured in the ENB's definition:

'an appropriately qualified and experienced first-level nurse/midwife/health visitor who has received preparation for ensuring that relevant experience is provided for students to enable learning

outcomes to be achieved and for facilitating the students' developing competence in the practice of nursing/midwifery/ health visiting by overseeing this practice. The role of the supervisor is a formal one and is normally included in the individual's managerial responsibilities' (ENB, 1993b).

According to Faugier (1992), the role of the supervisor is to facilitate personal and professional growth in the supervisee, and to provide support for the latter's development of autonomy. She proposes a 'growth and support' model comprising the following elements:

1. generosity of time and spirit;
2. rewarding supervisee' abilities;
3. openness;
4. willingness to learn;
5. being thoughtful and thought-provoking;
6. humanity;
7. sensitivity;
8. uncompromising rigour and standards;
9. awareness of personal supervisory style;
10. adoption of a practical focus;
11. awareness of differences in orientation between supervisor and supervisee;
12. maintenance of distinction between supervisory and therapeutic relationship;
13. trust.

Supervision is one of a triad of concepts relating to the support of students in workplace settings, the others being mentorship and preceptorship.

Mentorship

Mentorship is perceived as an important concept by the nursing and midwifery professions, as evidenced by the considerable number of papers published in the area. The English National Board (1993a) defines a mentor as

'an appropriately qualified and experienced first-level nurse/ midwife/health visitor who, by example and facilitation, guides, assists and supports the student in learning new skills, adopting new behaviour and acquiring new attitudes'.

Mentorship is seen by many writers as being a long-term relationship that extends throughout a student's programme, whereas others limit the concept to a relationship within a specific placement. In some systems, students are encouraged to choose their own mentors, and in others the mentor is assigned to the student. The former is preferable if possible, since it increases the likelihood of compatibility between mentor and student, an important factor in the relationship.

One of the controversial issues in mentoring is whether or not a mentor should also act as an assessor in relation to their students. Anforth (1992) argues that the role of mentor is incompatible with that of assessor, since it presents a moral dilemma between the guidance and counselling role and the judgmental assessment role. However, I find it difficult to understand why there should be a dilemma between these two aspects, since assessment should constitute an important teaching and learning strategy and not simply a punitive testing of achievement. If the mentor has an open, honest and friendly relationship with the student, assessment can provide a rich source of feedback and dialogue to further the student's development. At this point I should nail my colours to the mast with regard to mentorship: I use the term *mentor* to describe a qualified and experienced member of the practice-placement staff who enters into a formal arrangement to provide educational and personal support to a student throughout the period of the placement (Quinn, 1995). This support may involve a range of functions including teaching, supervision, guidance, counselling, assessment and evaluation. However, the mentor is not the only member of the practice-placement staff who carries out these functions, and other staff will undertake these according to the needs of the student and the practice area.

Preceptorship

From the foregoing discussion it is apparent that there is much overlap in the literature between the concepts of mentor and preceptor. Burke (1994) sees preceptors and students as having a short-lived, functional relationship for a specific purpose in a practice setting. Given my definition of mentorship above, I see preceptorship as a specific teaching and learning strategy rather than as a generic support system for students. My definition of a preceptor, therefore, is 'an experienced nurse, midwife or health visitor within a practice placement who acts as a role model and resource for a student who is attached to him or her for a specific time-span or experience'.

Preceptorship utilizes the principle of learning by 'sitting next to Nelly' but in a more systematic and planned way. A student is attached to the preceptor for a relatively long period of time such as a day or a week, and 'shadows' the preceptor throughout. The student's role is to observe the various interactions and decisions that the preceptor is involved with in the course of his or her work, and then time is made available for the student and preceptor to meet privately to discuss the events that have occurred. During these meetings, there is two-way dialogue about the various approaches adopted and the decisions made by the preceptor; and the student can ascertain the basis for such decisions. Clearly the person chosen to be the preceptor needs to have the confidence and interpersonal skills to be questioned about why one course of action was taken rather than another, and the system needs an equally confident student who will not be overawed by the power differential.

In management training, the preceptorship is often conducted in an institution other than the one in which the trainee works, and this has the advantage of avoiding a 'boss' relationship between preceptor and student. Preceptorship offers not only benefits to the students, but also to the preceptors, since the system helps the preceptors to clarify their reasons for making particular decisions or taking certain courses of action.

ROLE OF THE LECTURER-PRACTITIONER OR LINK-TEACHER

At one time in nursing, there were two types of nurse teacher: the nurse tutor, whose primary responsibility lay in classroom teaching, and the clinical teacher, whose primary responsibility was teaching in practice-placement settings. These roles have been unified under the title of lecturer/practitioner, a qualified teacher who has retained clinical competence and whose responsibilities include teaching, supervision and assessment of students.

The ENB commissioned a research project on the role of the teacher/lecturer in practice (ENB, 1998), in nursing and midwifery practice in both institutional and community contexts. The aims of the project were to map the national range and variations in the roles and responsibilities; to explore the factors promoting or inhibiting the role, and to identify the most effective model to meet criteria for clinical competence/credibility, promoting professional knowledge and scholarship. The main findings included:

- the most dominant model was that of 'link teacher';
- two thirds of respondents said there was no specific preparation for the role;
- the system is almost uniformly an un-managed system;
- students expressed a strong preference for lecturer/practitioners to work alongside them;
- practitioners felt they should continue to undertake practice assessments of students, but valued lecturer support in this activity;
- all respondent groups referred to the difficulties of being accountable to 'two masters'.

It is interesting to note that the dominant model is that of the link-teacher, whose role is to establish relationships with a small number of clinical areas for the purposes of liaison, trouble-shooting and staff development. The latter is primarily aimed at qualified staff in clinical areas, who will be acting as supervisors, mentors and preceptors to students undertaking practice placements.

Gerrish (1992) identifies three key roles for teachers in practice settings:

1. *Educational support for practice-based staff.* This includes advice about dealing with supernumerary students on pre-registration programmes, and support for staff acting as mentors to students.
2. *Tutoring students.* This includes facilitating the development of

students' autonomy as students, and their skills with regard to reflective practice.

3 *Facilitating good practice.* This includes awareness of current practice, providing a resource to unit staff, promotion of research-mindedness, and fostering a critical approach to practice.

Gerrish suggests that teaching in practice placements requires a commitment by the teacher, collaboration between education and service staff, and staff development for teachers on their new role in relation to practice.

Staff development for supervisors, mentors and preceptors

The careful selection of practice-placement staff for these important roles is crucial, and Burke (1994) suggests that personal characteristics, clinical expertise, teaching skill, and motivation are important. Courses of preparation may take the form of recognized courses such as Teaching and Assessing in Clinical Practice (ENB, 1997, 1998), City and Guilds of London Course 7307, or a Certificate in Education course. On the other hand, they may be specifically designed in-house courses of preparation, and these need careful joint planning between education and service, and also ongoing monitoring and quality assurance.

Encouraging student autonomy means a 'hands-off' approach which some experienced practitioners may find uncomfortable. There is also the potential for perceived threat on the part of practitioners who qualified some time ago, when supporting DipHE or undergraduate students. This may result in barriers arising between mentor and student, to the detriment of learning.

One very useful strategy for staff development is networking between practice-placement support staff. Networking can be formal or informal, and functions in much the same way as self-help groups by providing mutual support and sharing of experiences. Jinks and Williams (1994) describe a study of the effectiveness of an educational strategy for community nurses in relation to teaching, assessing and mentoring of pre-registration students. They found that half the sample felt their preparation had been adequate and this correlated with the taking of a formal course of teaching and assessing.

Clinical supervision

Clinical supervision is a relatively recent peer-support initiative for practitioners in clinical and community settings, and is defined by the Department of Health (DoH) as:

> '*a formal process of professional support and learning which enables the individual practitioner to develop knowledge and competence, assume responsibility for their own practice and enhance consumer protection and safety of care in complex clinical situations*' (DoH, 1993).

Table 16.2

Characteristics of clinical supervision (Grant and Quinn, 1998)

Purpose
Professional support and learning
Development of knowledge and competence
Responsibility for own practice
Enhance consumer protection
Help practitioner to examine and validate her practice and feelings
Pastoral support
Formative assessment
Ensuring standard of clinical and managerial practice
Maintain and support standards of care
To help the client
Improve quality of patient care
Improve staff performance
Reduce stress and burn-out

Process
A formal process
A practice-focused professional relationship
Should be developed according to local circumstances
Every practitioner should have access
Preparation for supervisors is important, and should be included in pre- and post-registration
    programmes
Evaluation is needed, and should be determined locally

Clinical supervision is described by the UKCC as 'an important part of strategies to promote high standards of nursing and health visiting care into the next century' (UKCC, 1996). Table 16.2 gives the main characteristics of clinical supervision.

Clinical supervision is carried out in two main ways: one-to-one supervision and group supervision.

One-to-one clinical supervision

This is the most common form of clinical supervision, in which an experienced nurse acts as the clinical supervisor for a less-experienced colleague. Practitioners normally choose someone with whom they have a good relationship to be their clinical supervisor, usually a colleague from the same area of work.

Group clinical supervision

In this approach, one supervisor is designated for the group, and the advantages claimed are that it exposes supervisees to alternative modes of helping, and an appreciation of the widespread nature of their concerns.

Implementing one-to-one clinical supervision

The introduction of clinical supervision is a very sensitive issue, and may be regarded with scepticism or suspicion by some practitioners. For example, prospective supervisors may see it as an unnecessary, time-consuming activity that diverts resources from direct patient/client care. Supervisees may be suspicious of the motives of managers in introducing clinical supervision, seeing it as a covert means of disciplining staff for inadequate practice.

Some practitioners may consider it naive to openly and honestly disclose important aspects of their professional practice to a clinical supervisor, particularly if they feel that such disclosure might adversely affect their future employment prospects. It is also possible that some models of clinical supervision may give staff the impression that it is a counselling intervention or, at worst, some kind of amateur psychotherapy.

Hence, one of the most important aspects of clinical supervision is the relationship between supervisors and supervisees. Mutual trust is required, and this could take some time to develop, particularly if there was no choice in the selection of the supervisor.

Negotiating the supervision contract

The first meeting between the clinical supervisor and supervisee tends to be the most difficult, since both parties may be unsure about how to proceed. It is helpful if this first meeting focuses on negotiating the supervision contract, as the process of negotiation will itself help to encourage the development of rapport between the two parties. Since the contract contains tangible aspects such as practical arrangements and record-keeping, it provides a less-threatening focus for discussion in the initial phase of the meeting when the parties are at their most anxious. A supervision contract is a useful way of clarifying the working agreement, as well as making for an easier relationship, since everyone knows where they stand. Table 16.3 shows the components normally included in a supervision contract.

Practical arrangements, i.e. time, place, frequency and length of meetings
Record-keeping arrangements
What will happen in the case of missed sessions
Confidentiality
What will happen in the case of incompetent practice
What communication if any will there be between the supervisor and the supervisee's manager
What access (if any) will the supervisee have to the supervisor between sessions

Table 16.3

Elements of a supervision contract (Grant and Quinn, 1998)

Practical aspects of supervision meetings

Practical arrangements for clinical supervision may not always be straightforward. For example, offices are rarely appropriate for clinical supervision, as constant disturbance can be expected from telephones and visitors. Cowes and Wilkes (1998) report that 'all members wanted to get away from their immediate working environment in order that privacy could be ensured and distractions minimized'.

Difficulty may be experienced in finding a suitably private room that is not already booked, particularly if several clinical supervision meetings are taking place on the same day. Over-running of a previous meeting is a common occurrence, resulting in erosion of the time available for the next meeting; one hour is a reasonable time allocation but timing will vary depending on local circumstances. The problem of room bookings is further compounded where supervision for practice nurses and health visitors takes place in rooms in GP surgeries, because the use of such rooms may be chargeable and this will impact on the overall resource provision for clinical supervision.

Given that both parties to clinical supervision are busy practitioners, it is likely that one or both will arrive late from time to time. When negotiating the supervision contract, it is useful to allow a margin for late arrival; for example, they might agree to wait up to half an hour for the other to arrive. This margin can help reduce panic reactions, such as driving too fast to get to the meeting on time. The time of day in which the meeting takes place will vary according to local circumstances, but many supervisors and supervisees prefer the end of the day, when patient/client demand may be less. The frequency of meetings varies widely in the literature, ranging from weekly to three-monthly.

Keeping records of supervision

It is important that both supervisor and supervisee keep records of clinical supervision for their personal professional profile, as evidence of professional development. Whilst these records are confidential to the individuals concerned, it is also necessary to keep a managerial record of clinical supervision which contains the minimum amount of information required by management in order to be able to confirm that supervision has occurred, and to enable the time to be costed. This would normally be the names of the supervisor and supervisee, the dates on which it took place, and the reasons for any cancellation. In cases of litigation by patients or clients, such records can provide evidence of the ongoing professional development of the practitioner involved.

TEACHING AND LEARNING STRATEGIES IN THE WORKPLACE

The principles of teaching and learning that have been expounded in this book are applicable to teaching and learning in the workplace. However, some teaching strategies are more appropriate for the workplace environment than others, and this section will explore a range of these.

Teaching on a one-to-one basis

Teaching on a one-to-one basis demands skills quite different from those used in the classroom setting; both teacher and student are more exposed to each other and the encounter takes place in the presence of other staff, patients and visitors. The need to appear competent and credible to all these groups, including the student, can add considerable pressure on the teacher, making it more difficult to allow the student to make decisions or to try out new approaches. On the other hand, there can be great personal satisfaction in helping to provide good quality nursing care whilst at the same time facilitating the growth of nursing skills in the student.

Much one-to-one teaching is opportunistic, i.e. the kind of sponta- neous teaching that occurs as part of everyday professional practice, with either students, qualified staff, or patients and clients. Opportunistic teaching can arise in a number of ways; for example, students may ask the teacher to go through some aspect or procedure with them, or simply ask questions about the care of specific patients. On the other hand, the teacher may herself initiate teaching by asking questions or by explaining aspects or procedures.

Teaching can also be initiated by the teacher if she perceives that a student or qualified member of staff is experiencing difficulty with procedures or understanding. Within a given workplace setting there will be some concepts that most students find difficult to understand, and the teacher is asked time and time again to explain these to each new student. It is a useful strategy to prepare an explanation in advance that can be 'wheeled out' as required, preferably using some kind of visual material. The guidelines on planning an explanation given in Chapter 7 will be helpful in this regard. Feedback on student learning is important even in spontaneous one-to-one teaching, so the teacher needs to use questioning to elicit the students' understanding of any explanations given.

Coaching

Coaching is a familiar concept in sport and athletics, where a skilled coach offers analysis and advice to help a sports-person or athlete to improve his/her performance. The term is also used in education, where it implies the offering of additional support and tutoring to help a pupil or student to prepare for examinations. Coaching can also be used as a management strategy for improving staff performance at work, and it is in this context that its relevance to clinical supervision becomes apparent.

Some NHS Trusts are using a self-study guide called the *Coaching Toolkit Programme* as part of the preparation for clinical supervision. The toolkit defines coaching as ' a person-to-person process which helps individuals to come to their own conclusions about the best way to achieve improved performance at work' (South and West Development Forum, 1996). This definition emphasizes the empowerment aspect of coaching; the onus is on the individual to decide how s/he will achieve improved performance. Within an organization, anyone can be a coach to anyone else, provided they have appropriate expertise and experience, and coaching is commonly used to help individuals to acquire new skills, take on new roles, apply learning gained from attendance at courses or study-days, and as part of annual individual performance review.

The key skills identified for coaching are fundamental skills that underpin any interpersonal encounter, including counselling and clinical supervision, and these are listed in Table 16.4.

The coaching toolkit uses a five-stage model with the acronym 'C.O.A.C.H.' to help make the coaching session more effective:

1. *Circumstance*. In this first stage the coach and the individual

Table 16.4

Coaching skills

Developing rapport and trust
Listening
Summarizing and reflecting
Self-disclosure
Questioning
Giving feedback
Using silence

attempt to get an overall picture of the current issue for the coaching session.

2. *Objective.* The coach helps the individual to formulate the objectives s/he wishes to achieve.

3. *Alternatives.* In this stage the possible range of options and alternatives are discussed.

4. *Choice.* During this stage, both parties come to a decision about which alternative is most appropriate, given all the factors.

5. *Handover.* This final stage is about how the choice is to be implemented, and the support required to do this.

Case-conferences

Ideally these should involve all members of the nursing team in discussion and evaluation of the nursing care of a particular patient. Medical staff have long used the case presentation method as a learning tool for students and qualified doctors, and the same principles apply to the use of nursing-care conferences. There is no standard format for such a conference, but it is usual for one nurse to present the patient's case and then for the whole team to be involved in the discussion. This helps the student to feel part of the nursing team as well as providing the skills in a public presentation of 'self'. Such conferences provide a useful holistic view of the patient and his or her problems, together with an opportunity to analyse critically the care that has been received, to the mutual benefit of both nurses and patients.

Handover report

Many qualified practitioner nurses view the handover report as a valuable opportunity to do some teaching. Handover is done normally in two ways:

1. verbal handover involving the entire nursing team meeting together in a room for a reasonable period of time during the day;

2. non-verbal handover is conducted at patients' bedsides using documents.

Verbal handover can be a useful teaching strategy if the ward manager or staff nurse often take time to ask questions about aspects of patients' conditions and care, and provided that the atmosphere is relaxed and informal. There are important trade-offs from a ward report in addition to the actual report itself, namely the fostering of team spirit and the development of public speaking ability and confidence in presenting information to peers. However, there are disadvantages of verbal handover, including nurses' reliance on memory, the amount of time consumed, and the fact that nurses are often called away before the handover is complete.

Kennedy (1999) reports on a study of non-verbal bedside handover in an elderly care setting. Using non-participant observation, the study investigated the early-to-late shift handover, and the key components of handover were identified as venue, grade of nurse, documents used, patient involvement, content of handover, whether the person handing over was the care-giver, and whether unnecessary people were present. The main findings were as follows:

- handover was quicker, and staff were available on the ward for other patients if needed;
- support workers played little part in the handover;
- staff were not confident about using care plans for the handover, as these could not be relied upon.

The study recommended that all qualified nurses should attend planning workshops, that bedside handover should continue and that patients should be included wherever possible, and that the role of the support worker should be reviewed in relation to communication and documentation.

Clinical rounds

Students can gain a great deal from accompanying a doctor or nurse on a clinical round. The former is useful for gaining insight into the role of the medical team in patient care, and it is interesting to listen to the discussion with regard to treatment. Students may find it valuable to accompany a nurse teacher on a similar round and to make comparisons of the needs of patients with similar conditions, and also to look at the difference in attitudes between such patients. Examples of pathology can be pointed out, for example oedema or inflammation, and the reasons discussed at the end of the round. Students should always carry a notebook to write down any queries or observations, but single sheets of paper must not be allowed, as they can easily be lost and other patients may read the confidential details.

Reflective practice diary

Reflective diaries or records are one of the key strategies in experiential learning and consist of brief written descriptions of situations that can be used as the basis for reflection later. The following examples are from the reflective diary of a health visitor who is undergoing training as a mentor.

Situation 1: student's first day on community placement

The first day of the student's placement was spent in discussion and negotiation of her learning contract in the light of my case load requirements. Since child protection is a major facet of my work, I made it clear to the student that this aspect must by law take priority over all other matters. Before commencing their community placement students are required to complete a community profile so that they have insight into the area. However, the student in question arrived at my office having completed a community profile on a completely different area to the one in which I work. This meant that the student had no information whatsoever about the area, so we had to negotiate a series of sessions in which I could explain the key aspects of the placement community. I also contacted her personal tutor in the college of nursing to emphasize how important it is for the student to undertake a community profile which relates to their placement.

Situation 2: student's first visit to a client's home

One of the items on my student's learning contract was to visit a family with a new baby. By accompanying me on the visit, the student was able to see and understand exactly what a health visitor does in such a visit. During a prior briefing discussion I explained the official standard for a new-birth visit, and asked the student to pay particular attention during the visit to how I taught the mother to look after the baby, and to compare my performance with that of the official standard. I wanted her to focus particularly on my use of verbal and non-verbal communication with the family, since interpersonal relationships are fundamental to the health visitor role.

On arriving back at the surgery following the visit, we had a debriefing session in which I challenged the student by asking her to evaluate my performance against the official standards, and how she would now approach her next new-birth visit in the light of what she had learned.

Situation 3: developmental assessment in the clinic

At age 18 months infants come to the clinic for assessment of physical and behavioural development, and this involves a variety of tests, e.g. hearing, speech, vision, motor movements, etc. I acted as a role model for the student, in that she was asked to observe and record carefully my relationships and involvement with the clients, with particular emphasis in this case on the practical aspects of testing. One of the objectives in the student's learning contract was to develop the skills of developmental assessment of infants, so I planned the learning environment with this goal in mind. During the clinic, the student was asked to observe me performing the developmental assessment on a number of infants, and was then encouraged to participate in the assessment of a number of infants. Once I was satisfied that she had grasped the essential points, I allowed her to conduct an assessment in partnership with me, but she was asked to take the lead, and to treat me as her student, showing me what to do. This was a very effective way of teaching, as it showed the student aspects which she needed to study further.

Critical incident technique

Critical incident technique (CIT) is a useful tool for identifying aspects of practice which the student felt were particularly positive or negative (Flanagan, 1954). These critical incidents can then be reflected upon and analysed to give new insights into practice. Critical incident technique was used by Benner (1984) in her study of acquisition of nursing skill, and she identified critical incidents as any of the following:

- those in which the nurse's intervention really made a difference in patient outcome;
- those that went unusually well;
- those in which there was a breakdown;
- those that were ordinary and typical;
- those that captured the essence of nursing; and
- those that were particularly demanding.

Subjects were asked to include the following information in their description of critical incidents:

- the context;
- a detailed description;
- why the incident was critical to the subject;
- what the subject's concerns were at the time;
- what they were thinking about during the incident;
- what they felt about it afterwards; and
- what they found most demanding about it.

Learning contracts

Learning contracts are an effective tool for developing student autonomy in practice placements. It is useful to meet with students prior to the placement to begin the initial contract negotiation, and this can be modified as required once the placement has commenced. The theory and components of a learning contract are discussed in Chapter 3 (p. 59).

Teaching a motor skill

Although it is possible to teach some motor skills by simulation in a nursing laboratory, such learning will still need to be consolidated in the workplace setting. Teaching motor skills involves the same principles as any other form of teaching, namely, an atmosphere conducive to learning that is free from threat or stress. There must be opportunity for feedback and analysis of the performance, and teachers must appreciate that learning a skill requires time and that individual students will differ in the amount of time they require. One point to be borne in mind is that nursing procedures involve more than motor skills; Gagne (1985) classifies procedures as intellectual skills or rules for determining the sequence of actions and thus students need to learn the procedural rules as well as the motor skills aspects.

When planning to teach motor skills, the teacher will have to consider the level at which the student must learn the skill. It is obvious that students cannot achieve the highest level of proficiency for every skill they learn; indeed, experienced nurses will vary in their relative degree of skill amongst the nursing procedures they practise. There will be some motor skills that students must learn to the highest level and others where an intermediate level is acceptable. A useful point of reference for levels of skills is the notion of taxonomies of motor skills; in Chapter 6 (p. 145), the taxonomy of Simpson (1972) is outlined in relation to curriculum objectives and this can provide guidance for the teacher. The taxonomy has seven levels as follows:

1. perception – concerned with perception of sensory cues;
2. set – concerned with readiness to act;
3. guided response – skills performed under guidance of instructor;
4. mechanism – performance becomes habitual;
5. complex overt response – typical skilled performance;
6. adaptation – skills can be adapted to suit circumstances; and
7. origination – creation of original movement patterns.

It would seem that many nursing skills learned by students will be geared at level 3 or 4 and that the higher levels may only be reached when the student has practised as a qualified nurse for some time. Skills at level 3 are commonly taught in specialist areas, where the student is allowed to perform under guidance having first been shown how to do a procedure. For example, the skills of dialysis may be taught at this level during a student's allocation to a renal clinical area, but there is no expectation that the student nurse will achieve a highly-skilled performance during the brief allocation period. The same can be said for other clinical specialisms such as intensive-care units, neonatal units and the like.

The teaching of motor skills involves the provision of information and the opportunity for practice under supervision. Table 16.5 gives a checklist for teaching a motor skill, and the key points are further elaborated below.

The provision of an atmosphere conducive to learning has already

Table 16.5

Checklist for teaching a motor skill

1. Provide an atmosphere conductive learning
2. Carry out a skills analysis to determine part-skills and elements
3. Determine the sequence of the procedure
4. Assess entry behaviours of students – these need not be taught again
5. Model the skill by demonstration at normal speed
6. Teach the sequence of the procedure
7. Teach the motor skill by either whole-learning or part-learning method
8. Allocate sufficient time for practice
9. Provide augmented feedback on performance
10. Prompt student to use intrinsic feedback
11. Encourage transfer of existing similar skills by pointing out similarity

been discussed and its importance noted. Skills analysis is a useful way of identifying the part-skills that comprise the total motor skill. Table 16.6 shows a task analysis for the motor aspects of the procedure of performing a surgical dressing.

These motor skills are further subdivided into part-skills and elements, and it can be seen that the elements consist of many previously learned entry behaviours, such as moving the bed table and

Table 16.6

The procedure of performing a surgical dressing

Total motor skill	Part-skills (tasks)	Elements*
1.0 Preparation of work area	1.1 Clearing space	1.11 Pushing locker away
		1.12 Moving bed table
	1.2 Screening	1.21 Holding curtain and pulling it round
	1.3 Closing windows	1.31 Pulling window cord
	1.4 Positioning patient	1.41 Asking if possible to lie recumbent
		1.42 Removing pillows
		1.43 Folding bedclothes
		1.44 Loosening clothing
		1.45 Covering with blanket
2.0 Preparation of equipment and trolley	2.1 Hand-washing	
	2.2 Cleaning trolley	
	2.3 Collecting equipment	
	2.4 Setting trolley	
	2.5 Taking to bedside	
3.0 Performance of dressing	3.1 Opening bags	
	3.2 Loosening dressing	
	3.3 Hand-washing	
	3.4 Opening packs	
	3.5 Removing dressing	
	3.6 Cleaning wound	
	3.7 Applying dressing	
4.0 Organization of trolley	4.1 Closing pack	
	4.2 Closing bags	
	4.3 Securing bags	
5.0 Ensuring patient's comfort	5.1 Attending to position	
6.0 Clearing of trolley and equipment	6.1 Removing from bedside	
	6.2 Disposal of soiled dressings	
	6.3 Disposal of instruments	
	6.4 Hand-washing	
	6.5 Clearing equipment	
	6.6 Cleaning trolley	
	6.7 Hand-washing	
7.0 Returning to patient	7.1 Assist with clothing	
	7.2 Assisting with position	
	7.3 Offering drink, newspaper, etc.	
	7.4 Removing screens	
	7.5 Returning tables, locker, etc.	
8.0 Recording and reporting	8.1 Writing report	
	8.2 Reporting verbally to nurse in charge	
	8.3 Comparing report with previous one	

*Elements are stated only for Section 1.0 of the total motor skills

pulling curtains. Determining the sequence of the procedure is important and it may be forgotten that students must remember this as well as the motor skills. Entry behaviours need to be identified, since they are already learned and hence do not need to be taught again.

Modelling of the skill is normally done by an actual demonstration, but in the classroom setting it can also be done by video, and it gives the students an overall impression of the skill they are aiming at.

There is some controversy as to whether skills should be taught in their entirety (whole-learning), or divided into part-skills, with each part being taught separately first and then combined into a whole – part-learning. The disadvantage of whole-learning in that it may be difficult to comprehend large units of procedures if taught together. However, part-learning may waste time because the student has to learn the part-skills first and then learn to combine them together. It may also be boring for the student if the part-skills are simple. The advantages of whole-learning are that it may be:

- more meaningful, as perceived as whole;
- more efficient, as students can identify the aspects which need further practice within the whole;
- more effective for students who already have a background in the skill;
- better for highly-motivated students; and
- better for older students.

The advantages of part-learning are that it may:

- help to motivate students, as each part-skill provides immediate achievement;
- by its small-step nature act as a reinforcement for learning;
- be better for younger students;
- be better for students lacking a background in the skill; and
- help to improve specific responses for part-skills.

Another area of controversy is that of massed practice versus spaced practice; massed practice involves continuous practice until the skill is learned, whereas spaced practice may spread the practice over a period of time, with rest in between. There is no evidence that one is better than the other, but there are obvious pitfalls associated with massed practice, such as boredom and fatigue. As we have seen earlier, feedback is a crucial aspect of motor-skills learning, without which no improvement can occur. The teacher needs to encourage students to become aware of the intrinsic feedback from their own muscles and joints, which informs them about the position of limbs and the action of movements. Information gained from their own observation of their actions will also help the students to learn a skill and here again the teacher may use questioning to ascertain whether each student is able to self-evaluate outcomes.

The main role of the teacher is in providing augmented feedback in the form of verbal guidance both during and on completion of the motor performance. The nurse teacher can teach for transfer of learning by using a variety of techniques to make the student understand the principles underlying the skill. Existing skills must have been well-learned if they are to transfer positively to the new skill, and the similarities need to be pointed out to the students.

Benner's model of skill acquisition in clinical nursing practice

Patricia Benner's book *From Novice To Expert* (1984) has become one of the most frequently quoted research studies in nurse education. Benner conducted paired interviews with beginners and experienced nurses about significant nursing situations they had experienced in common, in order to identify any characteristic differences between their descriptions of the same situation. Additionally, she carried out interviews, critical incident technique, and participant observation with a sample of experienced nurses, new graduates, and senior students, to ascertain the characteristics of performance at different stages of skill acquisition.

Using an adaptation of the five-stage model of skill acquisition developed by Dreyfus and Dreyfus (1980), she described the characteristics of performance at five different levels of nursing skill: novice, advanced beginner, competent, proficient, and expert. During her passage through these stages, the student relies less upon abstract rules to govern practice, and more on past experience. Nursing situations begin to be seen as a unified whole within which only certain aspects are relevant, and the nurse becomes personally involved in situations rather than a detached observer. It is important to note that Benner uses the term *skill* in its widest sense to mean all aspects of nursing practice, and not simply psychomotor skill performance.

Stage 1: novice
This level is characterized by rule-governed behaviour, as the novice has no experience of the situation upon which to draw, and this applies to both students in training and to experienced nurses who move into an unfamiliar clinical area. Adherence to principles and rules, however, does not help the nurse to decide what is relevant in a nursing situation, and may thus lead to unsuccessful performance.

Stage 2: advanced beginner
Unlike principles and rules, aspects are overall characteristics of a situation that can only be identified by experience of that situation. For example, the skills of interviewing a patient are developed by experience of interviewing previous patients, and the advanced beginner is one who has had sufficient prior experience of a situation to deliver marginally acceptable performance. Advanced beginners need adequate support from supervisors, mentors and colleagues in the practice setting.

Stage 3: competent
This stage is characterized by conscious, deliberate planning based upon

17 TEACHING PATIENTS, CLIENTS AND THEIR FAMILIES

In Chapter 16 a range of 'consumers' of nurse education were identified, including pre-registration students, post-registration students, health care support workers, and practitioners receiving informal, spontaneous teaching as part of their day-to-day professional practice. However, there is another significant group of people who do not come under the banner of nurse education, but for whom teaching by nurses, midwives and health visitors is an important part of their care, namely patients, clients and their families.

Each of the chapters in this book has focused on a particular aspect of nurse education, with a strong emphasis on a range of teaching strategies. These teaching strategies are essentially generic, in that they can be used for teaching adults in any educational setting, and with any subject-matter, so this means they should be equally applicable to the teaching of patients, clients and their families. However, there are some important differences between the teaching of students and that of patients, clients and families, and this chapter will explore a range of issues relating to the teaching of the latter group.

ISSUES AND CONTEXT

When considering the teaching of patients, clients and their families, it is useful to clarify what is actually meant by 'teaching'. Nurse-patient interactions involve a wide range of activities subsumed under the umbrella term 'communication', and these include social conversation, information-giving, asking and answering questions, explaining, and demonstrating skills. It is only social conversation that would not normally be included in the concept 'teaching', so it seems sensible to consider teaching as a fairly generic activity encompassing a variety of interaction activities that often overlap with the concept of 'professional practice'.

One of the similarities between teaching students and teaching patients, clients, and their families is that they both involve a wide range of contexts, including hospitals, clinics, GP surgeries, nursing homes, and patients/clients homes. Hence, the principles of teaching students in clinical and community settings, as discussed in Chapter 16, will be useful as a basis for teaching patients, clients and their families.

Sources of professional guidance

The UKCC Code of Professional Conduct governs the practice of every nurse, midwife and health visitor, and statement 5 of the Code reads:

'You are personally accountable for your practice and, in the exercise of your professional accountability, must work in an open and co-operative manner with patients, clients and their families, foster their independence and recognize and respect their involvement in the planning and delivery of care' (UKCC, 1992).

This statement applies to all aspects of care, including the teaching of patients, clients and their families, and it is interesting to compare it with the humanistic philosophy of adult education, which shares the same beliefs about openness, fostering independence, and student involvement.

The UKCC *Guidelines for Professional Practice* offer a number of helpful points about information-giving that can be applied to the teaching of patients, clients and their families (UKCC, 1996) including:

- the importance of giving clear information on which the patient/ client can make informed choices;
- the need to recognize patients/clients as equal partners;
- the importance of using language that is familiar to them;
- the need to ensure that patients/clients understand the information they are given;
- written communication is as important as verbal communication;
- patients/clients have a legal right to information about their condition, and registered practitioners providing care have a professional duty to provide such information;
- a patient/client who wants information is entitled to an honest answer, although selective information may be appropriate in rare circumstances;
- you always need to obtain the explicit consent of patients/clients before disclosing specific information.

This last point about confidentiality becomes an important issue when teaching members of a patient/client's family about aspects of their loved-one's care. The patient/client may not wish certain details to be disclosed to members of his family, so the teacher will need to ensure that confidentiality is maintained, and prepare her approach should the confidential issue be raised by the family.

Differences in assumptions underpinning the teaching of students and patients/clients

The teaching of students in nurse education is premised on a number of assumptions, and it is interesting to see if these assumptions are necessarily valid for the teaching of patients, clients and their families. Table 17.1 identifies a range of common assumptions that it would normally be appropriate to apply to nurse education students. Of course, there will be individual student variations within these categories, but we can expect that these assumptions would be more or less valid for most nurse education students. Similarly, the assumptions on the right-hand

related illness, the National Minimum Wage and the New Deal to combat unemployment, initiatives to reduce crime and fear of crime, reduction of air pollution to combat respiratory illness such as asthma. Partnerships at local level between health authorities and other relevant organizations are also seen as being vital components of the proposals.

Unlike the large number of targets in the *Health of the Nation* document, national and local targets are set in just four areas of major ill health:

1. heart disease and stroke;
2. accidents;
3. cancer;
4. mental health.

The green paper suggests four national targets to be achieved by the year 2010 in relation to these four areas: the death rate from heart disease, stroke and related illness in those under the age of 65 to be reduced by at least one third; accidents to be reduced by at least one fifth; death rate from cancer in those under the age of 65 to be reduced by at least one fifth; death rate from suicide by at least one sixth. The Government proposes a three-way National Contract for Health involving government, local agencies, and individuals, each taking responsibility for improving health. The focus for the drive against inequalities in health will be schools, workplaces and neighbourhoods, thus covering the spectrum of age-groups from children through to older individuals.

One of the innovations triggered by the green paper is the magazine *Target*, produced by the Health Strategies Unit and distributed to a wide readership in the NHS, local authorities, voluntary groups, schools and the private sector. The magazine aims to disseminate examples of good practice within the areas highlighted by the green paper, and contributions are invited from members of these groups.

Saving Lives: Our Healthier Nation

This public health white paper builds upon the Green paper *Our Healthier Nation*, and aims to save over 300 000 lives over the next ten years in England (DoH, 1999). The underlying philosophy is the mobilization of the public to meet the government's targets:

1. reducing coronary heart disease and stroke by two-fifths in people under the age of 75, saving some 200 000 lives;
2. reducing the death rate from cancer by one-fifth in people under the age of 75, saving some 100 000 lives;
3. reducing the death rate from accidents by at least one-fifth, and serious injuries by at least one-tenth, saving some 12 000 lives;
4. reducing the mental illness death rate from suicide and undetermined injury by at least one-fifth, saving some 4000 lives.

A healthy citizen programme is to be introduced consisting of three main elements:

1. expansion of the NHS Direct helpline to include an NHS Direct Online service for health information and advice, including self-help groups. This commenced in December 1999;
2. health skill programmes for self-help and helping others;
3. expert patient programmes to help patients to manage their own chronic illnesses.

First aid training is to be expanded, and health skills programmes for young people will be introduced on injury prevention and resuscitation. Defibrillators will be provided in public places, and training in their use will be introduced.

Health visitors are encouraged to 'develop a family-centred public health role, working with individuals, families and communities to improve health and tackle health inequalities'. This will be achieved by the health-visitor-led team delivering a range of care including advising and supporting parents, child health programmes, health promotion programmes, and developing community support networks.

Strategies for teaching patients, clients and their families

There are three main types of teaching intervention, depending on who does the initiating:

1. *Nurse-initiated teaching.* This has two components:
   (a) teaching that the nurse believes the patient requires, e.g. how to administer her own insulin;
   (b) teaching that the nurse believes the family requires, e.g. how to carry out eczema dressings on their child, or how to deal with an elderly patient following discharge home. This is termed *carer education*;
2. *Patient/client-initiated teaching.* This is teaching that the patient/client requests, e.g. 'How can I maintain my weight loss after I have been discharged home?'
3. *Family-initiated teaching.* This is teaching that the family requests, e.g. 'How can my husband reduce the risk of a recurrence of his heart attack?'

These categories can present dilemmas, such as whether the nurse should teach a seven-year-old directly, or teach his parent instead. In some circumstances, family members need to be taught how to supervise their loved-ones in such activities as taking their medication, or ensuring they do their exercises. This is not the only example of 'carer education'; some children are the sole carers for ill or disabled parents, and in this case the child needs to be taught how to care for the parent.

The issue of confidentiality is important in terms of teaching the carer; the nurse must ensure that the patient/client identifies what information he is willing to have divulged to the carer, and which must remain confidential.

Planning for teaching

When teaching patients, clients and their families, the teaching can be either planned in advance, or spontaneous, depending upon the context. Advance planning is always preferred, since it helps to eliminate errors and omissions. However, even spontaneous teaching can incorporate an element of advance planning; the principles of planning for teaching are discussed in detail in Chapter 7.

Giving information and explanations to patients, clients and families

When giving information to patients, clients and their families, the following tips may be helpful:

- Ascertain what they already know about the subject or issue, and then build upon that knowledge (this is the principle of Ausubel's Assimilation Theory of Meaningful Learning described in Chapter 4 (p. 91).
- Deal with the most important aspects of the topic or issue, and add those of lesser importance later.
- In order to avoid overloading the patient/client/family with information, proceed in a sequence of small steps, checking their understanding at each step (this is based upon the work of Skinner described in Chapter 5 (p. 114)).
- Avoid the use of medical terminology as far as possible, by translating it into layman's language.
- Observe them closely for signs of puzzlement, and if detected, help to clarify the point of concern.
- Observe them closely for signs of fatigue or distress, and if detected, discontinue the session.
- At the middle and end of the teaching session, ask the patient/client/relative to repeat back to you, in their own words, the gist of the information you have given them.

A detailed discussion of planning an explanation can be found in Chapter 7 (p. 184).

Using questioning with patients, clients and families

Questioning is an important strategy when teaching patients, clients and their families, and their types and purposes are outlined below:

1. *Open questions.* These are phrased so as to allow the patients to respond in any way they like, and are particularly useful for ascertaining patients' feelings.
2. *Probing questions.* These are used to follow-up a previous response by the patient, and allow the teacher to explore the response in more depth. However, their use requires skill and sensitivity on the part of the teacher, as they may provoke anger or distress in some situations.

3. *Factual questions*. These are used to check whether the patient has understood the teacher's points, and consist of simply asking him to repeat back certain items of information.

A detailed discussion of questioning can be found in Chapter 7 (p. 188).

One-to-one teaching with patients and clients

This is the most common form of teaching with patients and clients in hospital, and its success depends to a large extent on the interpersonal skills of the teacher. The pace of the teaching has to be judged carefully to ensure that the patient is keeping up with the information, and the atmosphere needs to be informal and relaxed. Patients with some conditions will tire easily, so the sessions should be kept short. Some of the advantages and disadvantages of one-to-one teaching are outlined in Table 17.2.

Advantages	Disadvantages
Patient gets the undivided attention of the teacher	Patient may feel 'under the spotlight'
Rapport can be established more quickly with just one patient	Patient may miss the support of other patients
Progress can be quicker with just one patient	Patient may feel that the teaching is going too fast for him
Teacher can check learning more easily with just one patient	Patient may feel embarrassed if he does not learn quickly

Table 17.2

Advantages and disadvantages of one-to-one patient teaching

Teaching small groups of patients and clients

Teaching in small groups can be a very useful strategy for teaching patients, clients and their families, and is used extensively in health promotion in the community. Group size is an important variable, and for maximum effect the number of patients should not be more than ten. Groups can be used for a variety of purposes, including collective exercise sessions, classes on a specific topic, discussions of health issues, and demonstrations of particular skills. Small group teaching requires a good understanding of group dynamics on the part of the teacher, as well as skills of facilitation.

The principles of small group teaching are discussed in detail in Chapter 14 (p. 353).

Using information materials for teaching patients, clients and their families

One of the important principles of teaching patients, clients and their families is the need to back up verbal teaching with written and pictorial materials. These enable patients to review the information they have been taught, and to refer to it again and again as required. It is also useful to have the same topic explained in more than one way, as this aids understanding. Information materials are available in a wide range of formats, from the simple pen and paper format produced by the teacher, through to the very polished materials available from health promotion departments. Information materials are often designed locally by groups of professionals to meet a specific local need, but it is important to ensure that the design and layout is reader-friendly and easy to understand.

Coulter *et al.* (1999) carried out an evaluation of patient information provided by a range of organizations including self help groups, consumer and voluntary organizations, professional bodies, health authorities and NHS trusts, drug companies, and private health insurers. The materials covered ten common conditions or treatments, and were reviewed by patients and academic specialists. The patients had personal experience of the health problems, and the academics were familiar with the research evidence. Focus groups were used to elicit the patients' opinions about the materials; the academic specialists used a checklist to review the materials independently, and the publishers of the materials were sent a questionnaire.

The findings included the following:

- Very few of the materials met patients' information needs adequately.
- Very few publishers had researched patients' information needs before they started.
- Specialists identified many inaccuracies and misleading statements, the most common fault being an over-optimistic view that empha-sized benefits and glossed over risks and side effects.
- Many materials were too basic and introductory, and some were too technical.
- Many materials contained advice that was not supported by evidence, with only two being based on systematic reviews.
- One-third of the materials did not include a publication date, and the specialist reviewers found that many were out of date.
- Focus group participants preferred a facilitative rather than prescriptive style, the use of picture and diagrams, a clear struc-ture and headings, and important sections highlighted.
- Participants preferred materials that actively engaged them, such as space to write down questions, or symptom diaries.

The authors offer the following checklist for the content of patient information materials:

1. Use patients' questions as the starting point.
2. Ensure that common concerns and misconceptions are addressed.
3. Refer to all relevant treatment or management options.
4. Include honest information about benefits and risks.
5. Include quantitative information where possible.
6. Include checklists and questions to ask the doctor.

7. Include sources of further information.
8. Use non-alarmist, non-patronising language in active rather than passive voice.
9. Design should be structured and concise with good illustrations.
10. Be explicit about authorship and sponsorship.
11. Include reference to sources and strengths of evidence.
12. Include the publication date.

Assessing patients, clients and their families' learning

Assessment of learning is an intrinsic component of the teaching process, regardless of the context in which the teaching takes place. However, when teaching patients, clients and their families, there are issues of which the teacher needs to be aware. When teaching students, there is an expectation on both sides that the latter's learning will be assessed from time to time; indeed, the student has no choice in the matter. Patients, clients, and their families are not students, and this needs to be taken into account when considering how to assess their learning following a teaching session. The most common method of assessing patients' learning is by the use of oral questioning, and this can usually provide sufficient feedback on their understanding. It is less common to find that patients' understanding is assessed by written methods, although the use of novel materials such as a quiz, or a sheet with spaces to fill in, may well be quite acceptable to patients, clients and their families.

Assessment of learning is discussed in detail in Chapter 8 (p. 200).

EXAMPLES FROM THE LITERATURE

In this section, examples of teaching patients, clients and their families has been selected from the literature to illustrate patient, client and family education in a range of contexts.

Teaching patients with diabetes

Brown (1997) explores the role of communication in promoting self-empowerment in people with diabetes. She cites Tones *et al.* (1990) on the components of self-empowerment:

- the provision of information;
- the clarification of beliefs and values;
- practising decision making;
- choosing health action;
- handling social and environmental constraints on the choice of health action.

She emphasizes the importance of open and honest dialogue between nurse and patient, and the use of open questioning to encourage patients to share their day to day experiences of living with diabetes.

In patient education it is important to ascertain any factors which might inhibit the patient's ability to learn the information, such as anxiety, or information that is too abstract to be given serious consideration at the time, e.g. the long-term complications of diabetes. Brown illustrates the situation where patients are not managing their condition effectively, and highlights the temptation for nurses to simply provide more and more information. She cautions: 'Information becomes education only when it is given in the context of the patient's life', pointing out that diabetes education needs to be ongoing.

The empowerment of patients with diabetes is also addressed by Parkin (1997) in the context of dietary management. She argues that patient education in diabetes has been based on the professional's perception of what the patient needs to know; a process of didactic persuasion is then implemented in an attempt to change the patient's behaviour. This often results in resistance on the part of the patient, and there is a risk of distorting the patient's own priorities by those of the professional. She sums up the position nicely: 'Knowledge alone will not result in behaviour change, but knowledge is important as behaviour change decisions cannot be made without it'. Parkin maintains that the empowerment approach is based on counselling skills, and the following points are made about the approach:

- The environment should be conducive to discussion, with privacy ensured.
- The discussion should begin with open questions to encourage the patient to talk, and to ascertain his needs and expectations.
- The use of silence can be helpful in getting the patient to 'open up'.
- Reflecting back the patient's comments can help the professional to see if she has correctly understood.
- Paraphrasing can be helpful to summarise the main points of the conversation.
- Self-care option are discussed, and the consequences of implementing these are explored.
- Changes in behaviour that are suggested by the patient are more likely to be followed through.

Teaching pain management to patients

Dealing with patients who are experiencing acute or chronic pain is very much part of the nurses' role, and nursing interventions can be divided into three broad categories (O'Hara, 1996):

1. teaching activities to enhance the patient's understanding of the significance and meaning of pain;
2. using measures to alter the sensory input of the patient's perception of pain;
3. helping the patient to develop skills in the self-management of pain.

The nurse can enhance the patients' understanding of his pain by teaching them about the cognitive, affective and behavioural factors that influence pain. Some activities of living, such as housework, may exacerbate pain, and others, such as taking a warm bath, may help relieve it.

Worries about the effect of chronic pain on their ability to work, and also on relationships with the family, may serve to exacerbate it. The frustration consequent upon chronic pain may cause patients' to become irritable or angry with little provocation, and this can also lead to an increase in tension within the family. Discussion of these factors with patients may well be helpful to them, by shedding light on their reactions and behaviour.

Another important aspect of the nurse's teaching role is that relating to the families of patients with chronic pain. Living with someone who has chronic pain can be very difficult for family members whose lives revolve around their loved-one's pain, and the following approach may help both them and the patient:

- Communication between the patient and his family is of paramount importance in pain management. The patient needs to explain what he is trying to achieve in his self-management of pain.
- Patients need to be honest with their families about their abilities, and learn to say 'no' to unrealistic expectations.
- Patients need to learn to ask for help when required, rather than trying to put on a brave face or suffering in silence.
- Patients need to learn how to communicate assertively rather than aggressively, so that a more positive response is evoked from people.
- Patients need to be prepared to challenge other people's views about what makes their pain worse.

Nurses may also be involved in teaching patients, clients and their families about the use of techniques such as relaxation and self-medication.

Teaching parents experiencing parenting difficulties

The two examples in this section demonstrate the use of small group strategies for client education in the community. One of the challenges confronting health professionals is how to deal with people who do not know how to be a parent. One would surmise that this should come naturally, but if the mother herself did not experience a nurturing relationship during her childhood, she may not be able to meet the needs of her child.

'Coping with Young Children'
Pritchard (1999) describes the development of a 'Coping with Young Children' group, the aims of which are:

- the prevention of child abuse and parenting breakdown;
- to develop parents' knowledge and ability in understanding their

children and develop strategies to manage children's behaviour effectively;

- to begin to address the parents' own needs, by exploring their own experiences, and gain insight into the links between this and their own child rearing practices.

Participants are parents experiencing severe parenting difficulties referred by social workers, health visitors and other members of the primary health care team. The courses run on one morning per week for sixteen weeks, followed by monthly sessions for six months. The venues include community centres and a Barnardo's family centre, and the course also includes home visits for individual work with parents.

The educational process consists of the following:

- A pre-group home visit is made to engage parents from the start, and to discuss the purpose of the group and the children' creche needs.
- A mini-bus is used if the parents have transport difficulties, and an orientation visit is arranged if the parents are unfamiliar with the venue.
- Members failing to attend are followed-up so that support can be provided.
- Friendships are nurtured within the group.
- Parents begin to address their distress in the secure and supportive group environment.
- Video is used for home recordings of situations that the parents find difficult, e.g. meal times, and each week a parent offers to show his or her video to the group, for comment and discussion.
- Facilitators provide guidance for the group, validating good practice and not colluding with punitive measures.

'Confident Parents, Confident Kids'

This multi-agency, Hampshire Parent Education Project has been successfully piloted in three geographical areas since 1997, and is being progressively extended to other areas. The initiative involves the Education Department and the Social Services of Hampshire County Council, the National Society for the Prevention of Cruelty to Children (NSPCC), and the Portsmouth Healthcare Trust.

The initiative was developed by a multi-agency team consisting of educational psychologists, an NSPCC team manager, a health visitor, a teacher, a representative from a family centre, and a special needs assistant. The impetus for the development was the rise in the numbers of children presenting with antisocial behaviour, and the need to support parents of such children from an earlier stage in the child's life (Crowther et al., 1999).

The course aims to increase parents' confidence in their parenting skills, by encouraging them to share both their positive and negative parenting experiences with other parents in a group setting, and to try out some of the ideas in their home setting. These can then be shared with the group during the weekly sessions; the group also serves as an informal support network after the completion of the course.

The course itself consists of eight sessions, each lasting two hours, and covers a range of topics including The Myth of the Perfect Parent; Play; Reducing Difficult Behaviour, and Looking After Yourself. The course requires a neutral, non-threatening venue, with creche and refreshment facilities, with ten participants as the optimum number for effective interaction. Both parents are encouraged to attend. One of the key aspects of the course is a home visit to each parent by the course leader before the commencement of the course, to encourage attendance and to address any queries or concerns. The visit also enables the course leader to identify any disabilities or difficulties the parent may have, so that these can be taken account of during the group sessions.

The course leader must be a professional with recent experience of work with early years, and who is committed to working in a joint agency context. The leader should also have experience of group facilitation, and a commitment to working in partnership with parents. Course materials are available for guidance on the running of each session, including specific techniques, and the use of a co-worker has been helpful.

The course is marketed in a variety of ways including word-of-mouth by parents and professionals, leaflets and posters in public venues, and newsletters; the course evaluations suggest that the course is well-received by parents.

Teaching for a healthy heart

One small group approach to this was devised by the Health Education Authority and called the 'Look After Your Heart' (LAYH), which is targeted at the general public.

The programme is run by specially trained tutors, and is offered in local venues such as leisure centres and hotels. The programme has three main components:

1. *Exercise and health.* This involves dynamic exercises that are graded according to the level of fitness of the participants, and is predicated on the acronym S.A.F.E.
(a) S stands for SAFETY:
   - the exercises are dynamic rather than static;
   - the pulse is monitored regularly;
   - perceived exertion is monitored.
(b) A stands for ACCEPTABILITY:
   - exercises are varied;
   - group support is present;
   - exercises are enjoyable.
(c) F stands for FITNESS-IMPROVING:
   - participants experience early benefits;
   - motivation is increased by early benefits.

(d) E stands for ECONOMY:
- no expensive clothes or equipment is needed;
- little time is needed, approximately half an hour three times a week.

Hence, safety is ensured by regular pulse-rate monitoring and perceived exertion monitoring. The exercises are varied, and utilize group support for motivation and enjoyment. They are not time-consuming, and can take as little as half an hour, three times a week.

Monitoring of the pulse rate is a very important aspect, and is carried out at the start of exercise, the *resting pulse*; within ten seconds of stopping, the *working pulse;* and at intervals of 30 and 90 seconds after stopping, the *recovery pulse*.

The difference between the working pulse rate and the 90 seconds recovery pulse rate gives an indication of improved fitness: the greater the difference, the faster the heart rate is returning to normal.

The exercises are designed to promote improvement in three areas, suppleness, strength and stamina. Suppleness is developed by gentle movements such as side bends, and knee bends; strength by press-ups, sit-ups and leg squats; stamina by jogging, running, bench-stepping, skipping, swimming, cycling, etc.

2. *Stress and relaxation.* This involves both information about the nature and management of stress, and also a basic relaxation programme of ten lessons covering all muscle groups.
3. *Healthy eating and other health topics.* This involves information about healthy eating, energy balance and weight loss, heart disease, cancer, and uses and abuses of drugs.

The LAYH programme operates on the basis of experiential learning. Rather than simply being told about the value of exercise, participants can undertake the actual exercise programme, and should see the benefits on their fitness levels quite early on in the programme. Similarly, undertaking relaxation on a regular basis is not something many participants will have experienced.

TEACHING CARERS IN THE HOME ENVIRONMENT

Following discharge from hospital, many patients require looking after by relatives or friends, and this is no easy task for people who are not professionally trained. Nurses need to be aware of carer's need for information about their role, and also about the support services available in the community. One of the most important points in caring for relatives is that the carer must look after their own health, as caring for sick or elderly relatives can be physically and emotionally exhausting.

Benefits of home care

Home care can confer benefits on both the carer and the relative being cared-for (Voluntary Aid Societies, 1997):

1. *For the relative*:
   - Being cared-for at home confers a degree of independence greater than that in an institutional environment.
   - A much more personal type of care can be given, as the carer knows the relative's personal likes and dislikes.
   - The home environment contains all the familiar home comforts, such as favourite books, pictures and furniture.
2. *For the carer*:
   - Providing support for the relative may enhance a closer relationship.
   - There is pride and satisfaction in knowing that the relative is receiving good care.
   - Looking after a relative develops organizational skills such as prioritizing and time-management.

Carer's needs

Carers need to be helped to recognize emotions, such as anger and guilt, and to identify the underlying reasons for it. They also need to be aware of the dangers of becoming isolated and lonely, and the need to actively maintain friendships and outside activities. It is essential that carers are made aware of the wide range of care professionals with whom they may have contact, including GP, social services, community nurses, chiropodist, and ambulance personnel. They will also need information on the types of benefits available to home carers, including Invalid Care Allowance (ICA), and disability benefits for the relative.

Caring for relatives dying at home

It is natural for most people who are terminally ill to want to be cared for at home, and whether or not this is feasible will depend upon the commitment of the carer, the suitability of the home environment, and the availability of local support services. Home care of a dying relative is very demanding, and the advice given in the previous section about the health of the carer is very much applicable here. In some areas, a care attendant is available to sit with the relative for a few hours; a 'tuck-in' service may be available to help get them to bed, or a live-in helper may be available to provide continuous care. Other short-term care is provided by day centres and day hospitals, and longer-term care by nursing homes or hospices.

Carers will need to understand the needs of a dying person and the fears they may have about dying, including fear of pain, suffocation or losing control over their lives (Mares, 1994). When the relative dies, the carer will need to know the procedures to follow, e.g. calling the doctor, contacting a funeral director, contacting other relatives and friends, contacting a minister of religious where appropriate, and registering the death with the Registrar of Births, Marriages and Deaths.

TEACHING PATIENTS, CLIENTS AND FAMILIES ABOUT SUPPORT GROUPS

Support groups or self-help groups are formed of people who join together because they have some life experience in common, such as problems with alcohol, experience of a particular disease or disability, or experience of bereavement or stillbirth. Support groups can help both those who have experienced these events, and their carers also. Contact details for support groups can be found in the local press, and in local libraries. The kinds of activities that take place in support groups include the following (Wilson and Myers, 1998):

- provision of information, e.g. by producing or obtaining literature, by invited speakers, by forming a library;
- social activities, e.g. dances, trips out;
- fund-raising;
- campaigning, e.g. publicity; lobbying health authorities;
- provision of services, e.g. volunteer helpers or physiotherapist.

The following list gives an indication of the range of support groups that exist in the community:

- Alzheimer's Disease Society;
- National Autistic Society;
- Cancer Relief Macmillan Fund;
- British Diabetic Association;
- Down's Syndrome Association.;
- British Colostomy Association;
- Royal Society for Mentally Handicapped Children and Adults (MENCAP);
- Age Concern;
- CRUSE (bereavement care);
- SANDS (Stillbirth and Neonatal Death Society).

REFERENCES

Brown, F. (1997) Patient empowerment through education, *Professional Nurse Study Supplement*, 13(3), 54–6.

Coulter, A., Entwistle, V. and Gilbert, D. (1999) Sharing decisions with patients: Is the information good enough? *British Medical Journal*, **318**, 318–22.

Crowther, C., Turner, C. and Smith, C. (1999) *Confident Parents, Confident Kids*, Hampshire County Council Education, Havant.

Department of Health (1999) *Saving Lives: Our Healthier Nation*, HMSO, London.

Faulkner, A. (1996) *Nursing: The Reflective Approach to Adult Nursing Practice*, Macmillan, Basingstoke.

Kemm, J. and Close, A. (1995) *Health Promotion: Theory and Practice*, Macmillan, Basingstoke.

Mares, P. (1994) *Caring for Someone Who is Dying*, Age Concern, London.

O'Hara, P. (1996) *Pain Management for Health Professionals*, Chapman and Hall, London.

Parkin, T. (1997) Patient control in dietary management, *Professional Nurse Study Supplement*, **13**(3), 57–60.

Pritchard, P. (1999) Helping parents with severe parenting difficulties, *Community Practitioner*, **72**(8), 248–51.

Tones, K., Tilford, S. and Robinson, Y. (1990) *Health Education: Effectiveness and Efficiency*, Chapman and Hall, London.

UKCC (1992) *Code of Professional Conduct for the Nurse, Midwife and Health Visitor*, 3rd Edn, UKCC, London.

UKCC (1996) *Guidelines for Professional Practice*, UKCC, London.

Voluntary Aid Societies (1997) *Carer's Handbook*, Dorling Kindersley, London.

Wilson, R.A. and Myers, J. (1998) *Self-Help Groups: Getting Started, Keeping Going*, 2nd edn, Wilson, Nottingham.

18

TEACHING INTERPERSONAL COMMUNICATION SKILLS

Interpersonal communication skills define our humanity, and underpin our personal and professional relationships with other people. They are particularly important to nurses, midwives and health visitors, whose role involves them in constant and intimate contact with patients/clients and their relatives. However, a number of research studies conducted in the 1980s suggest that nurses' communication skills are not as effective as they might be (e.g. Ashworth, 1980; Faulkner, 1980; Macleod Clarke, 1982). Faulkner and Maguire (1994), in a study of cancer patients, found that health professionals who are taught communication skills are better equipped to assess their patients and clients. The relative recency of interpersonal skills teaching in nursing is highlighted by Chapman and Fields (1996):

> '*Those interpersonal skills aimed at enhancing the psychological, emotional and social well-being of clients have, until recently, been largely neglected in that aspect of nurse education which sets the tone for professional socialization, the curriculum*'.

This omission has been addressed over the past two decades by the development of experiential learning techniques, which have become the method *par excellence* for teaching interpersonal communication skills in nursing, midwifery and health visiting.

This chapter begins with an overview of the principles of interpersonal communication, then addresses the planning and teaching of interpersonal communication skills, and concludes with a consideration of three important aspects: transactional analysis, assertiveness, and conflict.

PRINCIPLES OF INTERPERSONAL COMMUNICATION

Communication is the transmitting or imparting of signals or information to a receiver. In the case of interpersonal communication, both transmitter and receiver are human beings, although they need not necessarily be in direct physical contact with each other. Intention to communicate is not a prerequisite; indeed, signals are often conveyed despite the transmitter's attempts to prevent this, as in non-verbal leakage of anxiety during an interview. Communication is usually classified into two broad categories, verbal communication and non-verbal communication, as illustrated in Figure 18.1.

Verbal communication

This involves the use of words as in speech and writing, but there is more than simply the meaning of the words themselves to be considered

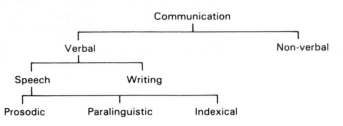

Figure 18.1

Classification of communication

in a communication. There are three aspects of speech that need to be considered: prosodic, paralinguistic and indexical aspects.

Prosodic aspects

These are aspects closely related to the meaning of the spoken words and include stress placed on syllables and the intonation of the voice. A rise in intonation at the end of a sentence usually indicates a question, even though the sentence is not in the interrogative form.

Paralinguistic aspects

These reflect the attitude or emotions of the speaker; very rapid talking may indicate anxiety and loud volume usually signifies aggression, depending on the context.

Indexical aspects

Regional accents and an individual's voice timbre are permanent features of the voice that convey information about the transmitter.

It is a good idea to use audiotaped voices when teaching these aspects of verbal communication; students can be asked to note down any particular aspects as outlined above and then compare with the rest of the group to see if common inferences were made.

Non-verbal communication

Non-verbal communication can be considered as a relationship language that conveys the correspondent's emotions, either consciously or otherwise. It is important to bear in mind that the meaning of any particular non-verbal signal will depend largely upon the context in which it is emitted, as well as the culture in which it occurs. Non-verbal communication is best taught using video or film sequences for students to analyse. It is interesting to turn off the volume on a film and watch the non-verbal elements in action. The main kinds of non-verbal signals used by humans are shown in Table 18.1.

Interpersonal effectiveness

Relationships with other people depend upon our effectiveness in communicating with them; interpersonal effectiveness has been defined as 'the degree to which the consequences of your behaviour match your intentions' (Johnson, 1978). Interpersonal effectiveness is dependent upon a series of prerequisites as outlined in Figure 18.2.

Table 18.1

Human non-verbal signals

Facial expression
Probably the first think we look at when we meet someone, facial expression is the main vehicle for signalling emotion. The mouth and eyebrows are capable of a wide range of variation in signals, as in surprise, smiling and anger.

Appearance
This conveys information about occupation, group affiliation and social class, although much is now dictated by fashion.

Gestures
These can be linked to a variety of emotions and social situations; clapping conveys appreciation to the recipient, a raised fist conveys solidarity or defiance. Many gestures are linked to speech, to give emphasis or describe spatial relationships.

Posture
This can convey passivity or assertiveness in social settings, according to the degree to which the body is held upright. A forward lean may indicate friendliness in some contexts and aggression in others.

Proximity and orientation
Proximity means the amount of distance between two persons during interaction and it seems that each of us has our own idea of personal space. If someone draws too close, we re-establish the space by moving backwards. Orientation is concerned with the angle between individuals, 90 degrees being the most common.

Bodily contact
This is the most intimate of non-verbal signals and involves such things as shaking hands, kissing and stroking. Many people are unhappy about being touched by persons other than their close friends and family, a point that comes out often when teaching interpersonal skills by experiential techniques.

Gaze
A person looks at another person much more when listening than when talking. Eye contact is mutual gaze and becomes uncomfortable if held for any length of time. Eye contact has been traditionally held as a gesture of sincerity.

One of these is self-awareness, which in turn is dependent upon feedback from other people; similarly, feedback is dependent upon a degree of self-disclosure that will only occur in an atmosphere of mutual trust.

Self-awareness

The notion of 'self' refers to all the thoughts, feelings and experiences relating to 'I' or 'me' and arises from both biological and environmental determinants. It comprises the way in which individuals see themselves – body image – and the way they feels about themselves – self-esteem.

Figure 18.2

The components of interpersonal effectiveness

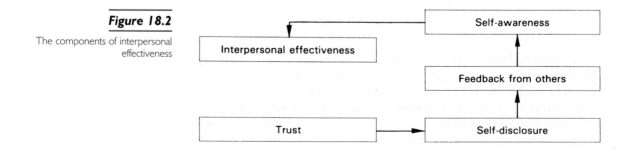

Our self-concept develops as a result of experiences and also by receiving feedback from other people. We tend to see ourselves in terms of a number of different roles, such as nurse, mother, athlete and so on, and during the course of development, the self-concept may be influenced by role models in real life or from the mass media. We are also influenced by what we think other people feel about us, the so-called 'looking-glass' self. Hence, we have a concept of what constitutes our 'self' and this concept is called self-awareness. Since the self is an entity that changes over time, we can never say that total self-awareness has been achieved. A useful device for conceptualizing self-awareness is the Luft Johari window (Luft, 1969), as illustrated in Figure 18.3.

	Known to self	Unknown to self
Known to others	Free self: open to self and others	Blind self: seen by others, but not by self
Unknown to others	Hidden self: seen by self, but not by others	Unknown self: Unseen by self and others

Figure 18.3

Self-awareness: the Johari window

The aim of self-awareness training is to extend the area of 'free self' and to reduce the other quadrants. There are two main ways in which we can become more self-aware: introspection and feedback from other people. Introspection involves looking within oneself and attempting to recognize and own our feelings and reactions. This needs considerable practice as well as a change in attitude, since socialization processes during childhood have tended to regard introspection as somewhat unhealthy. The ability to be able to recognize that one is feeling resentful during a conversation may well enable that person to guide the conversation in a more useful direction.

Burnard (1990) suggests a simple method of enhancing self-awareness through focusing on three hypothetical 'zones':

- Zone 1 involves outward focusing of attention on the outside world and our behaviour, and is synonymous with wakefulness;
- Zone 2 involves inward focusing attention with introspection of our thoughts and feelings; and
- Zone 3 involves fantasy such as day-dreaming and imagining.

Burnard suggests that it is important for nurses to be aware of their focus of attention and its shift between the three zones, since this will improve their abilities of observation and interpretation.

Meditation is a useful technique for getting in touch with one's emotions and the basic principle is that the person positions themselves in a relaxed, comfortable atmosphere and then concentrates on a single object or idea. Another interesting technique for self-awareness is the 'twenty statements test', in which the student is asked to write down twenty answers to the question 'who am I?' It is easy enough for the first ten, but much more difficult to think of another ten.

Feedback, self-disclosure and trust

Introspection alone is not sufficient for developing self-awareness; we need to be told by other people how they see us. Being able to give and receive constructive feedback is an important interpersonal skill, although one should avoid forcing feedback on someone else. When giving feedback to someone about a negative aspect of their behaviour, it is vital to avoid global condemnation of them as a person. By focusing on the specific behaviour and describing it clearly, one can provide constructive feedback without devaluing the person as a whole. It is more constructive to say 'It annoys me when you leave the treatment room untidy' than to say something like 'You are so unprofessional, leaving the treatment room in a mess like that'. Video recording provides the best way of seeing oneself as others see us and is often combined with role-play to provide feedback to students about their relationship skills.

PLANNING TO TEACH INTERPERSONAL COMMUNICATION SKILLS

Detailed planning is essential for teaching in this very sensitive field. Table 18.2 shows a three-stage model for planning and implementing this area of the curriculum.

Table 18.2

Planning model for teaching interpersonal communication skills

A.	Setting up the group	1.	Detailed explanation of purpose
		2.	Outline of current research
		3.	Negotiation of ground rules
		4.	Dealing with anxieties of members
		5.	Facilitating relationships
B.	Choosing a conceptual framework for the course	6.	Include all aspects of interpersonal communication, as in Figure 18.2
C.	Implementing the programme	7.	Consider the importance of warm-up
		8.	Emphasize the importance of briefing and debriefing after activities
		9.	Encourage the keeping of experiential diary throughout the course
		10.	Consider formative and summative evaluation

Setting up the group

The introduction of training in interpersonal communication skills needs to be preceded by careful and detailed explanation to students about the purpose and goals of the topic. Students may be wary of the notion at first and require opportunities for free and frank discussion about the nature of the sessions. This can allay many anxieties if done in a sensitive manner by the teaching team. Topics such as self-awareness may engender considerable anxiety in students, particularly if they fear humiliation or exposure of 'weakness' in front of a group. It is a useful idea to introduce some of the research findings about communication skills in nursing, so that students have some idea about the importance of this area and are motivated to learn the skills themselves.

Ground rules

One way of helping students to gain confidence with their peers is by negotiating ground rules for the conduct of the group; these ground rules identify the parameters of behaviour that the group agree upon and some common examples are given in Table 18.3

1. Members must address other members by name
2. Each member is responsible for himself/herself and must decide how far he or she wishes to go in any activity
3. Members must not speak on behalf of other group members, but should refer to 'I' when making statements
4. Members must treat the events that happen in the group as confidential, and not repeat incidents outside the group
5. Members should try to react honestly to other members, but without 'put-downs'.
6. Members must try to accept other members' expressions of feelings rather than discounting them

Table 18.3

Some ground rules for groups learning communication skills

'Worry box'

Another useful way of lowering anxiety is to use an exercise called the 'worry box' in the very first session on interpersonal skills. This exercise is designed to allow each group member to voice an anxiety they may have about the topic, but in an anonymous setting. Each group member is invited to write down on a slip of paper one anxiety or concern they feel about the learning of interpersonal skills. This is done without using names, and then the group leader collects all the slips into a box; after shuffling the slips the leader goes around the group and invites each member to take a slip from the box and silently read it. Each student is required to formulate a response to the anxiety voiced on their slip and this response should offer some supportive comment to the rest of the group. In this way, each group member receives some positive supportive comment from another member of the group and the exercise serves to illustrate that most group members have similar anxieties or concerns about the topic. It has the added advantage that no student is identified by name, hence avoiding the threat of disclosure in the early stages of group formation.

Initiating relationships in a group

It is of crucial importance to start helping students to initiate relationships with other group members right from the outset of the programme and there are many ways in which this can be accomplished. One way, which is both enjoyable and non-threatening is to have the students work in pairs to exchange aspects of themselves; each can be given a couple of minutes to do this and then they are asked to change partners and do another exercise. This can be repeated several times so that each group member meets most or all of the group. An example is given in Table 18.4.

Table 18.4

Exercise for initiating relationships in a group

This exercise consists of a number of pairings with group members. You are asked to choose partners whom you know LEAST WELL amongst the group. Please begin each partnership by INTRODUCING YOURSELF to your partner.

1. Choose a partner whom you know LEAST WELL. Each take a couple of minutes to DE-BAGGAGE, i.e. tell the other person of any frustrating incidents or 'hassles' you have experienced within the past week, e.g. difficult journeys, personal conflict, etc.
2. Choose another partner whom you know LEAST WELL. Each tell the other person about the following:

   If you were to imagine that you were a well-known book, which one would you be? Why did you choose this particular one?

3. Choose another partner whom you know LEAST WELL. Each take a couple of minutes to tell the other person about the following:

   If you were to imagine that you were a famous character from history, who would you choose, and why?

4. Remain with your present partner and join TWO OTHER PAIRS. In this group briefly discuss your feelings about the exercise

Choosing a conceptual framework

Many students find it difficult to see why the various activities used in interpersonal skills training are important, so it is vital that the nurse teacher spend time with the group explaining the overall framework for the programme of training in this field. Clearly, any programme of training must involve a selection from the enormous range of possible topics for inclusion, and a conceptual framework is useful to help delineate this selection.

Systematic network analysis

Figure 18.4 shows a systematic network-analysis of interpersonal effectiveness in nursing, and this can serve as a basis for the planning of the course content. It has been divided into the domains of knowledge, skills and attitudes, but obviously these are not separate categories, as each of the components is influenced by all three. However, it is useful for clarification, provided it is not seen as rigid or inflexible. An outline of the main components of this network is given later in the chapter.

Implementing the programme

Having decided upon a conceptual framework for the course and having carefully set up the group, the programme can then be followed according to the chosen sequence. This sequence should, in my opinion, be graded so that group trust and confidence can be built up gradually, and this implies the use of activities that are not highly threatening in the early phases of the programme. As confidence and trust develops, it

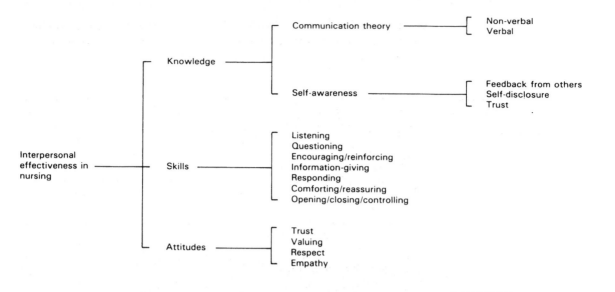

will be possible to introduce activities that call for greater personal investment and disclosure.

Figure 18.4

Systematic network-analysis of interpersonal effectiveness in nursing

Briefing and debriefing

Whether the student is pre-registration or post-registration, it is always very important for the teacher to plan carefully for briefing and debriefing.

Briefing

This is carried out prior to any learning activity or experience and consists of a careful and detailed explanation of the aims, goals or purposes of the activity in question. Briefing should also include any rules or other features of the activity and provide opportunity for questions by the students. In some cases, the teacher will not want to reveal the purposes of an activity beforehand, since this may spoil the discovery element in it; the teacher should, however, explain that he or she wants the participants to discover things for themselves so that they feel the activity is purposeful.

Debriefing

This is vital after every activity, as it is through such debriefing that learning takes place. Pearson and Smith (1985) suggest that debriefing consist of three stages:

1. What happened? This involves participants in describing their actions and experiences during the activity, and provides a non-threatening start to debriefing.
2. How did the participants feel? The teacher invites the main participants to say how they felt about the activity, then brings in the rest of the group. Emotional reactions or outbursts may occur during this stage.
3. What does it mean? During this stage the teacher helps the

students to discover the meaning and implications of the experiences and feelings they have had by encouraging them to generalize these.

'Ice-breakers' and 'warm-up' activities

Another useful concept prior to group activities is the notion of warm-up activities or 'ice-breakers'; these are brief activities, usually of a physical nature, which are designed to facilitate the relaxation of students so that they enter the main activity in a state of readiness, similar to the way in which athletes warm-up before a big race. Table 18.5 gives examples of simple warm-up exercises.

Table 18.5

Examples of warm-up activities

1. 'SWAN LAKE': Members are asked to imagine they are ballet dancers performing in front of an audience. They are asked to dance around the room for about two minutes.
2. DE-BAGGAGING: Members are asked to form pairs and to spend two minutes each telling the other person about any problems or hassles they had that day, such as getting to work late.
3. NAME BALL-GAME: Members of the group form a circle and the leader gives a large sponge ball to one of the members. The object of the game is for each member to throw the ball at another member, whilst at the same time shouting out that member's name. If correct, the recipient throws the ball to someone else; if incorrect, the recipient throws the ball back to the thrower at the same time giving his or her correct name. The thrower then throws it at the same person again, this time saying the correct name.

STRATEGIES FOR TEACHING INTERPERSONAL COMMUNICATION SKILLS

One very useful strategy for teaching interpersonal communication skills is the reflective diary. Students are to reflect on each experience and to enter this reflection into their diary as soon as convenient. Over the course of the training programme, the student will build up a valuable record of his or her feelings and reactions to the experiences encountered and in this way can monitor progress.

Giving and receiving constructive feedback

A systematic way of giving feedback to students about their group skills is to use interaction-analysis techniques.

Group interaction analysis

encouraged Group interaction analysis involves using a variety of observational techniques to record what is happening in a group and systems have been devised by many people (Bales, 1950; Turner, 1983). I prefer to use a simulated case study for the group discussion, with about eight students forming the discussion group. The remainder of the students are assigned different observational roles for recording what happens during the group discussion, as outlined in Table 18.6.

The eight students are asked to form a group and to discuss the material contained in the case study for about twenty minutes. This gives sufficient time for students to become really involved in the issues and also allows them to become accustomed to the video camera so that

Data	Method of recording
1. Number of contributions per individual	Each group member is given a tally for every contribution made. These are totalled up at the end
2. Length of individual contributions	Every five seconds a note is made of which group member is speaking
3. Flow of interaction across group	A map of group members' positions is made on flipchart, and the direction of interaction drawn as arrows from person to person
4. Group processes	Using a record sheet each group member is given a tally for specific behaviours such as questioning, etc
5. Group processes	The whole discussion is videotaped

Table 18.6

Roles of observers for group interaction analysis

eventually they forget it is there. After the discussion, each type of observation is discussed by the total group, including the replay of the videotape. The data from the record sheets is used to show participants which kind of behaviours predominated in their interaction with other members of the group. Table 18.7 shows the record sheet for group behaviours and Table 18.8 the descriptions of each behaviour.

Table 18.7

Record sheet for group interaction analysis

NAMES OF GROUP MEMBERS							
Behaviours							
Initiating							
Inviting-in							
Controlling							
Obstructing							
Building							
Summarizing							
Supporting							
Tension-relieving							
Monopolizing							
Evaluating							
Requesting information							
Questioning							
Timekeeping							

Table 18.8

Description of behaviours for group interaction analysis

Behaviour	Description
Initiating	Starting off discussion; starting a new line of discussion
Inviting-in	Inviting another group member to contribute
Controlling	Steering the course of discussion
Obstructing	Preventing another member from making a point
Building	Adding to a previous contribution from another member
Summarizing	Stating what the group has discussed so far
Supporting	Showing agreement with another member by verbal or non-verbal means
Tension-relieving	Making jokes or humorous comments when group is intense
Monopolizing	Dominating the discussion to the exclusion of other members
Evaluating	Giving opinions about the value of the discussion
Requesting information	Asking for facts or opinion
Questioning	Seeking further clarification from a specific member
Timekeeping	Monitoring the time available for discussion

Self-disclosure

In order to encourage feedback from someone, it is necessary to disclose a little about oneself. Mutual self-disclosure results in increasing trust and development of a relationship, provided that the disclosure is appropriate to the stage that the relationship has reached. People may choose to disclose a wide range of details about themselves, such as interests, aspirations, family relationships and so on, which help the other person to get to know them.

Self-disclosure inventory

A useful way of assisting students to learn about self-disclosure is that of a self-disclosure inventory. The student is asked to spend about 20 minutes completing the inventory on their own and then to join another student to discuss each other's responses to the questions. Finally, this pair of students joins with another pair and each person talks a little about their partner's inventory responses. Table 18.9 shows such an inventory; the questions can be answered at any depth, from the superficial to the profound, the students making the choice as to what they feel is right for them.

Trust

Underpinning all interpersonal skills is the concept of trust, which implies confidence that the other person will not let you down. In a trusting relationship, we can share thoughts and feelings without fear of the consequences and this is the hallmark of a meaningful relationship. Of course, it is not always appropriate to place one's trust in some other person, but it is an important concept when learning interpersonal skills in nursing. There are a number of trust exercises that can be useful for exploring this area, many of which involve physical trust. Students can be blindfolded and then led by another student around an obstacle

Question 1.	Please complete the following sentences: (a) I'm quite good at . . . . (b) I'm not very good at . . . .
Question 2.	How would other people describe you?
Question 3.	What are your present feelings about yourself?
Question 4.	Over the next five years what is your greatest wish?
Question 5.	Over the next five years what is your greatest fear?
Question 6.	Over the past year what do you consider has been the most successful achievement in your life?
Question 7.	Over the past year what has been the least successful achievement in your life?
Question 8.	In the space below, draw a sketch or cartoon to illustrate where you see yourself at this stage of your life.

Table 18.9

Self-disclosure inventory

course; two other examples of such trust exercises are shown in Table 18.10.

1. **'Blade of Grass'**: One group member is asked to stand with feet anchored to the floor like a blade of grass, with eyes closed. She is surrounded by a circle of group members. She is instructed to act as if she were being blown by the wind, swaying over in any direction but always keeping her feet on the same spot. The role of group members is to stop her falling over by gently pushing her back towards the other side of the circle. This continues for three or four minutes and then a debriefing session is held to discuss feelings and reactions.

2. **'Lump of Clay'**: One member is asked to lie on the floor and six other members kneel beside her, three on each side. They work in pairs, lining up with each other at the shoulders, hips and legs of the recumbent student. They kneed the student's body for two minutes, stroke it smooth for two minutes and then finish off by rapidly patting the body. De-briefing is carried out as before, with discussion of how it felt to trust other group members to handle your body.

Table 18.10

Examples of trust exercises

Effective listening skills

The ability to be able to listen to people is an important social skill in any setting, but in nursing it is particularly vital to the effectiveness of communication. Encouraging patients to talk about their worries and anxieties is a key function of the nurse, but patients can be so easily discouraged by a listener who is plainly not paying attention.

Passive and active listening

A distinction is often made between passive listening and active listening, the latter being preferred for effective communication. Active listening involves a high degree of concentration on the part of the listener with avoidance of interruption or judgement. The active listener is attending not only to the words that are being conveyed, but all the other accompaniments of speech outlined earlier. The tone of voice of the patient, the volume or loudness, any signs of emotion, can all convey important data to the nurse and may not be congruent with the words that are being uttered. Effective listening utilizes silence to the patient's advantage, giving time for them to formulate ideas, and the effective listener encourages the speaker to carry on talking.

Triadic exercises

Triadic exercises are very useful ways of teaching effective listening skills. Students form groups of three and take the following roles: one speaker, one listener and one observer. The speaker can choose any topic to talk about, such as where they went on holiday and the listener is instructed to behave in a way that indicates they are not listening very attentively. After a few minutes, the triad discusses how it felt to talk to someone who is not interested and then the exercise is repeated using effective listening skills. Students change roles after each exercise so that everyone has a chance to try out the three roles. Table 18.11 gives guidelines on effective listening skills.

Table 18.11

Guidelines on effective listening skills

1.	Convey attention to speaker	Give non-verbal signals by alert posture, gaze and eye-contact, nodding and smiling as appropriate
2.	Focus on total content of message	Listen to what is said, but attend also to any paralinguistic aspects such as anxiety
3.	Listen for cues from speaker	Cues are often indirect questions or key words that are repeated during a conversation, and signify concerns that are important to the speaker
4.	Observe and listen for incongruence	The speaker's non-verbal signals may convey a very different message from the words being spoken
5.	Make effective use of silences	Silences give the speaker opportunity to think about what to say next, or to reflect on what has been said. Avoid the temptation to fill these with questions or talk
6.	Convey acceptance of what is being said	Show the speaker that you are accepting what is being said without judging it in any way
7.	Make appropriate use of paraphrasing	It can be helpful to the speaker to have a paraphrase of what has been said, as a means of clarifying issues
8.	Make appropriate use of summarizing	Summarizing can help the speaker by reviewing what has been said; it also serves as a check for the listener as to the accuracy of the listening

Effective questioning skills

As well as being a skilled listener, nurses need to be skilled in the art of conversing with patients and colleagues and Macleod Clark (1984) has identified a number of sub-skills of verbal communication. These involve encouraging patients to communicate, questioning, responding and giving information. Nurses can encourage patients to talk by active listening, as outlined previously, and by the use of reflecting, which involves saying what the patient has just said, or a paraphrase of it.

It needs to be borne in mind that questioning has a very different role in normal social interaction from that used in educational settings. In education, the person asking the question usually knows the answer already, whereas in normal social interactions, the questioner is seeking information or data.

- *Cognitive questions* require the respondent to answer from his or her knowledge base and can range from recall of specific information to the evaluation of courses of action.
- *Affective questions* require the respondent to answer about his or her feelings and values.

These two major categories or domains of questions can be further subdivided in a variety of ways.

1. *Closed questions* involve a narrow range of response choices, such as 'yes' or 'no', or a specific factual answer such as name and address. They are useful for gathering data quickly.
2. *Open questions* allow the respondent to answer as they wish, without a framework imposed by the questioner.
3. *Leading questions* encourage the respondent to answer in a predetermined direction, e.g. 'You're not worried about your operation, are you?'
4. *Probing questions* follow-up previous questions, to try to glean more information from the respondent.

The questioning skills of nurses are extremely important when dealing with patients and clients and the literature suggests that they overuse closed questions and leading questions. Closed questions in themselves are not necessarily wrong, in fact they are very efficient in getting precise information and facts. However, if used to elicit feelings, they are much less appropriate than open questions; the latter are very important in following up cues emitted by the patient. There is some evidence that nurses tend to make few positive responses to cues emitted by patients, which means they are either unskilled in detecting such cues or else they are choosing not to respond to them.

Conversational skills

As well as questioning skills, there is a range of other conversational skills that are important to develop. The nurse needs to be able to encourage patients and clients to discuss their problems by giving full attention to them, using verbal and non-verbal cues, such as eye-contact, posture and orientation. The use of reinforcement in the form of smiles, head-nodding and touch can help the patient to continue talking and it is important to provide reassurance and comfort when the patient feels distressed or worried.

Student nurses may need much practice in the effective opening of conversations with patients and it is surprising to find that nurses often forget to do the normal social greetings before engaging in questioning or information giving. During the course of a conversation or patient interview, it is all too easy for the busy nurse to control the direction and content. In some instances this may be appropriate, particularly if the purpose is information-giving, but even here there is a danger in being too nurse-centred. Because nursing is a very busy and demanding profession, there is pressure to deal with issues quickly and efficiently and it is tempting to try to cut out any digressions during an encounter with a patient. However, it may well be that the patient has important things to discuss that he or she cannot easily raise directly and so they give hints or cues to these in an indirect manner. The experienced nurse will quickly spot such cues, particularly when they are repeated in the course of conversation and allow the patient to focus on them by the skilful use of open questioning.

Giving information to patients and clients

Some useful pointers for giving information to patients and clients are identified by Macmillan Open Learning (1996):

- Assess in partnership with patient/client what s/he wants or needs to know.
- Start with the principal points and offer secondary information later.
- Offer the information in a logical sequence related to what the patient/client wanted to know when you jointly made your assessment.
- Use uncomplicated language and sentences, avoiding jargon.
- Invite the patient/client to recap what you have said so you can clarify any difficulties or clear up any misunderstanding.
- Give the patient/client time to absorb the information; arrange another session for answering questions if necessary.
- Follow up verbal information with written instructions where appropriate.

Breaking bad news

One of the most demanding aspects of interpersonal communication that nurses have to face is the breaking of bad news to a patient, client or relative. Not only does the nurse have to deal with the fear and anxiety in the recipient, but also her own anxiety about that person's reaction to the news. The term *bad news* is a relative term; what is bad news for one person may not be a problem for another. For example, being informed that you have developed diabetes would probably be perceived as bad news, but being informed that you are paraplegic, or have a terminal illness is of a different order of bad news. Whenever a nurse has to convey bad news to patients or relatives, there are ethical and moral issues to be taken into account. For example, if a patient asks a nurse if he has cancer, she may give an evasive answer that avoids directly confronting the difficult issue. Another common issue is collusion between relatives and nurses to prevent a patient being informed about a life-threatening illness, in order to prevent their loved one from having to cope with the knowledge of imminent death. Kendrick (1998) considers that, by concealing the truth from a patient, the nurse is robbing him of the opportunity to reflect upon his life and to put his affairs in order. He further argues that lying or deceiving patients is only morally justified if it promotes good intent or prevents harm, such as when giving information over the telephone about someone who has just died. It may be morally justifiable to state that the loved one has collapsed and been admitted to hospital, but to omit on the telephone the fact the she has died. The justification is that the recipient may experience harm if told bad news over the telephone, particularly if they are on their own in their home.

Given the sensitive and painful nature of breaking bad news, it is good practice for institutions to have a written policy for this area. One such example is that of Loddon NHS Trust Child Health (1999), who have formulated comprehensive guidelines for breaking bad news to parents about their child having a disability. The following is a sample from the guidelines:

- The parents should be together to receive the news, and the infant should be present if possible.
- A consultant paediatrician, accompanied by a specialist health visitor, should break the news.
- The news should be broken as soon as possible, even if it has to include an element of doubt about the diagnosis.
- Parents should be allowed time to ask questions, which should be answered directly and honestly.
- Parents should be allowed time together in private after this interview.
- The child's name should be used throughout.
- Parents should receive a written summary of the salient points.

Transcript analysis

There are many ways of teaching effective conversational skills, and one of the most useful ones is the technique of 'transcript analysis'. This technique involves the student in making an audio or video recording of an interaction with a patient or member of staff and then making a written transcript of the recording. The transcript can then be analysed in terms of the communication skills that the student displayed in the interaction and provides a powerful tool for individual or group development.

Transcript analysis is used in the following sequence.

1. The student is asked to make a recording of an interaction with a patient or member of staff, using either audio or video recording. The interaction can be real or simulated, the former being preferred if at all possible. The recording should be of fairly short duration, five to ten minutes maximum, so that the task of writing a transcript is not too burdensome.
2. A written transcript of the recording is then made by the student to include any non-verbal accompaniments such as pauses or laughter. An example of a page of transcript is given in Table 18.12.
3. The student then subjects the transcript to a detailed analysis, checking for the effectiveness of communication in all aspects of

Table 18.12

Example of an audiotape transcript

Interviewer	Well, Carol, thank you for agreeing to talk to me about something that concerns you in the field of health education. Would you like to tell me what the topic is?
Respondent	The topic is head lice in schools, which is rife at the moment.
Interviewer	Er, would you like to tell me what it is that concerns you about it?
Respondent	Yes – until a few years ago the school nurse always used to inspect children's heads to see they were free from lice or nits, but recently, because so many children have now got head lice and nits, the school nurse feels it is no longer her responsibility, but the responsibility of the mothers to pick up and consequently treat head lice, and I feel because there are more head lice in schools now that it is the school nurse's place to educate the mothers, even if she doesn't look in the actual children's heads, which is time consuming, she shouldn't just leave it and say that there are so many children with head lice – she should make more of an issue out of it and have groups of mothers and have actual health education classes concerning head lice.
Interviewer	You seem to feel very strongly about that.
Respondent	Yes, yes. Because lots of mothers, quite well motivated mothers, look at their children's head recently and pick up that they've got head lice and realize that this has to be treated, not just for their own children's sake but for the sake of the other children who can easily become infested from their children, but it is the less motivated mothers, who don't bother to think that there's anything abnormal about having head lice, who never treat their children, who in turn keep causing the children who are being treated to become re-infested with the lice, and I feel that the school nurses shouldn't just wash their hands of the problem because it's too vast a problem to cope with, but should have health education classes and therefore try to motivate the mothers who don't understand the problem. Don't you agree that this is now an issue, because something is common in schools, the school nurses shouldn't say that you shouldn't do anything about, there's nothing you can do?
Interviewer	Well now, you use the word 'issue' – do you think generally speaking people see that as being a major issue?
Respondent	Yes, I think that probably it's becoming more and more obvious that they do. It's causing great concern – and probably great concern to teachers as well, who themselves are quite at risk – and the mothers, of course, are at risk from also getting head lice.
Interviews	Mm-mm. Mm-mm.
Respondent	Because it's well known that nits jump from child to child pretty quickly, but they also can live in brushes and combs just for a little while, obviously not for any length of time; and I think mothers need, really, to have it brought into the open that all kinds of children – dirty and clean children – can become infested with head lice or nits.
Interviewer	Mm-mm. Mm-mm.
Respondent	Lots of mothers don't know the difference between head lice and nits, and what they're actually looking for.
Interviewer	Mm-mm. Brought into the open? What were you thinking of.
Respondent	Because lots of mothers like to hide it, and they will probably find that their children become infested with nits and lice, rush off and treat it and don't like to tell anybody else their children have got it, and therefore the children that they have already been in contact with are at risk. Because the mothers probably feel ashamed. Though most mothers are aware of this problem now, still there's a stigma about nits.
Interviewer	Stigma. Mm-mm. What would you like to happen?
Respondent	I think that there should be more health education in schools regarding nits – not just an examination of the children's heads as there used to be, but more groups – groups of mothers with the school nurse, all talking properly about head lice. Having a film – even having real head lice, which are easily obtainable, to show the mothers what they actually do look like, and what they're looking for.
Interviewer	Mm-mm. So it seems to me you're saying that really it needs an intensive campaign to re-educate or educate . . .
Respondent	Yes, I think an intensive campaign is starting, apparently there was a programme on breakfast television, which not all mothers watch because breakfast television tends to be on at the time when mums are taking children to and from schools anyway. So that's the kind of programme they would miss, but probably . . . obviously the media are becoming aware that it is a problem, well then maybe it is coming more into the open – but then therefore some mothers will think it even more of a stigma. Don't you agree?
Interviewer	Have you thought of ways of how you could overcome that problem? In terms of publicity and so on, getting people to . . .
Respondent	Yes, as I've just said, I think the schools' nurses should not just wash their hands of the affair and say it's up to the mums and give them a vague little leaflet with a silly drawing of a creature with legs, of any kind of size, nothing relevant to the actual size of the lice . . .
Interviewer	Mm-mm.
Respondent	And I think that mothers should be encouraged to go to the school, if it's only just for a few minutes before the end of school, when they're actually there chatting about nothing much outside school anyway, they could be in the school for five minutes talking to the school nurse.
Interviewer	Mm. How do you see your own involvement progressing, and can a single heath visitor do very much to . . .

listening and conversation referred to above. The student is also required to evaluate his or her effectiveness overall and to identify any further skills development required.

4. The transcript is copied to other members of the interpersonal-skills training group and each group member's recording is played to the rest of the group for feedback and discussion.

The peer-group feedback can be extremely useful, as it gives the individual a range of opinions about the skills that were demonstrated and the things that require more training. If any group member feels they wish to criticize any aspect of an encounter, they must say what they would have done to make it better, thus ensuring that all feedback is constructive rather than negative.

Transactional analysis

Since its invention by Dr Eric Berne in the early 1960s, transactional analysis (TA) has mushroomed into a major psychological movement. Berne was a practising psychiatrist and his system derives from the analysis of the basic structural unit of social intercourse, the transaction. Transactional analysis is a tool that anyone can use as a teaching or learning device for understanding behaviour in interpersonal interaction. It has its own language and this is the keystone of the system, since the language used is that of everyday life rather than the exclusive 'language of the priesthood' characteristic of psychiatry. The analysis of social transactions can enable people to understand what happens when they are involved in interaction so that they can exercise freedom of choice in what they do, rather than feeling that events simply take over. The basic concept in the method is that of the ego state, which Berne describes as 'a system of feelings accompanied by a related set of behaviour patterns' (Berne, 1966). Each person has three such ego states in his personality: parent, child and adult.

Ego states

Parent
This is best explained using the analogy of Harris (1973). He describes this ego state as a kind of tape-recording of all the transactions which took place between the parents of an individual in the early formative years of his life. These data were recorded raw, without any modification such as interpretation of meaning and consist of all the rules, censures and 'dos and don'ts' of his first five years of life. Also recorded are the pleasure data from that period and all data are recorded as being true, even if this is not really the case.

Child
This consists of the recordings of the internal events that took place in the first five years, that is the feelings and emotional responses to the conflicts of these years. The recording can be said to have two sides, the

first a negative one, in which the feelings are of frustration, rejection, aggression, etc., and the second that of the positive feelings. These include the wonder of the first discoveries, the exploration, creativity and all the other feelings of happiness in early childhood.

Adult

This stage commences at the age of about ten months, when the individual begins to exert some control over his world. The thinking process is used to work out life.

> *'Through the adult the little person can begin to tell the difference between life as it was taught and demonstrated to him (parent), life as he felt it or wished it or fantasized it (child), and life as he figures it out by himself (adult)' (Harris, 1973, p. 30).*

The adult functions like a computer, examining both the parent and the child data against the reality of today, accepting or rejecting it as appropriate. Another function is that of estimating probabilities so that solutions can be devised if required. Creativity is also a major concern of the adult, and stems from curiosity.

The fundamental importance of these ego states lies in their influence on the individual during social interaction. At any point in a transaction one of these states will predominate, so that an individual may respond as a parent, adult or child. These states may vary during an interaction, and a person can be said to be 'in his or her child, adult or parent state'. Being in one's 'child' is not to be equated with being childish, since the child can be considered as the most valuable aspect of personality, contributing creativity and pleasure to life.

'OK-ness'

The language of transactional analysis includes another important concept, namely that of 'OK-ness'. A person who feels OK experiences feelings of approval towards himself, feelings of being alright. 'Not OK' means the opposite of this, and the vocabulary of transactional analysis is used to describe the four possible life positions for a two-person transaction:

1. I'm not OK, you're OK.
2. I'm not OK, you're not OK.
3. I'm OK, you're not OK.
4. I'm OK, you're OK.

The first position is universal for the early years of infant life and stems from feelings of inferiority towards the adult. This position of OK-ness is either accepted by the child, or is replaced by positions 2 or 3 during the third year of life. The new position is then maintained throughout life unless a conscious decision is made to change it to position 4.

Stroking

The first three positions are related to 'stroking', which is another major concept in transactional analysis. A stroke is the unit of social action, an exchange of strokes being a transaction. Stroking is wider than just physical contact, implying any action that acknowledges the presence of the other person. Berne states than an individual seeks recognition in the form of strokes, and that this stems from the need for physical stroking during infancy in order for survival. Strokes may be positive or negative, but both can function as survival value, in that any form of stroking is better than none.

In position 1, stroking is present from the parents, and the person who remains at this position tends to try to win approval and recognition from others, possibly by 'creeping'. The people from whom approval is sought tend to have a large parent, which forms the source of the strokes. Position 2 is the result of lack of stroking by the mother or father, leading to the viewpoint that no one is OK and an individual who remains at this position tends to reject all strokes that are offered and simply gives up, perhaps ending up in a psychiatric hospital.

Position 3 is described by Harris in terms of the child with non-accidental injury, who has concluded that his cruel parents are not OK. His source of stroking then becomes his feeling of peace when he is alone, and he rejects stroking from others. A person who is at this position tends to think that he is right, and that everything is the fault of other people. An example is the psychopathic personality, who displays no conscience about his behaviour. The fourth position, 'I'm OK, you're OK', is a position taken, a conscious, deliberate decision that is not controlled by past personal experiences, but by such things as values and philosophy. The most common position, however, is that of 'I'm not OK, you're OK', with most people falling into this category.

Transactions

Analysis of a transaction involves identifying the particular ego state that each of the transactors is in at any given time and this can be assessed by various clues, physical and verbal, which indicate the behaviour of parent, adult and child respectively. Transactions can be divided into two main types, complementary and crossed. Figure 18.5(a) shows the typical diagram used to illustrate transaction, and in Figure 18.5(b) we can see an example of a complementary transaction between parent and parent states. A complementary transaction is one where the lines of transaction are parallel; these complementary

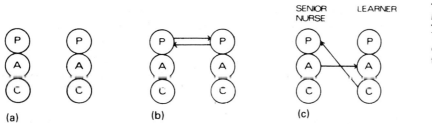

(a)　　　　　　(b)　　　　　　(c)

Figure 18.5

Typical transaction diagram / complementary transaction / crossed transaction

transactions are in agreement, and can continue indefinitely. Figure 18.5(c) shows an example of a crossed transaction indicated by the non-parallel lines on the diagram. Whenever a crossed transaction develops, communication comes to a standstill.

The kind of transaction illustrated in Figure 18.5(b) might take the following form:

Nurse teacher A: These DipHE nurses seem so superior, they need bringing down a peg or two.
Nurse teacher B: I quite agree, in my day we daren't say anything unless we were asked.

Both teachers are in their parent, using the sort of language that their parents used when they were small. Figure 18.5(c) might take the following form:

Senior nurse: Would you collect a sputum specimen for Mr Jones, please, nurse?
Student: Why do I always get the unpleasant jobs to do?

In this case, the senior nurse is addressing his or her adult to that of the student, but the student is responding from his or her child to the senior nurse's parent.

The aim of this analysis is to help people to make sure that their adult is in control of any transaction and this can be assisted by developing the ability to recognize one's parent and child and also to be aware of the child in other people. If the latter is achieved, then the other person's child can be cared for, stroked and allowed expression.

Categories of transaction

All transactions can be classified into one of six categories.

1. *Withdrawal* occurs when a person opts out mentally, whilst remaining physically present. For example, students in a group may allow their attention to drift to the events of the previous evening, rather than attending to the discussion.
2. A *ritual* is a series of socially defined actions, such as greetings, leave-taking and more formal things such as religious services.
3. An *activity* is a way of structuring time, usually in ways useful to the individual such as working, doing odd jobs, etc.
4. A *pastime* is a social way of passing the time and may take the form of chat at a party, with such topics as 'Do you know so-and-so?', etc.
5. A *game* is a very important concept in transactional analysis and Berne has devoted a whole book to the subject (Berne, 1966). He defines a game as 'an ongoing series of complementary ulterior transactions progressing to a well-defined predictable outcome'. Games always involve ulterior motives and a pay-off, and the following example of the best-known game will serve to illustrate the function of games.

Imagine the following transaction taking place in the office of a nurse teacher in a higher education institution:

Student: I can't stand living in the halls of residence any longer.
Teacher: Have you thought about taking a flat?
S: Yes, but I couldn't afford it.
T: What about sharing with some other students; that would save money.
S: Yes, but I don't know anyone who wants to move out.
T: Have you asked the residence manager if they have any addresses?
S: I don't get on with her; she doesn't like nurses.
T: Why don't you advertise on the student union notice board?
S: I don't fancy sharing with a stranger.
T: What about living back at home?
S: I couldn't go back home again, mum would drive me mad.

This game is called 'Why Don't You, Yes But,' and can be explained by reference to the child/parent interaction. The teacher here is in their parent state and the student in their child and the purpose is for the student to reject all the suggestions given until the teacher lapses into silence, defeated. This demonstrates to the student the inadequacy of the parent. In order for this game to be played, the teacher has to indulge in a game called 'I'm Only Trying To Help You'.

6. *Intimacy* is free of games, and occurs in the absence of fear. In this situation the transaction is conducted by the adult but allows the natural child to come through, with all its advantages.

Interpersonal conflict

Conflict is a very emotionally-charged term that implies a clash or disagreement between opposing issues or persons. Interpersonal conflict occurs whenever an action by one person prevents, obstructs or interferes with the action of another person (Johnson, 1983). Conflict is normally thought of as a negative phenomenon, but it can have many positive effects; change arises out of conflict, and much useful material can come out of disagreement amongst a group. Internal conflict within individuals can arise as a result of many factors, and has a profound effect on all their behaviour. Conflict can be created in an individual whenever there is a threat to his needs, status or prestige, but the most common source is that of power relationships between group members and between members and leader. This conflict stimulates mental-defence mechanisms for coping, and the result is such things as aggression, withdrawal and rationalization. An adaptive group meets conflict by discussing the issues and adapting goals, whereas a maladaptive group may fragment into small, competing elements.

De Bono (1985) suggests that people disagree for four fundamental reasons:

verbal cues such as upright posture and eye contact and the avoidance of incongruent cues such as smiling. 'I would prefer not to discuss this matter in front of the patient; can we go somewhere in private'.

Any of the three aforementioned forms of response may be quite successful in getting one's own way; indeed, the apologetic response can be extremely powerful in this respect. However, what really matters is how you feel after having made a response and it is here that assertiveness may offer something different. Even if an encounter results in 'failure', we may still feel good within ourselves if we chose an appropriate mode of responding. Selection interviewing is a good case in point. It is important that the applicant does not emerge from an interview feeling that he or she has 'sold my soul', particularly if they were unsuccessful anyway.

Teaching assertiveness is best done by triadic exercises and I usually begin by taking a few common social situations where assertiveness may be an advantage.

Saying 'No'

I introduce this topic by emphasizing that two beliefs are important when saying no. The first is that everyone has a right to say no and the second is that by refusing the request you are not rejecting the whole person. There are four basic techniques about saying 'No' (Turner, 1983):

1. *Cracked record*. This involves saying the same thing over and over again until the requester gives up, e.g. 'I don't want to discuss it at the moment'.
2. *Time-out*. We often feel that we have to make an instant decision when meeting a request. Time-out means taking a few minutes to think about the request and then letting the person know the outcome.
3. *No excuses*. There is no need to justify a refusal unless you want to, so it is better not to make excuses. Excuses often provide more ammunition for the requester to use in persuasion.
4. *No waiting*. Having turned down a request, it is common for an individual to remain with the requester trying to off-load any guilt feelings about the refusal. The best thing is to leave the requester as soon as you have said no.

Having given some guidelines to the students I then ask them to act out a scenario such as being asked to go out in the evening with another student. It is a good idea to begin with non-threatening everyday situations such as this, and then gradually progress to professional ones. One student is the requester, one the respondent and one an observer, and the role of the requester is to try to persuade the respondent to agree to go out for the evening. The respondent tries out the various techniques of saying no and then the triad members discuss their feelings and reactions.

Facing devaluation by other people

It is a fact of life that most people encounter negative criticism or devaluating comments from others and the following techniques are designed to help cope with this.

1. *Fogging*. As the name suggests, this involves putting up a 'fog' that absorbs all the comments that are directed against you. The first rule is to avoid denying the criticism or defending yourself and the second is never to counter-attack. It is virtually impossible to keep negative criticism going in the face of this 'fog', e.g. 'I can see that you must find my behaviour inexplicable'.
2. *Negative enquiry*. Asking for more information about the behaviour at issue can be a useful way of defusing criticism, e.g. 'What is it about my approach that makes you unhappy?'

Facing aggressive attacks from others

There are two basic points to bear in mind when dealing with an angry outburst:

1. Do not accept that you are the cause of the anger; it may well lie completely elsewhere, but it is likely to lie within the angry person.
2. You have the right to walk away from anyone shouting at you.

A possible sequence for dealing with outbursts is as follows:

1. Gain attention by repeating a phrase such as 'Please listen to me'.
2. Establish eye contact and hold it.
3. Have ready a phrase consisting of:
   (a) recognition of the anger;
   (b) your own reactions;
   (c) willingness to co-operate.
4. Encourage them to sit down.
5. Listen to what they have to say.
6. Move to joint problem-solving.

These situations can be practised in triads, with each member taking turns to be the actor and the respondent. Having had some practise with these examples, the members should be asked to bring real-life nursing examples to act out, as this makes the exercises more realistic and useful.

REFERENCES

Ashworth, P. (1980) *Care to Communicate, Royal College of Nursing, London.*
Bales, R. (1950) *Interaction Process Analysis: A Method for the Study of Small Groups*, Addison-Wesley, Cambridge, MA.
Berne, E. (1966) *Games People Play*, Andre Deutsch, London.
Burnard, P. (1990) *Learning Human Skills. An Experiential Guide for Nurses*, 2nd edn, Heinemann, Oxford.
Chapman, T. and Fields, H. (1996) Interpersonal and communication skills: a continuous curriculum challenge, in *Themes and Perspectives in Nursing*, K.

Soothill, C. Henry and K. Kendrick (eds), 2nd edn, Chapman and Hall, London.

De Bono, E. (1985) *Conflicts: A Better Way to Resolve Them*, Penguin, Harmondsworth.

Faulkner, A. (1980) The Student Nurse's Role in Giving Information to Patients, · Unpublished M. Litt thesis, University of Aberdeen.

Faulkner, A. and Maguire, P. (1994) *Talking to Cancer Patients and their Relatives*, OUP, Oxford.

Harris, T. (1973) *I'm OK, You're OK*, Pan, London.

Johnson, D. (1978) *Reaching Out*, 2nd edn, Prentice Hall, NJ.

Kendrick, K.D. (1998) Bereavement part 2: breaking bad news, *Professional Nurse*, **14**(2), 135–38.

Loddon NHS Trust Child Health (1999) *Managing Bad News: A Draft Guideline for Discussion*, Internal policy document, Loddon NHS Trust Child Health, Basingstoke.

Luft, J. (1969) *Of Human Interaction,* National Press, Palo Alto.

Macleod Clark, J. (1982) Nurse-patient verbal interaction: an analysis of recorded conversations from selected surgical wards, Unpublished PhD thesis, University of London.

Macleod Clark, J. (1984) Verbal communication in nursing, in *Communication*, A. Faulkner (ed.), Churchill Livingstone, Edinburgh.

Macmillan Open Learning (1996) *Professional Relationships: Influences on Health Care*, Macmillan Magazines, London.

Pearson, M. and Smith, D. (1985) Debriefing in experience-based learning, in *Reflection: Turning Experience into Learning*, D. Boud, R. Keogh and D. Walker (eds), Kogan Page, London.

Turner, C. (1983) *Developing Interpersonal Skills*, Further Education Staff College, Blagdon.

Teaching study skills

19

Students commencing a programme of study in higher education have two characteristics in common; they are adults with a greater or lesser amount of life experience, and they have had the benefit of some ten years of compulsory schooling. It would seem safe, therefore, to assume they had accrued a range of study skills over that period of time, but experience with higher education students shows they often have considerable weaknesses in this area.

The inclusion of study skills training is now an important feature of higher education; the diminishing resource base for teaching, combined with the ideology of student-centred-learning, has led to an increase in self-directed learning in most curricula for professional education. Also, many students entering nurse education are mature individuals who have may not have undertaken any study since leaving school, and even those students who enter with previously-acquired qualifications may find that the approach to teaching has shifted considerably since they qualified. Without the support of study skills workshops and advice, students may find it very difficult to pursue independent study in an efficient and effective manner.

LEVELS OF STUDY IN NURSE EDUCATION

It is self-evident that students need to be able to undertake independent study at a level appropriate to the award they are pursuing. Within nurse education there is the full spectrum of academic awards, from Diploma of Higher Education through to Doctor of Philosophy, but there are also in-house CPD programmes that may or may not carry academic credit. One of the characteristics of the progression from diploma level through to doctoral level, is an increase in students' independence and autonomy. Table 19.1 shows the characteristics of a range of levels of study in higher education, derived from the University of Greenwich level descriptors.

STUDENTS' LEARNING STYLES (COGNITIVE STYLES)

In Chapter 2 (p. 32) the differences in students' preferred ways of learning or processing information were discussed, and these differences were referred to as learning styles or cognitive styles. Research into learning styles has impacted on the literature of study skills, particularly the work of Marton and colleagues on deep and surface processing. Hartley (1998) points out that new teaching methods are being devised

Table 19.1

Characteristics of levels of study in higher education

Award	Levels CAT	Characteristics
Diploma of Higher Education (DipHE)	1,2	Extends and reinforces theoretical/practical aspects of knowledge
Bachelors degree with honours	1,2,3	Requires a capacity for sustained, independent, high-quality work
Masters degree	M	Requires ability to reflect on significance and inter-relationship of knowledge, and to formulate original ideas and innovative proposals, all with a fair degree of autonomy
Doctoral degree (PhD)	n/a	Requires ability to produce an independent and original contribution to the field of knowledge

to foster deeper learning in various subject disciplines, that are not normally included on traditional study-skills courses. However, he comments that the evidence from such methods suggests that they reduce surface learning but do little to develop deep learning, and he attributes this to institutional constraints.

MAKING EFFECTIVE USE OF THE LIBRARY

Since one of the main characteristics of undergraduate and postgraduate study is the ability of the student to work independently, the library is the single most important educational resource for this. If they are to benefit from their studies, students need to develop a thorough understanding of all the facilities afforded by a library.

Registration and induction

Library registration usually takes place at the same time as general registration for a programme, and student identity cards are issued that incorporate library access. In higher education, it is common practice for the library to provide an induction programme for new students, complemented by written guides to the various library facilities. The induction covers such aspects as the opening hours, the borrowing rights of students, any system of fines that may be in operation, and photocopying facilities. In addition, it should be pointed out that no food or drink is allowed into the library, and conversation reduced to the bare minimum to avoid disturbing other people's study.

Most libraries in higher education have a security system which is activated if a book is taken out of the library without the appropriate authorization. Multidisciplinary libraries are common within the health service and combine the resources for a wide range of health professions such as nursing, midwifery, medicine, and the professions supplementary to medicine. The periodicals or journals stock is usually very extensive in multidisciplinary libraries.

Classification systems

The Dewey classification scheme (Dewey decimal system) is the system favoured by university libraries to classify resources. It is divided into ten main classes:

000 Generalities;
100 Philosophy and related disciplines;
200 Religion;
300 Social sciences;
400 Language;
500 Pure sciences;
600 Technology;
700 Arts;
800 Literature;
900 General geography and history.

Within this main classification, there are more specific ones; for example, nursing is classified at 610, anatomy and physiology at 612, psychology 150–159, and education at 370. The Dewey classification is used not only for the main book stock, but for reference books, periodicals, oversize materials, pamphlets, and audio-visual media. When searching for specific subjects, students tend to concentrate on books, and may need reminding to look at the other resources shelved in different areas of the library

Searching the catalogues

The on-line public access catalogue (OPAC) is the fastest way to locate books and other resources; it operates via the internet and is accessed from the higher education institution's web page. The OPAC offers a range of options when searching for resources:

1. *Author and title*. This is the fastest search if both the author and the title are known.
2. *Author*. This will search for work by a specific author.
3. *Title*. This will find a specific titled item.
4. *Keyword*. A keyword is entered, such as bereavement, and a list of titles will appear that matches the keyword.
5. *Subject*. This is used to find the shelfmark, e.g. psychology.
6. *Class*. This is used to search for items within a Dewey decimal classmark, e.g. 610, nursing.
7. *Author and keyword*. This is used if the author is known, but only a general idea of the subject is known.
8. *Number*. This is the ISBN number unique to each book, and is the fastest way to search for a book.

The web OPAC will also show details of loans, fines, and reservations.

Books

Although the majority of the book stock of a library is available for loan, there are some categories that have restricted access. A short loan collection consists of books that are in very great demand, and the loan period for these is only one or two weeks in order to maximize their availability to all readers. A counter text collection also contains popular books as well as other materials, and is available for use in the library only. The reference collection contains materials that are not available for loan, including statistical sources, encyclopaedias, dictionaries and directories. If the library does not stock a particular book or other resource, it can be obtained via the inter-library loan service, and a charge may be levied for this service.

Periodicals

The term *periodical* applies to any journal, newspaper or magazine, and these are a valuable source of reference, particularly as they contain material that is published long before it reaches the textbooks. Current editions of periodicals are usually displayed prominently in the library, with back copies stored under the appropriate classification.

Databases

Most libraries will have a range of computer databases stored on CD-ROM (Compact Disc - Read Only Memory). A compact disc can hold the equivalent of a quarter of a million pages of A4 text or pictures, with very fast access to indexes and abstracts. One of the most frequently used in nursing is the Cumulative Index of Nursing and Allied Health Literature (CINAHL), which contains citations from a large number of journals. MEDLINE is the database of the National Library of Medicine, USA, and NERIS is a British educational database. BIDS (Bath Information and Data Services) Inside Information Service is a British Library product that gives access to the recent contents of the 10 000 most popular journals held by the Document Supply Centre. The service is accessed over the JANET (Joint Academic Computer Network).

The English National Board for Nursing, Midwifery and Health Visiting (ENB) has produced a CD-ROM that includes the ENB Health Care Database, and the text of all current ENB Circulars and Regulations, careers advice and the ENB News. The CD-ROM is available on subscription, and is updated every three months.

Other library resources

In addition to books, periodicals and databases, libraries hold syllabuses, prospectuses from educational institutions, student dissertations, and audio-visual materials such as videotapes.

Searching the literature

Most undergraduate and postgraduate programmes in nurse education require students to be able to undertake a literature search and review, particularly in relation to research projects. In some institutions and organizations, the library staff will undertake a literature search for students, but there may be conditions or restrictions attached to this service. Table 19.2 gives a checklist for undertaking a literature search.

Table 19.2

Undertaking a literature search

Before the search
1. Decide exactly what it is you want to know, i.e. the subject. Use dictionaries or encyclopedias if unsure of definition, and check synonyms and related terms
2. Decide on the limits of the search, for example how far back will it go? Will it be restricted to certain areas or aspects? How long will it take?

During the search
3. Consult the Web OPAC for the material held by the library on your subject
4. Consult the relevant CD-ROM databases on your subject
5. Consult other relevant abstracts and indexes on your subject
6. Consult other relevant bibliographies on your subject
7. Locate each of the references, using inter-library loan as appropriate
8. Read this material, noting the quality. For example, is there any obvious bias? Does it contain a bibliography? What is the quality of the index? Have there been previous editions? It is easier to start with the latest material first, proceeding to the earlier material
9. Complete a separate reference card for each reference, using a standard format such as the Harvard system
10. Complete reference cards for further references which might be given in the sources you locate

Bibliographies

There are two main types of bibliography, each of which contains references to work in a given subject area. The first kind is the retrospective bibliography, which gives a list of references up to a particular date, for example, Thompson's *Bibliography of Nursing Literature 1960-70*. The second kind is the serial bibliography, which is published at regular intervals; for example, *Nursing Bibliography* (monthly) and *Current Literature on Health Services* (monthly). The *British National Bibliography* is published weekly and contains every publication in Britain since 1950.

On-line information services are remote databases such as the *International Bibliography of the Social Sciences* (IBSS).

Abstracts

These consist of summaries of publications in certain fields, for example *Hospital Abstracts*, *Nursing Research Abstracts*, *Research into Higher Education Abstracts*.

Indexes

Indexes contain references for articles on a particular subject, culled from a variety of journals; for example, *International Nursing Index*, *British Education Index*.

Citing and listing references

It is a general requirement throughout higher education that students correctly cite and list the references used in their written work. This applies to all forms of material to which reference is made in the student's work.

Book references

Students should be encouraged to use a standard format or citation style in their work, such as the Harvard system or the numeric system. Harvard referencing for a single book is shown in Table 19.3, and referencing for a chapter in a book is shown in Table 19.4. The purpose of underlining and italics is to show which element of the citation is a separately-published unit.

Table 19.3

Harvard system for book references

Author's surname and initials
Indication of editorship, where appropriate
Year of publication
Title, in italics or underlined
Edition
Publisher
Place of publication

Example:
Quinn, FM (ed.) (1988) *Continuing Professional Development in Nursing: A Guide for Practitioners and Educators*. Stanley Thornes, Cheltenham

Table 19.4

Harvard system for book chapter references

Author's surname and initials
Year of publication
Title, in single quotation marks
Editors initials and surname
Title of book, in italics or underlined
Publisher
Place of publication

Example:
Hinchliff, S (1988) 'Lifelong learning in context', in FM Quinn (ed.) *Continuing Professional Development in Nursing: A Guide for Practitioners and Educators*. Stanley Thornes, Cheltenham

In the numeric system, each citation is numbered in the sequence it appears in the text, and the full citation is given against the appropriate number in the listing at the end.

Example.
'Quinn (7) suggests that the main purpose of problem-solving groups is to encourage critical thinking'. In the reference listing, the full reference would appear as follows:

> 7. Quinn, F.M. (1995) *The Principles and Practice of Nurse Education*, 3rd edn, Stanley Thornes, Cheltenham.

Journal articles

For journal articles, slightly different details are needed to help the reader locate the information. The use of italics is also different from the convention used for book references, as shown in Table 19.5.

| Author's surname and initials |
| Title of article |
| Title of journal in full, in italics |
| Volume number or date |
| Page numbers of article/extract (first and last) |

Example:
Quinn FM, Phillips M, Humphreys J and Hull C (1997) 'Professional development for nurses: a national open learning partnership'. *Open Learning*, **12**, 1, 45–51

Table 19.5

Harvard system for journal references

Further examples of the style of reference appear at the end of each chapter of this book.

Citing electronic sources

Citations of material from the internet are as given in the example below:

ENB *Review of the Framework for Continuing Professional Development* http:/www.enb.org.uk/33frame.htm

EFFECTIVE READING SKILLS

The student may gain a great deal of information by simply handling a book and noting some of the features of it. An idea of its content can be ascertained from reading the publicity description found on the back of the book or the flaps of the dust jacket. In addition, a preface or foreword will indicate the target audience and often the aim of the author, but it should be remembered that a foreword by an eminent writer, although usually a good recommendation, should not be taken as the sole criterion of the excellence of a book.

A glance at the bibliographical page will indicate the author, title and date of publication and if the book is into a second or subsequent edition, this may indicate success. The contents page can be scanned for an idea of the main sequence of the book and it is important to examine the index to see the kind of content included.

Approaches to reading

Students will approach reading in different ways, depending upon its purpose. Brown and Atkins (1988) identify six approaches:

1. *Scanning*. This approach is used to find a specific piece of information.
2. *Skimming*. This is used to obtain an overall impression of an article or chapter.
3. *Surveying*. This is used to ascertain the overall structure of an article or chapter.
4. *Light study reading*. This is reading with no specific purpose other than general background study.
5. *Directed reading*. This is focused reading for a specific purpose, e.g. to grasp concepts, theories, etc.

6. *Deep study reading.* This is active reading in depth, e.g. to discover meanings, to consider and evaluate arguments, etc.

Pre-reading and follow-up reading

It is very useful for students to do some relevant reading prior to each group meeting , if at all possible. They will be in a much better position to contribute during the session, and will also have a good insight into the topic under discussion. It is equally valuable to do some follow-up reading each week after the unit meeting, as this will help them to consolidate their learning and also offers further perspectives on the topic.

Processing texts

Understanding of written texts can be thought of as a constructive process in which the reader first tries to classify the information into fact, narrative and so on. Two levels are then identified, microstructure and macrostructure (Kintsch and Van Dijk, 1978): microstructure is the structure of sentences, propositions and words, and macrostructure is the global meaning of the text, which is obtained by combing the microstructure. There are four rules for isolating the macrostructure:

1. *Deletion*, the taking out of irrelevant properties;
2. *Generalization*, substitution of lower-order concepts by higher-order ones, e.g. substituting furniture for tables and chairs;
3. *Selection*, removal of properties already stated in the text, i.e. removal of repetitive ideas;
4. *Construction*, the creation of a general concept where none is apparent.

These rules are under the control of schema; these are said to be the basic building blocks of the human information-processing system and can be defined as 'large, complex units of knowledge that organize much of what we know about general categories of objects, classes of events and types of people' (Anderson, 1980). When attempting to understand text, students try to select appropriate schema that will account for the material under consideration. The end result of these rules is that a summary or gist of the material is made and this equates with understanding it. These rules can be taught to students to help them to process texts in nursing and the teacher can test each stage to monitor progress.

Another helpful approach to reading texts is to teach students to use procedures or algorithms, two of which are outlined in Table 19.6.

Readability tests

It is useful to apply tests of readability to textual materials as a rough guide to their difficulty or otherwise, one of the most common being the 'Flesch formula for reading ease' (Flesch, 1974). This consists of testing a random sample of passages from the text and applying a formula to calculate reading ease. The formula is:

SQ3R procedure (Robinson, 1946)
SURVEY: student tries to get an overview of the main points in chapter
QUESTIONS: each main point stated in form of a question
READ: student reads the passage to find out answer to questions
RECITE: answer recited out loud without using the book
REVIEW: whole chapter reviewed to give overall impression

MURDER procedure (Dansereau, 1978)
MOOD: getting the right mood for study
UNDERSTANDING: reading for understanding
RECALLING material
DIGESTING material
EXPANDING knowledge by self-enquiry
REVIEWING mistakes

Table 19.6

Examples of algorithm procedures for reading texts

$$RE = 206.835 - 1.015SL - 0.846WL$$

where RE is the reading ease, SL is the average sentence length and WL is word length. The procedure is as follows:

1. Test a minimum of three, randomly selected passages of 100 words each, avoiding introductory ones and beginning with a new paragraph.
2. Calculate the SL by taking the number of words in the sample and dividing by the number of sentences.
3. Calculate the WL by counting the number of syllables in each word of the 100-word sample.

The reading ease score is interpreted as in Table 19.7

Level of material	Reading ease score
Very easy	90–100
Easy	80–90
Fairly easy	70–80
Standard	60–70
Fairly difficult	50–60
Difficult	30–50
Very difficult	0–30

Table 19.7

Interpretation of reading ease score: Flesch formula

EFFECTIVE NOTE-TAKING

Bligh (1998), in a review of studies on note-taking as an aid to memory, concludes that the evidence supports the position that note-taking during a lecture does aid students' memory of the lecture content. He also notes the evidence that note-taking for revision can improve performance. Therefore, on balance it appears that note-taking is to be recommended if it is done effectively, i.e. recording the key points rather than trying to write down everything word-for-word. At degree level, it is more important to note key references given in the unit, so that the original source can be accessed later, avoiding reliance on secondary sources. Table 19.8 gives some advantages and disadvantages of note-taking.

Advantages	Disadvantages
Provides a permanent record for later review. Material is encoded in student's own words. Material is actively processed by the student. Aids memory of lecture points. Aids performance in revision.	May be inaccurate. Student may miss part of lecture whilst writing notes. May inhibit student's own processing activities if structured by teacher.

Some teachers prefer to give notes in the form of handouts, so that accuracy is ensured and nothing is missed during the lesson. On the other hand, giving printed notes means that the students do not have a chance to encode material in their own words, a major disadvantage. It also means that students' own unique processing activities are suppressed. Perhaps the best compromise is for the teacher to use incomplete handouts that contain the key headings and sub-headings of the lecture, but with sufficient space for the student to write in their own notes.

Systems for note-taking

If students wish to take notes from teaching sessions, there are a number of systems for this.

The standard system

The standard system consists of writing down the key headings and sub-headings, with outline descriptions under each one as in Table 19.9

Table 19.9

Standard system of note-taking: bronchial carcinoma (Source of data: Crompton *et al.*, 1999)

Incidence	Commonest fatal cancer in developed world Commonest cancer in men, accounting for half the total cancer deaths in men Second most common cancer in women, after breast cancer
Aetiology	90% accounted for by cigarette smoking Risk is 40 times greater for smokers over non-smokers Passive smoking accounts for some 5% Urban residents have higher incidence than rural Industrial products, e.g. asbestos, chromium
Pathology	Cell types: squamous cell; adenocarcinoma; small-cell; large-cell Narrowing; obstruction; cavitation; infection Direct spread to pleura; mediastinum; chest wall; brachial plexus Lymphatic spread to supraclavicular and mediastinal lymph nodes Metastatic spread to liver, bone, brain, adrenals
Clinical features	Local: cough, haemotysis; breathlessness; pleural pain; chest pain; Horner's syndrome; Pancoast's syndrome General: pneumonia; anorexia; weight loss; lassitude; symptoms due to metastases, e.g. epileptic seizures, jaundice
Investigations	Radiology; bronchoscopy; biopsy; sputum cytology; thoracotomy
Management	Surgical resection (not possible or appropriate in 85% of patients); radiotherapy; chemotherapy; laser therapy
Prognosis	80% die in first year, 56% 5-year survival

The pattern system

The pattern system uses only main concepts, which are connected by lines showing the interrelationships, as in Figure 19.1.

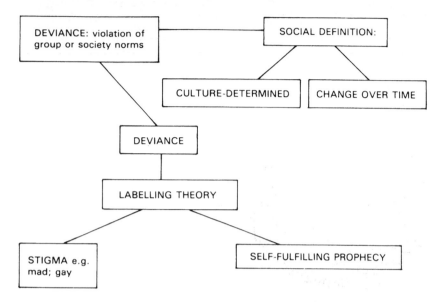

Figure 19.1

Pattern style of note-taking: labelling theory

The Cornell University system

This system is best used with loose-leaf A4 size paper, on which the student rules a two-inch margin on the left-hand side. The system uses five Rs, namely record, reduce, recite, reflect, review. Notes are recorded during the lecture, using only the right-hand side of the paper. As soon as possible afterwards, the learner underlines the key words in the notes and then enters cues in the left-hand column, which will stimulate recall of the ideas in the notes. It is often a difficult exercise to think of appropriate cues, so the learner is required to reorganize and work through the material, which in itself encourages remembering. The third component is reciting the main material, using the cues in the left-hand column. The main material is kept covered and the learner recites out loud their own version of the lecture material. After this, the learner reflects on the content of the lecture and at this stage may add their own ideas and conclusions. The final stage is review, which should be done at regular intervals to assist long-term retention. An example is given in Table 19.10. This system has the advantage of avoiding the rewriting of notes, which is wasteful of time.

Bligh (1998) offers advice to students on effective note-taking:

1. Organization should be familiar with the way lectures are organized.
2. Abbreviations should be used and you should develop your own system of shorthand for frequently-occurring concepts.
3. Layout should be neat and flexible. Plan your notes so that information from other sources can be added later.

Table 19.10

Cornell system of note-taking: acute pyelonephritis (Source of data: Davison et al., 1999)

Cues	Notes
Infection	*Aetiology*: ascending infection via ureters; blood-borne infection
E.coli; Proteus	Most commonly *E.coli* (75%) and Proteus
Inflammation; Abscesses	*Pathology*: renal pelvis inflamed; small abscesses common
Loin pain; fever	*Clinical features*: sudden onset of loin pain; fever; vomiting rigors
Urinalaysis; blood culture;	*Investigations*: urinalysis reveals pus cells; red cells; organisms,
IVU	blood culture; intravenous urogram
Appendicitis, etc.	*Differential diagnosis*: acute appendicitis; cholecystitis; salpingitis
Antibiotics; IV	*Management*: antibiotics; intravenous therapy if severe
Rest	*Nursing*: bed rest until afebrile and pain-free; assistance as required
ADL	with activities of living

4. Note questions and problems rather than facts.
5. Keep a notebook for thoughts and ideas about the subject, for use any time.
6. Review notes immediately after the lecture, and add any further points.
7. Familiarize yourself with the subject before attending the lecture, so that your mind is prepared.

PARTICIPATING IN GROUP DISCUSSION AND SEMINARS

A key aim of units at undergraduate and postgraduate level is to foster students' critical thinking abilities, and one way of doing this is to encourage them to participate actively in discussion and debate. They should be encouraged to venture opinions to the group, even if they are not entirely sure of their knowledge. The value of participation lies in stimulating other members of the group to challenge contributors' ideas, and students should try to keep an open mind about the issues they confront, even if they feel strongly one way or the other; this will allow them to evaluate the issue more objectively.

Not everyone likes group work, and students may feel that the same few people always dominate the discussion, so that others cannot get a word in. Unit leaders need to be alert to this, and be prepared to take steps to encourage the more silent members to contribute. Students must be encouraged to participate in group discussions during the units; it really is important that they experience the process of constructive criticism.

Seminar presentation involves speaking to the group on a particular topic, either chosen by the student or allocated by the tutor. Students may feel that this is a nerve-wracking experience, especially if they have not done anything like it before! Tutors can give guidance and tips to help students with seminar presentations, as shown in Table 19.11.

PLANNING TO STUDY

Studying at higher education level needs to be carried out frequently and regularly in order to achieve the required learning outcomes of the programme. This is easier said than done, particularly where studying is

1. Prepare your material carefully, i.e. ensure that any visual materials are written large enough to be seen.
2. Make a brief plan of the presentation, so that you have the sequence in front of you (it is very disconcerting for you to lose your place).
3. Ensure that you have thoroughly understood the content of your material, you may be questioned about it by group members!
4. Prepare the classroom carefully beforehand, i.e. make sure that everyone can see the chalkboard/screen, etc.; ensure that the overhead projector is aligned carefully, with a full-size image on the screen (if unsure how to do this, ask your tutor)
5. Remember, the aim of the seminar is that the group *learns* something from your presentation, i.e. do not bombard them with masses of information; use overhead projector or handouts for key points; allow sufficient time for note-taking.
6. Allow opportunities for *discussion*, i.e. the seminar is *not* about giving information, but should stimulate thinking and debate; keep formal information to a minimum; posing questions for the group to answer can stimulate debate.
7. Try to make your presentation serve two purposes, i.e. for the seminar and also as the basis of your unit assessment. This will ensure that you take the necessary care over the reading and preparation of the topic.

Table 19.11

Guidance for students' seminar presentations

done on a part-time basis. Study time often conflicts with work responsibilities and family commitments, and there may well be associated guilt if studying is seen to take the student away from her/his children. It is therefore very important to plan carefully for study, so that a sensible balance is struck between these conflicting demands.

Planning study time

Like most other activities in life, studying is facilitated by planning. A carefully prepared plan of study can eliminate the somewhat haphazard approach that tends to be common among students. To be really effective, study must be seen as a natural part of the student's life, just like meal times and other routines. Another aspect is the temptation to escape from the chore of study by using certain devices that may or may not be unconscious. For example, day-dreaming is a common occurrence during study and also frequent trips to make coffee, or some other ploy that takes one away from the 'unpleasant' situation. Boredom is another problem against which the student must fight, and it is good advice to suggest that he or she uses a pencil to make notes at regular intervals, thus aiding concentration and providing a feeling of 'getting somewhere'. Joining with a small group of students to examine a common problem can be a motivating activity from time to time and gives different perspectives to an aspect of study

When planning for study it is important to include regular breaks so that fatigue is avoided. Stretching one's legs every hour or so will help keep concentration and make the subsequent study more efficient. It is unlikely that a period of study longer than about three hours will be useful at any one time and even this length may prove difficult. An interesting suggestion is given by Bandura (1977), which he terms 'self-reinforcement'. It involves setting oneself certain study goals and allocating a reward that is conditional upon attainment of these goals. For example, students might decide to study a particular section of a textbook until they could describe its content in their own words. The reward that they allocate could be a walk in the park, which can be taken only when the objective has been achieved.

Organizing the environment for study

It is important that books and materials can be left lying in the same place, since having to put them away and then take them out on another occasion can be very demotivating. A comfortable chair is crucial, with good support for the lumbar spine and the room should be at a comfortable temperature with adequate ventilation to offset fatigue. Daylight is the best form of illumination, but in the evenings it is good to have two light sources with adequate shading to prevent glare. Many students automatically switch on music when commencing study, as this makes the task less of a chore. However, music is a source of distracting input that will interfere with studying, so it is better to save music for the five-minute breaks in studying every hour or so.

STRATEGIES FOR EFFECTIVE STUDY

There are a number of strategies that can help students to study more effectively, including rehearsal, mnemonics, and self-assessment.

Rehearsal

This is the silent repetition of sentences or words over and over again as a way of remembering them. It is a particularly important metacognitive strategy for retention of material and there are two closely related concepts that need to be considered also. Review involves going back over material that one has previously read and recitation is actually saying the material out loud.

Mnemonics

These are memory aids that involve mental strategies, the best-known ones involving rhymes such as 'Thirty days hath September, April, June and November ...'.

Table 19.12 shows the classification of disease and its application to the causes of haematuria. A very useful mnemonic for remembering the classification of disease is CTINMADII, pronounced 'see, tin, mad, eye eye'. Each letter stands for a cause of disease and is often called the 'pathological sieve'. It can be seen that any disease or disorder can be recalled using this device, provided the student can remember the examples of each condition.

Mnemonics can be visual, as in the case of imagery. Evidence suggests that by forming a mental picture or image we can remember items much better. For example, one can picture items associated with aspects of the home; one item may be hanging in the hall, another on the sofa. A more practical example in nursing is the use of images of patients one has nursed in the past. The student should try to recall a patient who had nursing problems and picture the care given. Narrative is a closely related idea, which consists of making up a story that links

Cause	Definition	Application to haematuria
Congenital	Present at birth	Haemophilia
Traumatic	Injury	Ruptured kidney
Infectious	Due to microorganisms	Cystitis
Neoplastic	Tumours	Papilloma of bladder
Metabolic	Disorder of metabolism	Renal calculus
Allergic	Due to hypersensitivity	Glomerulonephritis
Degenerative	Due to ageing	Not applicable
Iatrogenic	Doctor-induced	Anticoagulants
Idiopathic	Cause unknown	Haematuria of unknown origin

Table 19.12

Classification of disease and an example applied to haematuria

all the words one wishes to remember. In the example given above of classification of disease, the narrative might go as follows: 'A man went to SEA in a TIN because he got MAD when he and his partner didn't see EYE to EYE'.

Self-testing

Self-testing can be a useful strategy for increasing retention of material and evidence for this is offered by Rothkopf (1970) and Rothkopf and Johnson (1971). Rothkopf maintains that learning from written materials involves two processes, the first one being the study and inspection behaviours of the student. He calls these 'mathemagenic behaviours', i.e. behaviours that give birth to learning. The second process is the actual acquisition of learning of the subject matter. Rothkopf maintains that the study habits of students are fluid and can be constantly modified during study. He tested these ideas in a series of experiments involving the use of inserted questions into texts and found that the greatest facilitative effect on learning occurred when the questions were inserted after the material to which they related, i.e. post-questions. The implications for students are that the regular testing of study materials by the use of post-questions may well enhance learning.

TACKLING ASSESSMENTS AND EXAMINATIONS

Assessments and examinations tend to be perceived by students as the most important aspects of a programme of study, and this is understandable, given the consequences of failure. Advice about tackling assessments and examinations can help relieve some of the anxiety students experience, and possibly improve their performance.

Approaching coursework assessment tasks

The most important single step in tackling the assessment is to read the assessment specification carefully. It is, unfortunately, a relatively common occurrence to find that a student has been referred on an assignment because he or she has not conformed to the assessment specification for that unit. No matter how scholarly or erudite an assignment is, it will not gain a pass grade unless it meets the specification for the unit. It is no good having 'the right answer to the wrong question'. When a student has thoroughly understood the assignment brief (if in doubt, it can be checked with the unit leader), she should ask herself the following questions:

1. Assuming that there is a choice of assignments, is it sufficiently motivating to pursue in preference to other relevant topics?
2. Is it manageable in terms of time and resources available to meet the deadline for handing in?
3. Are there sufficient references available to be able to demonstrate skilful use of the literature?

Reading for the assessment

When writing assignments it is vital to demonstrate the ability to use the literature with insight. Textbooks are a good starting point by providing an overview of the topic. Students should always check the date of publication, especially in books that have been reprinted several times. It is easy to misinterpret a current reprint date and assume that the book is quite new, whereas it may be several years old and therefore possibly out of date. Journals offer up to date articles on specific aspects of a topic, and usually contain an abstract from which the students can quickly tell whether or not the article is relevant to their study. Journal articles are also important as a source of criticism of other articles or theories. Journals often run consecutive editions containing 'blasts and counter-blasts' from contributors with opposing viewpoints, and these provide fascinating insights into critical, analytic argument. The literature of philosophy is often overlooked by nursing students, but can be extremely useful in providing insights into issues such as values, beliefs, judgements, freedom of choice, etc. The mass media, i.e. newspapers, radio and television, is also a useful source of reference. There are many excellent articles/programmes relating to health matters, and these tend to address current, controversial issues.

Effective writing for coursework assessments

It is the coursework assessments, along with clinical assessments and examinations, that enable students to demonstrate achievement of the learning outcomes of their programme. Most students will require some help with the formulation of their assignments, particularly if they have not had recent experience of study.

Composing an essay-type assignment

Composing an essay involves four main processes (Humes, 1983):

1. *Planning*. This takes more time than any other process, and includes not only the initial planning before commencement of writing, but the constant planning that goes on throughout the composition. Planning includes the organization and generation of content and the sequencing of goals.
2. *Translating*. This is the transformation of thoughts into written

form and consists of complex mental activities such as attending to syntax and structure.

3. *Reviewing*. Writers engage in retrospective activities to check if their written ideas are actually what was intended. It also serves to re-orientate the writer for the next section.

4. *Revising*. This covers editing of the written material and usually results in the production of a second draft, although much editing can occur during the initial draft.

Essay-type assignments vary enormously in their approach, from the standard essay question to case studies and problem-centred assignments. However, it is possible to draw a few general guidelines for students to consider. Essays must be written in prose, not in note form, with sentences of appropriate length and the sensible use of paragraphs. Great store is attached to legibility and clarity of expression in all educational systems, so careful planning is required beforehand. Even under examination conditions it is important to do a brief plan before attempting to write an answer to ensure that all the main aspects have been considered for inclusion.

The length of an assignment must be clearly indicated by the teachers and any minimum and maximum length strictly adhered to. It is quite unfair to state that an assignment has a maximum of 3000 words and then to accept ones that are perhaps twice this long. Students who stuck to the limit are then, in effect, penalized as the others will have included much more material in their work. Strict attention must be paid to the wording of the assignment; there is an ever-present temptation to interpret the question or title in the way the student would like it to be phrased, rather than how it actually is phrased. Students should use fluorescent highlighter pens to identify the key words in the question or title, since these dictate the form of response required. Table 19.13 gives a list of common terms and their meaning.

ANALYSE	Literally, breaking-up the issue into its constituent parts and describing them in detail
ASSESS	Estimate the pros and cons of the issue and give a judgement on these
COMPARE AND CONTRAST	Show the similarities and differences between the concepts
DEFINE	Show the exact meaning of the concept
DESCRIBE	Give a picture of an object or event without judgement
DISCUSS	Give viewpoints from both sides and then round off with own conclusion based on these
LIST	Write down in tabular form with minimum words
OUTLINE	A general overview without fine detail
STATE	Present the points briefly without elaboration

Table 19.13

Common terms used in assessment

It is well worth spending time initially on designing the overall structure of the assignment, as a good assignment can be weakened by a poor or incoherent structure. Whilst there is no ideal or standard structure, it may be helpful to offer the student a basic pattern as shown in Table 19.14.

Table 19.14

Typical structure of an essay assignment

1	Title
2	Introduction
	Focus of assignment
	Problem or issue
	Context
	Literature review
3	Main body
	Description
	Analysis/argument
	Synthesis/argument
	Evaluation
4	Conclusions
	Review of issues
	Student's opinions in the light of the foregoing discussion
	Recommendations if appropriate
5	References
	Use standard system of referencing, e.g. Harvard
6.	Appendix
	Useful for documents that could not be included fully in the text for want of space, but which would provide useful information for the reader

Word processing

Word processing is the answer to students' problems when editing the final draft for submission. With this technology, they can move paragraphs around, or insert and delete until they are happy with the result. Handwritten assignments do not easily allow for alterations without a great deal of re-writing, so it might be worth their while to acquire word processing skills. Tutors can offer useful advice and tips on editing, as shown in Table 19.15.

Table 19.15

Tips for students on editing their assignments

1. Check the number of words (do a spellcheck on word processor); it is normal to accept 'plus or minus 10%' of the required word length, i.e. if the assignment is 2500 words, then an acceptable range would be 2250–2750 words. If you go outside these boundaries you may well find that your marks are adversely affected. It is more difficult to write concisely, and therefore students would be unfairly advantaged if they were allowed to exceed the word length by a significant amount.
2. Avoid 'padding' your assignment with materials that are not strictly relevant to the topic. Students are often tempted to include material in the appendix just because it is readily available from their institution. Any material in the appendix must be referred to in the main text, and must have a substantial contribution to make to the assignment.
3. Carry out a final check against the unit assessment specification to ensure that all aspects have been addressed.
4. It is imperative that careful attention is paid to the procedures for handing-in of your assignment.
5. Always keep a copy of the assignment. In the very best systems there is always the possibility of a mishap, and an assignment may occasionally go astray. It is heartbreaking if this occurs and you have not kept a copy.

Revising for examinations

Examinations are virtually confined to pre-registration programmes in nursing and midwifery education, and are often perceived by students as the most stressful aspect of a course. It is crucial that students commence revision as early as possible if stress is to be minimized, and the regular review of lecture notes will help. Again, planning is the key to effective revision, with objectives and deadlines for each week, but in the case of examination revision, motivation is of paramount importance. The use of study groups for revision can provide excellent motivation and in addition, the presence of other students who feel equally ignorant can be very reassuring. Frequent changes of stimulus can help combat staleness and the use of a learning resources centre with audio-visual aids may provide a welcome change from reading. It cannot be over-emphasized that cramming is a very inefficient and risky business, as the high levels of stress that develop close to the examination act to impair the learning performance.

Examination technique

Sitting for an examination requires a degree of self-control, since panic can so easily undermine an otherwise well-prepared candidate. If the examination consists of an unseen paper, the candidate will not be allowed to take any resources into the examination room other than those for writing and drawing. The instructions for filling in the answer book should be noted. On the first scan of the paper, the student should carefully note the number of questions to be answered, the parts from which they should each be selected if relevant, and the amount of time to be allocated to each. It is wise to allocate an equal amount of time to each question, including an allowance at the end of the examination to go back over and check the answers. The students should be advised to scan the questions and to select the one which they feel most confident about. Once writing begins anxiety levels should fall, and the students will be able to choose subsequent questions in a more rational frame of mind. Students should be advised to make a brief plan before commencing a question, as this can ensure that all necessary elements of the answer have been considered. This plan can then act as a prompt when the writing begins to flow. It is important that a careful watch is kept on the time, as it is all too easy to overrun on the easier questions, leaving a shortfall for the more difficult ones. During the last five minutes or so, the student should read through all answers, adding brief points that were missed the first time. As a final check the student should ensure that all papers are properly identified according to the instructions.

Undertaking objective tests

Objective tests seem to have gone out of fashion over the past few years, but some institutions may still use them. Students should be given careful guidance about how to approach objective tests:

1. Read the instructions for the test carefully, especially those concerned with completion of the answer sheet.
2. Check the procedure for changing an answer.
3. Check if the test has a correction-for-guessing built into the marking, as this will make it advisable to avoid guessing.

4. Work quickly through the test, completing only those items which can be answered easily.
5. Return to the beginning and attempt the next level of difficulty, again leaving the items which require a great deal of thought.
6. Finally, spend the remaining time on the difficult items; keep a careful watch for negative items, as these may easily be overlooked.

REFERENCES

Anderson, J. (1980) *Cognitive Psychology and Its Implications*, Freeman, San Francisco.

Bandura, A. (1977) *Social Learning Theory*, Prentice-Hall, Englewood Cliffs, NJ.

Bligh, D. (1998) *What's the Use of Lectures?* 5th edn, Exeter, Intellect.

Brown, G. and Atkins, M. (1988) *Effective Teaching in Higher Education*, Methuen, London.

Crompton, G.K, Haslett, C. and Chilvers, E.R. (1999) Diseases of the respiratory system, in *Davidson's Principles and Practice of Medicine*, 18th edn, C. Haslett, E.R Chilvers, J.A.A. Hunter and N.A. Boon (eds), Churchill Livingstone, Edinburgh.

Dansereau, D. (1978) The development of a learning strategies curriculum, in *Learning Strategies*, H.F. O'Neil (ed.), Academic Press, New York.

Davison, A.M., Cumming, A.D., Swainson, C.P. and Turner, N. (1999) Diseases of the kidney and urinary system, in *Davidson's Principles and Practice of Medicine*, 18th edn, C. Haslett, E.R Chilvers, J.A.A. Hunter and N.A. Boon (eds), Churchill Livingstone, Edinburgh.

Flesch, R. (1974) *The Art of Readable Writing*, Harper and Row, New York.

Hartley, J. (1998) *Learning and Studying: A Research Perspective*, Routledge, London.

Humes, A. (1983) Research on the composing process, *Review of Educational Research*, 53(2), 201–16.

Kintsch, W. and Van Dijk, T. (1978) Toward a model of text comprehension and production, *Psychological Review*, 85, 363–94.

Robinson, F. (1946) *Effective Study*, Harper, New York.

Rogers, C. (1969) *Freedom to Learn*, Charles Merrill, Ohio.

Rothkopf, E. (1970) The concept of mathemagenic activities, *Review of Educational Research*, 40, 325–36.

Rothkopf, E. and Johnson, P. (1971) *Verbal Learning Research and The Technology of Written Instruction*, Teachers College Press, New York.

20

TEACHING AND SUPERVISING RESEARCH

In nursing, midwifery and health visiting, research is acknowledged as a central component of professional education, and there are a number of levels at which the concept may be addressed. Research appreciation, or basic research literacy, is the most fundamental level and aims to provide students with a basic grounding in the concepts and approaches to research. It is mainly a theoretical introduction, but may include some experiential activities such as undertaking a literature review or formulating a research proposal. Research appreciation is characteristic of academic level 2 programmes for both pre-registration and post-registration education in nursing. The next level is characteristic of honours degree programmes, both pre- and post-registration, and requires students to undertake some form of research project, usually involving fieldwork, and which contributes significantly to students' final honours classification. At taught masters degree level, a research project requires a more specific focus, and greater depth and originality, than an honours degree project. Master of Philosophy (MPhil) and Doctor of Philosophy (PhD) degrees consist almost entirely of a research project, and are 'taught' by supervision rather than lectures; hence the term 'research degrees' for this level.

It is likely that both teachers and practitioners of nursing will encounter students who are undertaking research projects of one kind or another, so the skills involved in supervising such students are important ones to acquire.

Within nursing, midwifery and health visiting, research is considered important for a range of reasons:

1. *Research and teaching*. Research and teaching are the two sides of the same higher education coin; in other words, research generates the subject-matter for teaching, while teaching provides the experiences that generate research. It is this symbiotic relationship between research and teaching that characterizes the British higher education sector, which includes nurse education. Before the binary divide between universities and polytechnics was abolished, it was suggested that, in the existing universities, research by academic staff took priority over the teaching of students. Within the polytechnics, the opposite was said to be the case, i.e. teaching took priority over research. Whilst this distinction did not hold true for some institutions on both sides of the binary divide, it is accepted that there was a more than a grain of truth in the generalization.

2. *Research and funding*. Research is not only linked closely to

teaching, it also generates income for the institution. The four-yearly cycle of the research assessment exercise (RAE) is conducted by the UK Higher Education Funding Councils, and the quality rating that each unit of assessment receives within an institution determines the amount of research funding it receives. (The RAE is discussed in detail in Chapter 21, p. 548). The term *research* itself covers a variety of activities such as patents, inventions, productions in performing and visual arts, and curriculum, teaching and assessment materials where these have been developed through research and have been published.

3. *Research and the profession.* One of the hallmarks of a profession is the possession of a distinct body of knowledge, and this is created by research. There has been considerable debate over the years about whether nursing has a sufficiently distinct body of knowledge, or whether it simply draws upon a range of other disciplines; this debate is also relevant to the teaching profession. However, the nursing profession has made major strides in developing a nursing research base for practice, characterized by the growth of organizations such as the Royal College of Nursing Research Society. The advent of the concept of evidence-based practice is likely to further reinforce the pivotal role of research in nurse education.

4. *Research and prestige.* In the world of academe, there is little doubt that research is considered more prestigious than teaching, and this has probably always been the case. Practical teaching is much like practical nursing, in that it seems to equate with the lowest rung on the professional ladder, with each subsequent promotion taking the practitioner further and further away from everyday teaching, and more and more into administration. Indeed, some higher education institutions use the term *easement* or *remission* to describe the reduction in practical teaching hours for those lecturers who take on other duties, usually of an administrative nature. These terms, by their very nature, evoke images of release from a prison sentence, and can only serve to reinforce the notion that everyday practical teaching is a job for those who lack the ability to move any further up the career ladder!

TEACHING RESEARCH IN NURSE EDUCATION

Although the nursing profession has long espoused the importance of research and its inclusion in nursing, midwifery and health visiting curricula, the integration of the professions into higher education raised questions about the ability of nurse teachers to actually teach research (ENB, 1993).

The research culture in nurse education

Prior to the move into higher education, colleges of nursing, by and large, had not developed a research culture. This is not a criticism;

nurse education evolved outside the higher education sector and was not therefore exposed to research culture that pertained in higher education institutions. The question of nurse teachers' ability to teach research led the English National Board for Nursing, Midwifery and Health Visiting to undertake a research project (LeVar and Steadman, 1996) with the following aims:

- to identify and report on the level of existing skills of nurse and midwife teachers to teach research and related aspects of Board approved curricula;
- to identify any action required to improve the current position.

The study comprised a review and analysis of published statistics on teaching staff, a review of documents, and interviews in three institutions, and questionnaires to all provider institutions for nursing and midwifery education. The findings from the analysis of published statistics showed 'a focus on obtaining higher degree qualifications across the whole teaching force'. The review of institutional documents showed that 'the submissions analysed met the Board's guidelines, were well constructed and imaginative, and included a variety of teaching/learning strategies to enable the students to achieve the learning outcomes'.

The outcomes and recommendations of the study included the following points:

- The quality of research teaching was satisfactory, but continuing development was required.
- Teachers of research should have engaged in research themselves, and possess a higher degree.
- There was evidence of action to promote a research culture in the institutions surveyed, including encouragement to study for higher and other degrees, and to engage in staff development for research.
- Institutions need to work towards a position where all teachers of research possess a higher degree, and have time and opportunity to be actively engaged in research.
- Institutions need to review the steps they currently take to promote a research culture.

The central importance of a research culture was further addressed in the ENB Research Culture Project (Crow *et al.*, 1997), which aimed to offer practical assistance on the role of the Board in commissioning research, offer insight into acquiring research funding, explore the development of a research culture, and seek evidence of research needs. Participants were drawn from institutions that had recently moved into higher education, and the recommendations included the following:

- Staff replacement costs and pump priming for educational programmes in research methods were seen as vital to support future development.
- The ENB should concentrate on auditing the opportunities for research development.

The role of a professional organization, the Royal College of Nursing (RCN), in supporting research and development was explored by McMahon and Kitson (1997). Sixty-six nurses (researchers, educators, managers, and practitioners) from the four UK countries were interviewed about their role in research and development, about what helped or hindered these activities, and what they saw as the role of the RCN in research and development. The findings on the factors that assist or prevent research and development activity included:

- the importance of skills and experience in project management and obtaining funding;
- a full-time funded post with time out for continuing professional development (CPD) was seen as a major enabling factor;
- the climate of competition in the NHS worked counter to nurses' R&D endeavours;
- individuals and support structures enabled nurses to deliver the R&D component of their role, e.g. local networks, clinical nursing leaders, collaborators, etc.

Participants in the study saw three main aspects to the R&D role of the RCN:

- commissioning research;
- disseminating and implementing findings;
- providing an infrastructure for R&D, e.g. library, information and networking, etc.

Ethics and nursing research

There is normally an ethical dimension to most research projects, but in nursing research ethical issues are of particular importance, given the potential vulnerability of sick patients and clients. A useful list of ethical principles for research in the clinical area is given by Wagstaff and Gould (1998):

- non-maleficence, i.e. the research should do the patient no harm;
- the consent of participants, or proxy consent, must be obtained;
- informed consent has several sub-components, including the need to disclose to participants any dangers of the research, and the importance of such consent being voluntary;
- justice, i.e. patients should not be overburdened with requests to participate in research;
- privacy, i.e. patients' privacy should be protected.

Proposals for research involving patient and clients must be approved by the institution's Research Ethics Committee before the research can commence.

OVERVIEW OF THE RESEARCH PROCESS

Research is a rational process of scientific enquiry directed towards a question or problem and resulting in extension of the total sum of knowledge. It is a way of making sense of the world through explanation, but the definition makes clear that it is not just ordinary enquiry such as that of casual observation. Research is scientific and science is characterized by objectivity and the empirical nature of its explanations (Kerlinger, 1979). *Empirical research* is a term used to describe the systematic, controlled gathering of evidence that characterizes science, including behavioural sciences. Objectivity means that the explanations are independent of the experimenter's own bias and this is ensured by the detailed reporting of every step in the research so as to enable another scientist to replicate the study. The publication of research exposes it to the scrutiny of the scientific community and this provides a measure of quality assurance.

THE SCIENTIFIC METHOD

The above criteria are the foundations of the scientific method of enquiry, a process of investigation consisting of a logical sequence of steps as shown in Table 20.1.

1　Defining the problem or question
2　Reviewing the literature
3　Formulating a hypothesis
4　Designing the study
5　Carrying out pilot study
6　Collecting the data
7　Analysing the data
8　Drawing conclusions and making recommendations

Table 20.1

The scientific method

Defining the problem or question

The research process begins with an observation about some phenomenon, or perhaps a feeling about something, and from this germ of an idea a research project may develop. We need to distinguish scientific problems from two others kinds, engineering problems and value problems. An engineering problem is concerned with how to do certain things such as 'how to reduce the incidence of pressure sores', whereas a value problem is concerned with what is good and which is best. A scientific problem has an advantage over these other kinds of problem because it is formulated in such a way as to render it capable of being tested. Scientific problems are to do with relationships between variables, and there are three criteria for a scientific problem as shown in Table 20.2.

Students usually have difficulty in choosing a research topic and it is helpful to advise them to identify a broad area of interest, and then

1.　It must be stated in interrogative form, i.e. in the form of a question.
2.　It must state a relationship between variables.
3.　It must imply empirical testing.

Table 20.2

Criteria for a scientific problem (Kerlinger, 1979)

focus down to clearly defined questions to which answers can be found. These answers may be empirical or literary. They also need to consider why the topic is worth investigating and what the likely benefits will be. If the student wishes to attempt to solve a concrete, practical problem in the immediate work setting, then this is considered to be an example of action research, which is typified by a requirement for specific knowledge for a practical problem in a specific situation (Bell, 1993).

Reviewing the literature

A literature review is carried out in order to gain an understanding of the theoretical background to the research project. In addition, a review of the literature will indicate whether previous work has been done in the same area. Even if this is the case, the student may wish to replicate a previous study and compare the results. Another advantage is that there may be methods of measurement in other studies that could be used. A search of the literature is often done in two stages: a general overview of the secondary sources, such as textbooks, CD-ROM, etc., and a specific review of the primary source material in written research reports.

Nelson (1998) discussed the distinction between conventional reviews and systematic reviews of the literature, pointing out weaknesses of the former such as bias or deficiencies that can lead to unreliable or misleading results. Systematic reviews, on the other hand, use the scientific method approach to ensure rigour, and the articles for review should be treated like subjects in a research project, i.e. clear criteria must be set for inclusion or rejection of articles for the review.

Formulating a hypothesis

A hypothesis is a supposition or conjecture about the relationship between variables that is couched in declarative rather than interrogative form. The hypothesis must be testable and therefore requires to be stated in operational terms that specify which operations are necessary to measure the variables. A hypothesis is usually stated in the null form, which is a negative statement that uses the form 'will not'. The null hypothesis is preferred in practice because it is easier to test statistically and adds a measure of objectivity to the acceptance or rejection.

Designing the study

In designing the research study the student must consider the type of research design that best meets the aims of the project.

Experimental research design

This is a type of research in which the situation to be studied is artificially controlled by the experimenter. Some form of treatment is administered and the effects observed, whilst maintaining other variables at a constant level. By systematically altering the treatment and observing the results, the experimenter may come to the conclusion that a cause-

and-effect relationship exists. The treatment may involve such things as administration of a drug, and is termed the independent variable because it is independent of the results of the experiment. The dependent variable is the observed changes in the subject's performance following treatment by the independent variable. The dependent variable is dependent upon the way in which the independent variable is manipulated, hence the independent variable is the antecedent and the dependent variable the consequence. This relationship is often stated as: 'If p, then q'. However, in the experimental situation, it is important to have a control group of matching individuals who are not given the treatment, but who are assessed on the same test as the experimental group. This has the effect of dealing with irrelevant variables that might confuse the findings, and allows the experimenter to assume that any difference in the experimental group is due to the treatment rather than to other factors. There are, however, confounded variables that the experimenter needs to consider; it is possible that there is another, unknown, variable that is acting to produce the effect, rather than the independent variable.

There are two vital aspects to be considered when designing an experiment: internal and external validity. Internal validity is concerned with aspects of credibility within the design itself, including such things as changes due solely to the passage of time, the effects of a test being affected by prior tests, and changes due to other events occurring between the independent and dependent variables.

External validity refers to the generalizability of the results and can be affected by such things as pre-testing causing sensitization of subjects to the phenomenon in question and thereby affecting results. There is also a notion called ecological validity, which questions the applicability of laboratory-based research to the real world.

One-way and two-way experimental designs

In experimental research there are two types of design – 'one-way' and 'two-way' – named according to the number of independent variables employed. Figure 20.1 shows a one-way experimental design; this uses only one independent variable and is often referred to as the 'classic design'. It consists of an experimental group and a control group: the experimental group is treated by the independent variable, whereas the control group receives no treatment. Both groups are subsequently tested for changes in the dependent variable (Figure 20.1(a)). Additionally, a pre-test can be given prior to the treatment to establish the existing level of the variable under study (Figure 20.1(b)). One of the limitations of one-way designs is the reliance on a single variable, which in the social sciences is rarely useful, since most behaviour is the result of many variables working together.

Two-way designs allow the use of more than one independent variable and are also termed *factorial designs*. Not only can the effect of each variable be measured as a separate entity, but also the effects of any interaction between them; these are called the main effect and inter-

Figure 20.1

One-way experiment design (a) without pre-test and (b) with pre-test

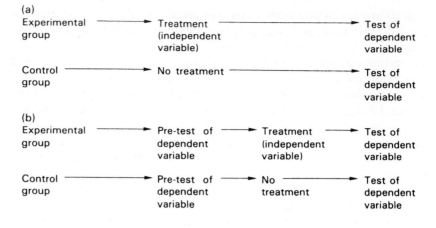

action effects respectively. Interaction effects can be described as: 'If p, then q, under condition r'.

The use of experiments, then, brings a degree of control that is important in determining the effects of the independent variable, but the student needs to be aware of the disadvantages in using them. Table 20.3 shows some of the pros and cons of this method.

Table 20.3

Advantages and disadvantages of experimental research

Advantages	Disadvantages
A high degree of control over potential confounded variable	Independent variables used in laboratory may not be as strong as naturally occurring ones
Situations are flexible to test a variety of aspects	Laboratory setting may lead to loss of ecological validity
They can be replicated by other experimenters	There are ethical difficulties in some areas where experiment is not acceptable
Hypothesis is used as a predictor for relationships between variables	By focusing on objectivity and control, the experiment may lose valuable subjective data
Data is generated which is objective and can be subjected to statistical analysis	It is not always practically possible to use experiments
Independent variables can be manipulated to demonstrate effects on dependent variable	

Non-experimental research design

This is research in which the researcher is unable to manipulate variables or to randomly allocate subjects and conditions. It is also termed *ex post facto* because it is research after the event, i.e. after the variables have already affected the subjects. For example, a postgraduate student may wish to ascertain if a correlation exists between pre-operative visits by an anaesthetic nurse, and perceived post-operative anxiety in surgical patients. Both experimental and non-experimental research make the assumption 'if p, then q', but non-experimental research uses surveys as its means of enquiry. In this method, a population is sampled to determine aspects of certain variables such as distribution and relationships, the latter being referred to as correlation. Correlation means literally the correlation between two sets of values, such as pre-operative visiting and perceived anxiety in surgical patients, and occurs in two dimensions, magnitude and direction. Magnitude is the strength of correlation on a scale of between −1 and +1, with 0 being no relationship, +1 meaning that a high score on one variable is accompanied by a high score on the other and −1 meaning that a high score on one variable is accompanied by a low score on the other. Magnitude is expressed as a 'coefficient of correlation' and direction is indicated by the plus or minus sign.

The simplest form of survey is the case study, which is a single study of an individual or organization. The main weakness from a research point of view is that the results cannot be generalized. Descriptive surveys are used to collect information from a representative sample of individuals in order to make generalizations. Opinion polls are examples, and this form of survey does not attempt to explain the information in any way, so if one wishes to know if there is any relationship between variables, then an explanatory survey is required.

Another form of non-experimental research is ethnographic research which utilizes the technique of participant observation. This involves the researcher in sharing the experiences of the subjects in order to gain insight into phenomena.

New paradigm research

The term 'new paradigm research' was coined by John Rowan and Peter Reason to describe a group of approaches that constitute a new paradigm in human research (Reason, 1988). According to the authors, traditional or normative research tends to alienate subjects from the work of the researcher, from other subjects, and from the products of the research. In new paradigm research, no distinction is made between subject and researcher, the aim being to work with people rather than on people. It is an approach that emphasizes action rather than intellectual problems, and this is exemplified in a technique called 'co-operative inquiry' (Heron, 1985). This approach makes no distinction between researcher and subject, with each individual taking both roles. It is used in conjunction with experiential learning, emphasizing the importance of reflection in the validation of experience. A group of student nurses may wish to enquire into some aspect of nursing, and they begin as co-researchers reflecting and clarifying the purpose and methods they will use. The study is then undertaken co-operatively by members of the group, and then the experience of this is reflected upon in order to help them to understand the meaning and implications of the study with a view to further modification of the original idea.

Sampling

This is a crucial aspect of research design and students usually need much help sorting it out. Sampling is the term given to the selection of the subjects for research, and implies that they are taken from a 'whole'. Sampling is necessary in research, in order to be able to generalize the results beyond the group that was investigated. The term 'population' implies any group of people or observations that includes all possible members of that category. A sample taken from a population must be representative of the characteristics of the population that is being studied. Samples are used because it is not usually possible to study every member of a particular population, so it is important to remember that the results of any one sample cannot be generalized beyond the population from which it was drawn. Measures of characteristics of a population are termed parameters and of a sample, statistics. There are a number of designs of sampling, the simplest being random sampling.

1. *Random sampling*. In this method, each member of the population has an equal chance of being selected, as in drawing names out of a hat. A more sophisticated method is to use computer-generated random numbers. Random samples allow results to be generalized to the rest of the population from which the sample was drawn, but it must be remembered that such generalization is never totally accurate, there being some sampling error always. This means that we must talk about inference and probability rather than certainty, and in simple random sampling the error diminishes as the sample size grows.

2. *Systematic sampling*. This is another type, in which the sample is taken from some kind of list at fixed intervals, for example, every fifth one. In this type, some members of a population have no chance of being selected and the randomness will be affected by the frame from which the names were taken. If this was done by simple random sampling, then the systematic sample will be equivalent. However, if the list is in some form of rank order, this would affect the representativeness.

3. *Stratified sampling*. This involves the researcher in dividing the population into layers or strata, on the basis of such characteristics as sex, social class, educational attainment, etc., according to the variables under study. A simple random sample is then taken from each stratum. If the sample is proportionate, i.e. reflects the proportion of subjects in the population, then this method is more representative than simple random sampling.

4. *Cluster sampling*. This involves the selection of natural groups on a random basis, and can be used where the size and cost of sampling a population in a simple random manner would be too great.

The decisions that the researcher must make with regard to sampling design are affected by a number of factors and Fox (1969) has put forward this adage: 'No data are sounder than the representativeness of the sample from which they were obtained, no matter how large the sample'. There are constraints on availability of time, finance and the facilities and assistance required, and non-response may alter the representativeness. The design of the sampling should be within the scope of the researcher, and compromise may have to be reached between this need and the type of sampling employed.

Measuring instruments or tools

Selection of instruments is a crucial stage in the research process, and the student needs to consider such points as the validity and reliability, practicality and so on, and whether or not the instruments are already available, or have to be designed. The following section outlines three common instruments used in survey research: questionnaires, interviews, and focus groups.

The questionnaire

This consists of a sequence of questions that the respondent is required to answer. There are two main areas in which it can be used: opinions and attitudes. When designing a questionnaire, it is important to produce a specification of the subject area that is to be measured, and also to consider the practical aspects such as:

- whether the questionnaire will be posted to the sample, or administered on a group or individual basis;
- what the sequence of questions will be; and
- will it use open or closed questions.

Open questions allow the respondent to answer in his own words, but are difficult to analyse, while closed questions give the respondent a limited number of choices from which to select his responses (Oppenheim, 1966). This makes analysis much easier and is recommended for most types of questionnaire.

The sequence of questions is important, as the initial questions should put the respondent at ease so that some kind of rapport is developed. The more searching, personal questions can be left until later in the sequence, when the respondent is convinced of the seriousness of the questionnaire. Wording of the questions is crucial and every effort must be made to eliminate ambiguity and possibility of bias. Leading questions are those that contain an implicit value as to what the behaviour in question ought to be. Prestige bias is the term given to responses which reflect distortion of the facts due to a prestige element. Questions that contain two elements are best avoided and it is essential that the questions are subjected to a pilot study, so that any of these problems can be resolved before the main data collection commences.

The interview

Interviews have a number of advantages over questionnaires, although questionnaires or schedules are used in an interview. The presence of an interviewer ensures that the respondent understands the purpose of the study and any misunderstood questions can be explained. The respondent's non-verbal communication can be noted, and the interviewer can be instructed to probe further into the responses to a question.

However, there is a danger of bias when using an interview technique, because the interviewer may introduce his or her own attitude without being consciously aware of this. The interviewer's responses, manner and other non-verbal cues may influence the response of the individual being questioned. Research students need to be made aware of the practical constraints on the use of this technique, particularly the problems of finance, training in interviewing technique, and the time involved in collection of data. There is a spectrum of interview techniques, ranging from the totally structured to the totally unstructured interview.

Focus groups

The use of focus groups is a technique derived from social science and market research, and the aim is to bring together a homogeneous group of individuals to share their opinions, attitudes, perceptions and feelings about a given topic. For example, a health visitor may wish to use focus groups in her research into the factors that influence teenage smoking. She would select a group of 8 to 12 teenagers who smoke, choose a venue conducive to the process, and conduct a focus group session of approximately one hour. The aim might be to ascertain teenagers' opinions about why they smoke, and the pressures they perceive as maintaining their smoking behaviour. Conducting a focus groups requires group facilitation skills such as establishing a supportive, non-threatening climate for the discussion, briefing participants on the aims of the group, encouraging participation and sharing of opinions, and summarizing from time to time. (Group facilitation is discussed in detail in Chapter 14, p. 353.) It is helpful to record the focus group discussion if appropriate, as this aids data analysis later on.

Focus groups have become firmly established as a qualitative research technique in both the education and health fields, and the following advantages are claimed:

- The researcher is sure of the response rate, as the participants are physically present during data collection.
- It is less costly to the researcher than postal surveys or individual interviews, requiring only about an hour to conduct. However, in nursing there is a hidden cost to the service, i.e. an hour of lost working time for each participant.
- It is said to generate data that is more 'ecologically valid' than some other forms of data collection, i.e. there is no prior categorization of responses by the researcher; participant's opinions are expressed in their own words.
- The presence of other group participants can allow members to speak more freely and honestly than they may be prepared to do in a one-to-one encounter.
- A skilled facilitator can ensure a psychologically-safe environment for discussion of sensitive topics.
- The researcher is able to seek clarification from participants on

their contributions, and to seek the views of other participants on individual contributions.

Carrying out a pilot study

Students should be strongly encouraged to undertake a pilot study to check out their methodology, as this will pay dividends in the data collection phase. A pilot study is really the main study done on a smaller scale, the purpose being clarification of procedures and methodology. The questionnaire should be tried out on a sample of people representative of the population to be studied, and the size of the pilot will be influenced by the time available and the size of the sample to be studied in the actual survey, but 10% seems a reasonable number for groups larger than 50. This pilot trial-run must go through all the stages in the research design, so that no aspect is omitted that might turn out to be a problem in the real survey. The results of the pilot study must be carefully evaluated and any improvements introduced into the final version. In the case of questionnaire design, the improvements made to questions mean that those questions need to be piloted again in the revised form.

Data collection

The actual collection of data will vary according to the instruments used, but some basic principles should be borne in mind. The research student should be encouraged to conduct the data collection with due consideration for other people. Access to a sample depends upon the goodwill of the people concerned and is not a question of the researcher's right to be there. The student must also bear in mind that other researchers may wish to approach an institution for access to a population and that the conduct on his or her research may well affect the kind of reception that subsequent inquiries receive. The approach must be made in ample time, so that arrangements can be fitted around the normal routine. Research students may forget that the prime purpose of an institution is not to provide a population for research, but to go about its business as efficiently as possible. In this sense, all research is at best an intrusion and at worst a nuisance. The sample must be put at their ease during the collection of data and the guarantee of anonymity assured. It is often necessary to take great pains to explain that results will not identify any individual, since many surveys may involve the statement of attitudes towards an authority or employer. At the end of the study, the student should send a written acknowledgement to the people involved in assisting the researcher, although it is not possible to thank individually the members of the sample.

Data analysis

Having obtained the data during the collection stage, the next step is to subject it to analysis. Research is classified into quantitative research, which is about collecting facts that are analysed using statistics, and qualitative research, which is more concerned with gaining insights, and data is analysed by qualitative methods.

If the research has used a qualitative approach the data analysis is likely to be partially or entirely qualitative, whereas a quantitative approach would require quantitative analysis using statistics.

Qualitative analysis

Statistical methods of analysis are not ruled out totally when analysing qualitative data; for example, students commonly use percentages to illustrate aspects of subjects' responses. However, there are severe limitations to statistics when attempting to analyse a wide range of qualitative data such as textual transcripts and the like. Qualitative analysis utilizes techniques such as network analysis, textual analysis, conversational analysis, and grounded theory to gain insight into phenomena.

Grounded theory is a common approach in social science research and is one of many styles of qualitative analysis of data. It is designed specifically for generating and testing theory, and theory should be grounded in qualitative data (Strauss, 1987, p. 22):

> *'Grounded theory is a detailed grounding by systematically and intensively analysing data, often sentence by sentence, or phrase by phrase of the field note, interview or other document; by constant comparison, data are extensively collected and coded, thus producing a well-constructed theory'.*

Quantitative (statistical) analysis

Statistics is invariably an area that causes students to become anxious, since the formulae can appear intimidating if the student does not have a good mathematical background. Teaching statistics need not be the dry presentation of figures and sums that characterizes students' views of statistics. I use the very first session of a research unit to involve the students in a carousel exercise (see Chapter 14, p. 381) that generates data for subsequent statistical analysis. This has the effect of motivating students because the self-generated data is relevant to them. Henshaw (1992) describes experiential methods of teaching statistics, utilizing existing quantitative and qualitative data that nurses are already familiar with, e.g. TPR charts, fluid charts, accident reports and the like.

However, statistical analysis need not be difficult and the amount required will depend on whether the research project is largely quantitative or qualitative. There is a danger that the raw data may be transcribed in error when being transferred, so it is essential to double-check the results. Accurate records must be kept and the original raw data should be kept until the study has been completed. The use of a computer for calculations can save considerable time, and there are statistics packages available such as Statistical Package for the Social

Sciences. The term *statistics* is used in three main ways (Guilford and Fruchter, 1973).

1. Statistics is a branch of the science of mathematics which deals with numerical data such as amounts, relationships, etc., in a sample.
2. Statistics is commonly used to describe numerical details in reports or records, particularly vital statistics such as births, marriages and deaths.
3. A statistic is a particular value, for example the average of a group of data. (The correct term for average is arithmetic mean).

Research information is termed *data* which is the plural form of datum, a numerical detail or fact. The original data gathered during research are termed raw data, since they have not yet undergone any kind of processing following collection. Processing of data is important in providing clarification, although there is inevitably some loss of fine detail which is referred to as degradation of the data.

Percentage
Percentages provide a useful method of comparing data on an equal basis, the assumption being that data are considered in terms of so many out of 100, i.e. so-and-so per cent. If we want to calculate, in terms of percentage, five cases out of ten then one can simply write 5 out of 10 as a fraction, and multiply by 100 per cent:

$5/10 \times 100$ per cent $= 50$ per cent

Percentages must be interpreted with caution when using a small number of cases. For example, in a group of 20 cases a change in one case would result in 5 per cent, whereas in a group of five cases a change in one case would be equivalent to a 20 per cent change. There are two further concepts that are closely related to the percentage – proportion and ratio.

Proportion
This is a part, or fraction of 1.0. For example, out of 60 student nurses commencing a course, 6 withdrew in the first year. The percentage of withdrawals is 10 per cent and the proportion of withdrawals is 0.10.

Ratio
This is a statistic denoting a relationship between parts and is expressed as a fraction. The ratio a to b is the fraction a/b, and the baseline is 1.0. For example, out of 40 students, 35 passed their assessment and 5 failed. The ratio of successful students to unsuccessful students in 35/5, i.e. 7:1.

These two latter concepts, ratio and proportion, are very closely related. In fact, a proportion is a particular kind of ratio that is limited to the relationship of a part to the total. A ratio, on the other hand, involves the relationship between parts.

Measures of central value

Central value is commonly called the *average*, but there are really three different measures of this concept, namely the *mean*, the *mode* and the *median*.

Arithmetic mean

To obtain the mean or average of a group of scores, the scores are added together and then divided by the number of scores.

Mode

The mode is defined as the score that occurs with most frequency in a set of data.

Median

The median is the point in a set of ordered scores that divides it into halves, so that exactly half the scores are less than the median and exactly half are greater than the median value. Calculation of the median value involves the use of a frequency distribution, so we need to examine this concept before returning to the median.

Frequency distribution

A frequency distribution is a table that separates the data into certain classes and shows how many data fall into each class. Frequency distributions can be plotted for both un-grouped and grouped data, the latter conveying much more clearly the information it contains.

Table 20.4 shows a frequency distribution on a set of un-grouped data which consists of a list of each of the average scores followed by the number of times each one occurred in the results. Table 20.5 shows the same data plotted in a frequency distribution, but using grouped data, i.e. scores that have been classed into score intervals rather than

Table 20.4

Frequency distribution of un-grouped data

Score	Frequency	Cumulative frequency	Cumulative percentage
84	1	20	100
82	1	19	95
81	1	18	90
78	2	17	85
77	2	15	75
75	1	13	65
74	2	12	60
73	1	10	50
72	1	9	45
71	1	8	40
70	1	7	35
69	1	6	30
66	1	5	25
65	1	4	20
63	1	3	15
61	1	2	10
58	1	1	5

Score interval	Frequency	Cumulative frequency
82–84	2	20
79–81	1	18
76–78	4	17
73–75	4	13
70–72	3	9
67–69	1	6
64–66	2	5
61–63	2	3
58–60	1	1

Table 20.5

Frequency distribution on grouped data

individually. This distribution shows much more clearly the arrangement of the scores and renders the data capable of being converted into a visual form of display. There are conventions for deciding upon the number of intervals and also the size of each interval, the former being from 10 to 20, and the latter being selected from 2, 3, 5, 10 and 20. When making calculations on an interval it is important to bear in mind that in statistics a score is never seen as an exact point on a scale, but as something occupying a whole interval, from half a unit below to half a unit above. Thus, with our data, the interval 58–60 really extends from 57.5 to 60.5, and a single score such as 84 really extends from 83.5 to 84.5.

Graphic display of frequency distribution
Figure 20.2 shows two methods of presenting the information contained in the frequency distribution. Figure 20.2(a) is called a histogram and Figure 20.2(b) a polygraph, both illustrating the information in a visual way, conveying maximum meaning.

Having discussed the concept of frequency distribution, we can now return to the calculation of the median. This was defined as the point that separates the top half of the ordered scores from the bottom half, so for the data in Table 20.5 we need to separate the top ten scores from the bottom ten scores, i.e. the half way point. If we examine the frequency distribution we can see that the third column is headed cumulative frequency and is derived by adding up the frequencies from the bottom to the top. We need the point below which ten cases fall, so we check up from the bottom of the cumulative frequency column until we reach the point we require. Unfortunately, in these data there are nine cases up to interval 70–72, and the next interval contains four cases. Now we require only one more case to make up our ten, so this must be taken from the next interval, i.e. 73–75. As we have already seen, this interval contains four cases, so we need to extend one quarter of the way into the next interval to reach our extra case. The interval 73–75 really has as its exact limits from 72.5 to 75.5, i.e. a total of three units. We need to extend one quarter of three units, i.e. 0.75 of the way into the next interval. This 0.75 is thus added to the lower limit of the category, giving a median of

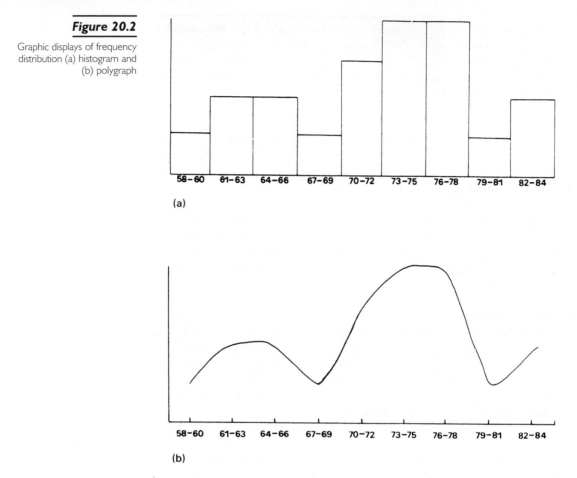

Figure 20.2

Graphic displays of frequency distribution (a) histogram and (b) polygraph

(a)

(b)

$$72.5 + 0.75 = 73.25$$

This can be checked for accuracy by working down from the top in a similar fashion, but subtracting the figure from the upper limit of the interval that contains the median. If, when calculating the median, the required number of cases works out exactly right in an interval, then the upper limit of that interval is taken as the median.

Percentiles

Another useful concept for processing data is that of percentiles. A percentile is the point below which a given percentage of scores fall. For instance, the 80th percentile is the point at which 80 per cent of scores fall below and 20 per cent fall above. The reader will see that the median is also the 50th percentile, as 50 per cent of the scores fall above and 50 per cent below. Percentiles allow a comparison to be made on two sets of data, by providing a common unit of measurement. The calculation of percentiles is quite straightforward, as is shown in Table 20.5. We must add a fourth column to the frequency distribution, namely the cumulative frequency percentage, which is obtained by taking each frequency in the second column and calculating what percentage of the total frequency it comprises. Now, the total frequency for all scores is 20, so commencing at the bottom of the column we can see that a frequency of one is equivalent to

$1/20 \times 100 = 5$ per cent

The next frequency up is also one, so this 5 per cent is added to the first 5 per cent, giving a cumulative percentage of 10 per cent. This is carried on for all the percentages in the list, until the final one arrives at 100 per cent. Reading across the table, it is easy to see that a score of 69 is at the 30th percentile, as 30 per cent of the scores fall below it and 70 per cent fall above. Similarly, a score of 81 is at the 90th percentile. In addition to percentiles, the term quartiles is also employed. The first quartile contains the scores up to the 25th percentile, the second up to the 50th percentile, the third up to the 75th percentile and the fourth up to a hundredth.

Scales of measurement

So far we have seen how raw data can be converted into processed data by using such statistics as the percentage, measures of central value, and frequency distribution. However, we need to examine another important aspect of statistics, namely scales of measurement.

There are four of these used in statistics, and they form a hierarchy of levels, with the higher ones subsuming the lower.

Nominal scale

This consists merely of names or labels for the data it contains, with no further details of quantities. The only criterion is that the classes be mutually exclusive, i.e. no member of the data can belong to both classes, e.g. gender of patient (male/female), nationality (English, Scottish, Welsh, ...).

Ordinal scale

This scale involves data in rank order but it does not assume that the distance between intervals is equal, e.g. satisfaction level (poor, satisfactory, good, excellent).

Interval scale

This scale does assume that the intervals between data are equal, and is thus termed the interval scale: the distance between scores 63 and 73 is the same as that between 74 and 84, namely ten. In the interval scale, e.g. when recording temperatures, however, a score of 80 is not twice that of a score of 40, because the zero point is arbitrarily defined rather than being an absolute zero.

Ratio scale

The highest form of measurement scales is the ratio scale, which does possess an absolute zero point. Most measures in the physical sciences possess an absolute zero point, so that one can safely assume that 10 litres is twice as much as 5 litres. In the behavioural sciences, however, the ratio scale is of little use, as it is very rare indeed to find a subject with zero characteristics.

Variability

The mean can be a useful measure, but is limited when dealing with more than one set of information. For example, two groups of subjects could obtain the same mean for a test, but the range of scores could be quite different. This could occur if the first group had a large number of high and low scores, with few in the middle, while the second had mostly middle-range scores. It is therefore useful to have a measure of the dispersion or variability of the scores. There are three main measures used to indicate variability: the total range, the semi-interquartile range and the standard deviation.

Total range

This is a very crude indicator of the dispersion of a set of scores, as it relies on the two extreme scores. It is calculated by subtracting the lowest score from the highest and in our data (Table 19.2), the range is 84 minus 58, i.e. 26.

Semi-interquartile range

The semi-interquartile range (Q) measure is closely related to the median and is one half of the range of the middle 50 per cent of scores. The middle 50 per cent of scores lie between the 25th and 75th percentiles and this range is referred to as the interquartile range, since these two percentiles separate the top and bottom quarters of the scores. The interquartile range is 77.5 minus 66.5, i.e. 10, and the semi-interquartile range is one half of this, namely, 5. This figure shows the average distance from the median to the 25th and 75th quartiles, and indicates the range of variability of the scores.

Standard deviation

This is the commonest and most reliable form of dispersion and is based upon the deviation of each score from the mean. The standard deviation is calculated using the following procedure:

1. Find the mean score for the group of data.
2. Calculate the amount by which each score 'deviates' from the mean, by subtracting each score from the mean.
3. Square each of these deviations, by multiplying each one by itself. (Note that if a deviation is negative, its square will be positive.)
4. Find the sum of these by adding them all together.
5. Divide this total by the number of scores.
6. Extract the square root of this figure, which gives the standard deviation.

The standard deviation is probably best explained by referring to the concept of the normal distribution, which is a mathematical concept consisting of a bell-shaped distribution curve. Many human characteristics are distributed this way, such as height, weight and intelligence. Figure 20.3 shows the normal distribution curve and its relationship to the standard deviation.

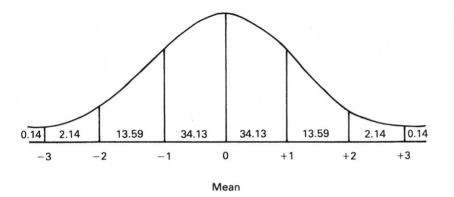

It can be seen that 68.2 per cent, i.e. about two-thirds of all the scores fall between minus one and plus one standard deviations from the mean. Approximately 95 per cent will fall between minus two and plus two, and virtually all cases will fall between minus three and plus three standard deviations. Thus, the full range of the normal distribution covers six standard deviations (99.72 per cent of the scores) and this fact provides a simple test of the normality of the distribution. If we divide the total range of scores by the standard deviation then the result should be approximately six. If it is less, then the distribution is more compressed than normal, and if greater, then the distribution is elongated.

Correlation

Correlation concerns the extent to which one set of measurements is related to another and is the basis upon which causation is inferred in statistics. It is measured using the correlation coefficient (r), which is a single number indicating the extent to which two variables are related. This figure varies from plus one, which means perfect positive correlation, to minus one, which means perfect negative correlation. In the former, high scores on test A are always accompanied by high scores on test B, whereas in the latter high scores on A are always accompanied by low scores on B. The main requirement for computing a correlation is that the data must arise from the same source.

The actual calculation of a correlation coefficient can be done using a variety of formulae, the most common one being Pearson's product moment correlation coefficient. The formula for this is somewhat complex at first glance, but is fairly straightforward to calculate:

$$r_{XY} = \frac{\sum xy}{N\sigma_x\sigma_y}$$

where r_{XY} is the correlation between a learner's score on test X and the score on test Y. xy is obtained by first multiplying deviation x by deviation y for each learner. All these products are then added up to give Σ_{xy}. N is the number of scores in the test. σ_x is the standard deviation of all the X scores. σ_y *is the standard deviation of all the Y scores.*

Probability

Probability is an important concept in statistics, as it is used to estimate the odds against a result occurring by chance. If the probability value is higher than a certain figure, then the results are said to be statistically significant, which means that the odds are in favour of the result being true. Probability is defined by Guilford (Guilford and Fruchter, 1973) as 'the ratio of the number of ways in which that favoured event can occur to the total number of ways the event can occur'. By favoured event he means the event in which one is interested, for example the ratio

(Ways in which a coin can land 'heads' up) : (Total number of ways the coin can land)

The ratio is 1/2, or 0.5 and this comes midway on the range of probability, which extends from zero to 1.0. Zero implies that there is no chance whatever of the event happening, and 1.0 implies absolute certainty that it will occur. Another example is the probability of getting a six when throwing a dice, i.e. 1/6 or 0.17. Probability is also additive, so that chance of either a five or a six coming up is 1/6 + 1/6 = 1/3 or 0.33. Probability levels are actually fixed in practice for statistical tests, at three levels:

- probability of 0.05, or five chance occurrences in 100. Odds against 19-1;
- probability of 0.01, or one chance occurrence in 100. Odds against 99-1;
- probability of 0.001, or one chance occurrence in 1000. Odds against 999-1.

Generally, the lower the probability, the greater the confidence that can be placed on the result. Values higher than 0.05 are considered to be 'not statistically significant'.

Interpretation of data, conclusions and recommendations in the research report

It is important to advise students that their research project should be written up as they go along, and not all left until the research has been completed. For example, the literature search needs to be done early so as to influence the methodology of the study, so the student can begin to write this chapter quite early on in the project. Although it depends upon the exact nature of the research project, the following sequence of chapters might be suggested to the student:

1. *Abstract*. This is a short (300 word) summary of the research project, i.e. what it is about, what the student found out, and what the implications are.
2. *Introduction and context of the study*. This should include: the context in which the study is based, e.g. community nursing, midwifery practice; why the student chose the topic/issue; and what problem/issue the student is attempting to address.
3. *Review of the relevant literature*. This chapter should critically review the literature relevant to the project and should inform the design of the study.
4. *Design of the study*. This chapter should include methodology, sampling, data collection, and methods of analysis of the data.
5. *Analysis and results of the study*. This chapter presents the data collected, in the form of summary tables, pie-charts, etc.
6. *Discussion of findings*. This is the key chapter, in which the student demonstrates critical thinking, analytical and interpretative skills. Findings should be discussed in depth, and attempts made to explain them. The discussion should address any aspects that appear to conflict with the literature. The student has to take responsibility for what he or she writes by weighing the evidence and arguing the case.
7. *Conclusions and recommendations*. This chapter summarizes the arguments, and identifies the implications of the results for professional practice.
8. *References*. These are very important indeed as they indicate the range and depth of the student's reading.
9. *Appendices*. These are for material that, whilst being relevant to the study, is not necessary to include within the main body of the text, e.g. examples of raw data, specimen materials, etc.

RESEARCH DEGREE SUPERVISION

Research degree supervision is one of the most demanding of all activities for lecturers in higher education.

There are three kinds of research degree, master of philosophy (M.Phil), master of science by research (MSc) and doctor of philosophy (PhD), although the latter is also termed D.Phil by some institutions. While both awards require a critical investigation and evaluation of an approved topic, the main difference between them is the requirement that a PhD must result in an independent and original contribution to the field of knowledge. There are two routes to a PhD, the first by submission of a thesis, and the second on the basis of a candidate's published work. For the award of a PhD by submission of a thesis, students normally register initially for an MPhil, and then subsequently transfer to PhD registration provided that their work is considered to be of an appropriate standard to allow transfer. However, possession of a masters degree may allow direct entry to PhD registration.

Funding for research degrees

Within the UK there is no automatic entitlement to funding for research degrees, so students have to seek funding from whatever sources they can. Students studying part-time can usually fund themselves from their own resources; full-time students normally have to apply for one of the following:

- a studentship from one of the research councils;
- a bursary from a higher education institution;
- other sources of research grants, e.g. NHS Executive Research and Development Project Grant Schemes.

Full-time studentships and bursaries are applied for in much the same way as one would apply for a job, include shortlisting and interviews, and there is considerable competition for these.

Admission requirements

The following sections are based upon the regulations of the University of Greenwich, but are fairly representative of the procedures used in other higher education institutions.

Unlike registration for other awards, registration for research degrees has to be approved by the institution's research degrees committee. The normal entry qualification for a research degree is the possession of a first or second class honours degree, and the minimum period of registration for each award is normally as follows:

1. MPhil: Full-time 18 months; part-time 30 months;
2. PhD: Full-time 24 months; part-time 36 months.

Registration can normally be backdated for up to six months from the date of application.

The process of study for a research degree

The research degree process consists of two main aspects, the design and implementation of the research project, and a programme of related studies in research methods and knowledge related to the topic of study. The former involves the drafting and implementation of all stages of the research proposal under the supervision of at least two supervisors, and culminating in the production of a thesis for examination. During the ongoing stages of the project, students are encouraged to submit and deliver research papers to conferences, and to engage with other research students within the department or school.

Formal structures

The research degrees committee of the institution is the body responsible for approving students' research proposals, and for monitoring on an annual basis the progress made by each student, including the frequency of meetings with their supervisor. The committee has the power to withdraw a student's registration on the grounds of lack of academic progress.

Research degree students normally have two or three supervisors; the first supervisor will supervise the student frequently and regularly, and take academic leadership of the project, while the second supervisor takes on the management of the research student. The supervisory team must have successfully supervised at least three candidates to successful completion, and for PhD students, at least one member must have successfully supervised at PhD level. One member must have sufficient experience so as to act as advisor to the rest of the team.

Research students' are examined by two to three examiners, at least one of which is an external examiner with considerable experience of examining research degree candidates at the appropriate level. The balance between internal and external examiners depends upon a judgement of the relative experience and expertise within the team. The examination consists of two phases, a preliminary assessment of the thesis, and the defence of the thesis by the student. The preliminary assessment serves to inform the examiners of each other's view, and to set an agenda for the defence meeting. The result can be one of the following: an unqualified pass, a pass with conditions, a fail with opportunity to re-submit, and a fail with no opportunity for re-submission.

Principles of supervision

Given that research degrees consist largely of independent work by the student, the role of the research supervisor has a disproportionate importance in comparison with the normal tutoring role on taught programmes. Needless to say, supervisors require good interpersonal communication skills and the ability to establish rapport with students, and while these qualities are required in any tutorial setting, they are particularly crucial in a tutor/student relationship lasting anywhere between two and six years!

The research supervisor's role consists of a range of support activities including the following:

- weekly or fortnightly supervisory meetings with the student, depending on whether they are full or part-time;
- negotiating with the students' their work schedule and deadlines for submission of written work;
- reading and offering critical comments on students' written work;
- record-keeping;
- notifying supervisory team members on the outcomes of supervisory meetings;
- producing progress reports for the department and the Research Degrees Committee;
- conducting an annual appraisal of the student;

- advising the student on research-related activities within and outside the institution;
- advising the student on submission of conference papers and publications.

Christopherson (1992) suggest that there are two main aspects to supervision of students' research projects. The first and most important concerns the abilities of the supervisor to challenge and motivate the student with a steady stream of ideas. The second involves the mechanics of facilitating the progress of the student. He cites the following common reasons for non-completion of research projects.

1. *A slow start.* The student needs to work hard in the initial stages to avoid slippage in the deadlines.
2. *Perfectionism.* Some students are never satisfied with their results and are constantly trying to improve them. Taken to the extreme, this will prevent the project from ever being completed.
3. *Distraction.* It is relatively easy for a student to be distracted by some aspect of the project, such as computer analysis of data, and as a result, spend too much time on this aspect to the detriment of the overall project.
4. *Inadequate collation of data.* This may be detected during the writing up of the project, and results in a need for further analysis which then delays the writing stage of the project.

Supervising research students does not always go smoothly; Cryer (1997) identifies the three most common dilemmas in supervision:

1. *Originality versus conformity.* This first dilemma is how far should the supervisor encourage students to aim for originality, or for conformity. Originality is considered an important aspect of research, particularly at PhD level, but Cryer identifies arguments against encouraging student to aim for original work:
   - Funding bodies impose a tight timescale for completion of projects, and this militates against creativity and inspiration.
   - It is difficult to get acceptance for very novel ideas, and there is evidence that innovative work is sometimes difficult to get accepted for a PhD.

   Cryer's advice is for supervisors to equate originality with publishability, in that it can be deemed to have originality if it is worthy of publication.

2. *Control versus autonomy.* This is about how the supervisor strikes a balance between close guidance of students' work and allowing them the freedom to work independently. Cryer sees the role of the supervisor as gradually moving the student from dependence towards independence, and stresses the importance of discussing the process with the student. Independence does not mean that the student works alone, rather, it involves the student in taking the lead and using the supervisor as a sounding board.

3. *Copy editor versus guardian of standards.* This relates to the 'passing' of theses, and concerns the balance between correcting students' 'written English' and academic aspects. Cryer points out that it is the research students themselves who decide when they are ready to submit their theses; the supervisor can only advise them on the readiness for submission. Clearly, the academic quality of the thesis is the main focus of the supervisor's attention, but students often need practice in academic writing. It is helpful to get research students to submit chapter drafts at regular intervals, so that advice can be given on students' writing ability.

One of the common problems encountered by research students is when two supervisors offer what seems to be conflicting advice. One view is that it is good for students to be challenged by the conflicting views of their supervisors, while others feel it is unreasonable to put the onus of dealing with this problem onto the student. One way around this is for the supervisory team to meet regularly so that issues are addressed and resolved. Another common issue is whether or not research students should be required, or merely encouraged, to perform public presentations of aspects of their research to peers and academic staff in the institution. Again, opinions differ on this point, with some arguing that compulsory presentations can be very stressful to the student, while other feel that presentations performed in a supportive environment can facilitate the students' socialization into the role of researcher.

REFERENCES

Bell, J. (1993) *Doing Your Research Project*, 2nd edn, Open University Press, Buckingham.

Christopherson, D. (1992) *Research Student and Supervisor: An Approach to Good Supervisory Practice*, Magdalene College, Cambridge.

Crow, S., Rogers, J. and Larcombe, K. (1997) Developing a research culture in education and practice, *Nursing Standard*, **12**(7), 34–5.

Cryer, P. (1997) *Handling Common Dilemmas in Supervision*, SRHE and THES, London.

English National Board for Nursing, Midwifery and Health Visiting (1993) *The Board's Response to the Strategy For Research in Nursing, Midwifery and Health Visiting: The Report of the Taskforce*, ENB, London.

Fox, D. (1969) *The Research Process in Education*, Holt, Rinehart and Winston, New York.

Guilford, J. and Fruchter, B. (1973) *Fundamental Statistics in Psychology and Education*, McGraw Hill, Tokyo.

Henshaw, A. (1992) Statistics: a painless injection, *Nurse Education Today*, **12**, 142–7.

Heron, J. (1985) The role of reflection in a co-operative enquiry, in *Reflection: Turning Experience into Learning*, D. Boud, R. Keogh and D. Walker (eds), Kogan Page, London.

Kerlinger, F. (1979) *Behavioural Research: A Conceptual Approach*, Holt, Rinehart and Winston, New York.

LeVar, R. and Steadman, S. (1996) *Teaching Research in Nursing and Midwifery Curricula*, ENB, London.

McMahon, A. and Kitson, A. (1997) Supporting R&D: the role of a professional organisation, *Nursing Standard*, **12**(12), 35–9.

Nelson, E.A. (1998) The value of systematic reviews in research, *Professional Nurse*, **14**(1), 24–8.

Oppenheim, A. (1966) *Questionnaire Design and Attitude Measurement*, Heinemann, London.

Reason, P. (1988) *Human Inquiry in Action*, Sage, London.

Strauss, A. (1987) *Qualitative Analysis for Social Scientists*, Cambridge University Press, Cambridge.

Wagstaff, P. and Gould, D. (1998) Research in the clinical area: the ethical issues, *Nursing Standard*, **12**(28), 33–6.

PART FIVE

CONTINUING PROFESSIONAL DEVELOPMENT

CONTINUING PROFESSIONAL DEVELOPMENT: THE UNIVERSITY CONTEXT

21

Within all sectors of education, continuing professional development is acknowledged as being essential for maintaining and improving the quality of educational provision. It is not therefore the exclusive province of individual teachers, but must take into account the goals and strategies of the latter's department and the institutions in which they work. Hence, there will be variations in the nature of continuing professional development (CPD) according to the priorities of the teacher's department, e.g. some departments may see their main priority as developing more staff as active researchers; others may wish to develop open and distance learning materials for their programmes. It is normally the case that funding for staff development is linked to these departmental/institutional priorities, and in this way teachers are 'encouraged' to undertake appropriate staff development within the stated priority areas. The importance of CPD to the work of the institution is underlined by its inclusion in the agenda of annual staff appraisal interviews.

The terminology related to CPD can be confusing, as there is a variety of terms in current use for what is essentially the same concept; continuing professional development, staff development (SD), continuing professional education (CPE), and lifelong learning. The first three are normally applied to formal learning in an institution, whereas the latter is a more generic term that includes learning outside the formal education system. There are two main reasons why CPD is an important concept for nurse teachers:

1. The design and delivery of CPD programmes and activities are significant areas of work in nurse education.
2. Nurse teachers are required to maintain their own continuing professional development.

In relation to point 2, the UKCC Code of Professional Conduct (UKCC, 1992a) states that registered nurses, midwives and health visitors are required:

> *'to act, at all times, in such a manner as to:*
> *(a) safeguard and promote the interests of individual patients and clients;*
> *(b) serve the interests of society;*
> *(c) justify public trust and confidence; and*
> *(d) uphold and enhance the good standing and reputation of the professions.'*

Continuing professional development has a major role to play in maintaining this requirement, and paragraph 3 of the UKCC Code specifically relates to CPD: 'maintain and improve your professional knowledge and competence'. The importance of CPD is further underlined in paragraph 3 of *The Scope of Professional Practice* (UKCC, 1992b):

> *'Foundation education alone, however, cannot effectively meet the changing and complex demands of the range of modern health care. Post-registration education equips practitioners with additional and more specialist skills necessary to meet the special needs of patients and clients'.*

The teacher's role in nursing, midwifery and health visiting is performed in two distinct, yet inter-related contexts, i.e. the university department and the workplace. The requirements for CPD cover both these settings, and for the sake of clarity the former is addressed in this chapter and the latter in Chapter 22.

This chapter begins with an overview of CPD in nursing, midwifery and health visiting, and a review of government policy with regard to lifelong learning. It goes on to explore a range of university-focused CPD strategies including staff appraisal, research and scholarly activity, writing for publication, the research assessment exercise, and the Institute for Learning and Teaching.

CPD IN NURSING, MIDWIFERY AND HEALTH VISITING

Obviously, CPD has important implications for both professional nurses and for the general public. The public has a right to be safeguarded against malpractice and to be protected from charlatans, and they have an expectation that nurses will possess up-to-date knowledge and skills appropriate to the specialism in which they practice.

A nurse's motivation to undertake continuing professional development may arise from a range of different needs. The most obvious one that springs to mind is the UKCC PREP standards, to which all registered nurses must conform if they are to continue on the register of nurses. The PREP standards are discussed in detail in Chapter 22. There are also more altruistic motives such as a desire to improve the standard of practice, and other less altruistic ones such as gaining further qualifications to enhance promotion prospects, or a desire to increase personal status by the acquisition of bachelors, masters or doctoral degrees. There is even the possibility that some nurses may see CPD as providing evidence of safe practice in cases of litigation by patients or clients.

Many qualified practitioners can be classified as post-registration students, as they are pursuing formal courses as part of their CPD. For the majority of these nurses, their studies will be undertaken whilst they are in full-time employment.

The position with regard to study leave and funding for CPD has worsened considerably over the recent past, and the best that many can expect to gain is partial funding. Study leave to attend formal courses is even more difficult to obtain, and in cases where it is granted the demands of service mean that it may not always be possible to take it. Hence, the demand for more flexible approaches to study has led to the development of open and distance learning programmes which allow post-registration students to study in their own time, and without the need for attendance at an institution.

Another significant development in the delivery of CPD for nurses is the accreditation of prior learning (APEL). This has enabled experienced practitioners to identify learning gained within the workplace, to provide evidence of such learning in a portfolio, and to use the credit thus gained to contribute towards the final award. For many nurses, this has meant a considerable reduction in the time taken to gain a higher education award.

GOVERNMENT POLICY ON LIFELONG LEARNING

This section will highlight aspects of four government documents that relate to lifelong learning and staff development.

The Fryer report

The first report of the National Advisory Group for Continuing Education and Lifelong Learning was published in late 1997 (DfEE, 1997). Its terms of reference were:

'To advise the Secretary of State on matters concerning adult learning as required, and with particular reference to extending the inclusion in lifelong and work-based learning to those groups and individuals whose increased participation will contribute to improvements in employability, regeneration, capacity building, economic efficiency, social cohesion, independent living and citizenship generally; and to make proposals in respect of:

(a) the preparation of a Government White Paper on Lifelong Learning;
(b) the strengthening of family and community learning;
(c) the contribution of further and higher education to adult learning, having regard to relevant recommendations of the Kennedy Committee on widening participation in FE and the National Committee of Inquiry into the future of HE;
(d) initiatives for development in the context of the University for Industry;
(e) the development of Learning Towns and Cities'

Clearly, there are implications for the nursing and midwifery professions arising out of the report, since it is aimed at all sections of society. The report highlights the lack of a lifelong learning culture in the UK, and the fact that education and training is considered inadequate to meet competitive challenges. According to the report, only 14 per cent of employees participate in job-related training, while one third say they have never been offered such training by their employer.

The report proposes a ten-point agenda for the development of a lifelong learning culture, as shown in Table 21.1.

Table 21.1

Ten-point agenda for lifelong learning (DfEE, 1997)

1. Development of a strategic framework for the promotion of lifelong learning
2. A campaign to revolutionize attitudes to lifelong learning
3. A commitment to widening participation and achievement in learning
4. Increased emphasis on home, community and workplace as places of learning
5. A need for simplification and integration of qualifications and learning pathways
6. Development of effective partnerships, planning and collaboration to provide lifelong learning opportunities for all
7. Provision of information, advice and guidance for people to access lifelong learning and to begin to take some responsibility for developing their own learning
8. A need for new data, targets and standards to underpin the new strategy
9. Effective use of the new technologies of communication and information to support lifelong learning
10. A need to ensure that funding and finance stimulate a far-wider group of participants, and do not constitute barriers to lifelong learning

Section 10 of the report focuses on promoting lifelong learning at the workplace, which includes:

1. job-related learning, i.e. specific learning to improve job performance;
2. transferable-skills learning, i.e. to produce a more responsive and flexible workforce;
3. personal development learning, i.e. knowledge and skills to help people make employment or career changes, and to facilitate their personal fulfilment.

The learning age: a renaissance for a new Britain

In February 1998, the government downgraded its lifelong learning plan from a white paper to a green consultation paper, and this was published as *The Learning Age: a renaissance for a new Britain* (DfEE, 1998a).

Whilst no direct reference is made within the green paper to continuing professional development, the document has implications for everyone:

> *'Learning is the key to prosperity – for each of us as individuals, as well as for the nation as a whole. To realize our ambition, we must all develop and sustain a regard for learning at whatever age'.*

Within the green paper, the government acknowledges the Fryer report's call for the development of a new culture of lifelong learning, and identifies the benefits for individuals, businesses, communities, and the nation.

The paper sets out a number of initiatives through which the government's strategy for lifelong learning will be carried forward.

University for Industry

The University for Industry (UfI)

> *'will act as the hub of a brand new learning network, using modern communication technologies to link businesses and individuals to cost-effective, accessible and flexible education and training'.*

The UfI will provide information and advice about courses via enquiry desks in towns, telephone, fax, email and website. As well as delivering learning packages to individual's homes through a variety of media, the UfI will have learning centres to which its students can go to access courses and materials. These learning centres will be operated by a wide range of providers, including further education colleges, universities and private sector institutions, and the UfI will be backed up by extensive advertising and publicity.

Learning Direct

This is a new national helpline to provide free, confidential, impartial and up-to-date information about the availability of provision, and can link the individual with a range of agencies such as further education, higher education and private sector providers.

Individual learning accounts

This is a national system, the aim of which is to provide an incentive for adults to undertake training. It is based on the principles that investing in learning is a shared responsibility, and that the individual is in the best position to decide what and how they need to learn. The accounts will be available to all, and will enable individuals to save and borrow to invest in their own learning. Following consultation, a framework will be constructed for the delivery of individual learning accounts.

Learning at work

The green paper highlights the variable spread and quality of training in the workplace and the need for workplaces to become centres of learning; this will be encouraged by a legislative framework. Investors in People (IiP) will become the standard for staff development in both public and private sectors, and a national skills task force will be established to assess future skill needs, strengthen partnerships at local level, disseminate information on changing skill needs, and tackle skill shortages in collaboration with other agencies such as the new employer-led national training organizations (NTO).

The Dearing report

The Dearing report was published in summer 1997, and its terms of reference were:

> *'To make recommendations on how the purposes, shape, structure, size and funding of higher education, including support for students,*

should develop to meet the needs of the United Kingdom over the next 20 years, recognizing that higher education embraces teaching, learning, scholarship and research' (Dearing, 1997).

This very comprehensive report makes 93 recommendations, a number of which have important implications for the continuing professional development of both practitioners and teachers of nursing.

Recommendations 9, 13, 14, 15, 47 and 48 refer specifically to staff development, and three main aspects are covered:

1. the need for institutions to review, update and make available to all staff their policies with regard to staff development;
2. the need for institutions to review the impact of communications and information technology on the role of staff, and ensure that the necessary support and training is made available;
3. that an Institute for Learning and Teaching in Higher Education (ILT) be established for the purpose of accrediting programmes of teacher-training, the commissioning of research into teaching and learning, and the encouragement of innovation. All new full-time academic staff should undertake ILT-accredited teacher-training as part of their probationary period of employment.

Higher Education for the 21st Century. Response to the Dearing Report

In February 1998 the Government published its response to the Dearing report (DfEE, 1998b). This section of the chapter will address the response to the recommendations relating to staff development that were highlighted in the previous section.

The government welcomed the recommendations on the need for institutions to review and update their staff development policies, and to make these available to staff, and encourages institutions to follow-up these recommendations. They also welcomed the recommendations on the need for training and support of both staff and students in communications and information technology, and identified the importance of the Institute for Learning and Teaching in the kitemarking and development of these materials. With regard to the recommendations concerning the ILT, the government stated that the Institute would be established by September 1998; its functions should be the accreditation of programmes of training for HE teachers, the commissioning of research and development into effective teaching and learning practice, and to stimulate innovation. The issue of accredited teacher-training is also welcomed:

> *'the government's long-term aim is to see all teachers in higher education carry a professional qualification, achieved by meeting demanding standards of teaching and supervisory competence through accredited learning or experience'.*

STAFF APPRAISAL/INDIVIDUAL PERFORMANCE REVIEW

We spend about one-third of our adult lives at work and as well as providing money for living, it also functions as an important vehicle for the expression of our individuality. There is little doubt that it is social relationships that make or break the working environment, rather than the nature of the job *per se* and it is a sad reflection on the management style of senior personnel that so many people fail to derive job satisfaction from their work. It is important to appreciate the holistic nature of work to the individual; it is intimately related to self-development, social position and identity and not simply a collection of performances to be evaluated. The concept of staff appraisal needs to be carefully defined in order to be distinguishable from other related concepts such as assessment and review of performance. Appraisal, in its literal sense, is the estimation of value or quality, and it is this emphasis on value that makes it more global than assessment. I see appraisal as being a humanistic concept in which individual's aspirations, perceptions and needs are considered, as well as their performance in the job. Hence, performance evaluation is a necessary part of appraisal, but there is much more to it than that.

Purposes of appraisal

Appraisal is used for a variety of purposes within educational management and these can be broadly classified into those that are aimed at the person being appraised and those that are aimed at management. In the former category, appraisal is used to encourage staff development, self-evaluation, team awareness and review of performance. From the management point of view, appraisal is used to clarify the organization's objectives, to improve communication, to develop staff resources and to evaluate the performance of the organization. I like to think of appraisal as a system in which staff can provide feedback to management and management can provide feedback to staff, in terms of ambitions, growth and development and perceived needs. The process of appraisal centres around two questions:

1. Are you contributing to the growth and development of the organization? and
2. Is the organization contributing to your own growth and development?

There is one purpose that I have omitted, but which is commonly suggested, namely, discipline. Indeed, appraisal may be a euphemism for a procedure that ends in disciplinary action. My own feeling is that this should not be used as a system for disciplinary action, since it undermines the whole purpose of appraisal, i.e. the development of the individual. Clearly, disciplinary action may be required in some cases, but the procedure should be distinct from appraisal. Equally, an appraisal interview should not form the basis for an employer's reference, as this may inhibit free and frank discussion during appraisal.

Implementing appraisal

In order to have maximum benefit to both appraisee and appraiser, the appraisal interview needs careful planning, and confidentiality must be ensured. The following sequence may be useful:

1. *Preliminary reflection.* A week or two before the appraisal interview, each party should take time to complete an initial form that focuses on key aspects of the appraisal such as those illustrated in Table 21.2. This ensures that each party has given consideration to the various aspects of appraisal and should mean that the interview itself can be used to best advantage.

Table 21.2

Aspects for preliminary reflection by the appraisee

1.0   *The previous year: performance*
1.1   Outline the main aspects of your job in order of priority
1.2   On a scale of excellent to poor evaluate your performance on each of the aspects you have identified, in relation to agreed objectives and standards
1.3   Identify any factors which facilitated your performance on the above aspects of your job
1.4   Identify any factors which hindered your performance on the above aspects of your job

2.0   *The previous year: development*
2.1   Identify ways in which you have developed professionally over the previous year
2.2   Identify ways in which you have developed personally over the previous year
2.3   Identify any opportunities that seemed to have a particularly beneficial effect on your development
2.4   Identify any opportunities which you would have liked in order to develop professionally or personally

3.0   *The coming year: performance*
3.1   What aspects of your job would you particularly like to develop?
3.2   What aspects of your performance would you like to improve?

4.0   *The coming year: development*
4.1   Identify your development needs over the coming year
4.2   Which of the above would be your highest priority?

5.0   *Action plan*
From the foregoing information, write down your action plan for the coming year, identifying each aspect in priority order

2. *The appraisal interview.* There are a number of points to be made about carrying out an appraisal interview. Sufficient time must be allowed, so that two-way feedback can occur without a feeling of having to move on quickly. Considering that the appraisal interview may be the only time the appraisee has the opportunity for in-depth interaction with the manager, it is not unreasonable to allocate an entire morning or afternoon. There must be no interruptions by telephones or callers, and instructions must be given to this effect. Provision of refreshment is a useful idea, as it avoids the loss of continuity occasioned by a visit to the common room for this.

Needless to say, the appraiser must approach the appraisal with as much objectivity as possible, and it is sometimes difficult to discuss the weaknesses of a respected colleague. On the other hand, the appraiser must be able to accept criticism of her own management of a team without becoming defensive. It is also important to ensure that the appraiser actually knows the performance of the person being appraised. If the appraisee is a teacher, then the appraiser may wish to observe the appraisee's teaching. However, peer observation of teaching is a sensitive area, and may be resisted by the appraisee's professional organization or trade union. However, with the advent of the Institute for Learning and Teaching, it is likely that peer observation of teaching will become much more established in higher education.

The career development aspect of appraisal is very important, and much time should be given to the discussion of the continuing professional development of the appraisee.

3. *The action plan.* At the end of the interview both parties should agree on an action plan for the appraisee that clearly states the actions which are to be undertaken over the coming year with regard to job performance and personal or professional development. This may involve taking further courses of study, gaining new experiences, attempting new techniques for teaching or undertaking research. When the appraiser has completed the appraisal form, both parties should sign it. One copy is given to the appraisee, and forms the basis of the following year's appraisal. A further copy is retained by the personnel department.

The development of appraisal can cause great anxiety amongst staff, particularly if they are suspicious of the motives for its introduction. Indeed, it has been referred to as 'an overt system of espionage by consent!' and this indicates the fear of information being used against the provider. Separating appraisal from discipline and references can go a long way towards reducing anxiety, but in the final analysis the system will be judged by the personal qualities and skills of the appraiser, including her sensitivity and trustworthiness.

RESEARCH AND SCHOLARLY ACTIVITY

As part of their contract of employment, academic staff in higher education are required to engage in research and scholarly activity (RSA); this is a generic term that covers a range of activities contributing to the continuing professional development of staff members. Research and scholarly activity takes place in two main ways:

1. as an ongoing activity throughout the teaching year; and
2. as self-managed activity separate from time-tabled teaching weeks and annual leave entitlement.

Research and scholarly activity should inform the individual's teaching, so the nature of the activity is normally negotiated between the staff member and her/his manager. However, during the annual staff appraisal system, teachers are normally required to demonstrate how they have used their RSA time.

The following are typical RSA activities:

- writing books;
- contributing chapters to books;
- writing papers for academic and professional journals;
- presenting papers at conferences;
- writing open and flexible study materials;
- undertaking research projects.

The most significant imperative for undertaking research and scholarly activity is the cycle of Research Assessment Exercises (RSE) conducted by the four UK higher education funding councils.

RESEARCH ASSESSMENT EXERCISE

The RAE is a mechanism for allocating research funding to institutions based upon the quality of their research, and is conducted by the four UK Higher Education Funding Councils every four to five years. The funding councils are as follows:

- Higher Education Funding Council for England (HEFCE);
- Scottish Higher Education Funding Council (SHEFC);
- Higher Education Funding Council for Wales (HEFCW);
- Department of Education for Northern Ireland (DENI).

Research assessment exercises were conducted in 1992 and 1996, and the next is scheduled for 2001. The purpose of the RAE is:

> 'to enable the higher education funding bodies to distribute public funds for research selectively on the basis of quality. Institutions conducting the best research receive a larger proportion of the available grant so that the infrastructure for the top level of research in the UK is protected and developed' (RAE, 1999a).

The RAE process

The process involves peer review of an institution's research active staff. In order to be considered research active, a member of academic staff must have had a minimum of four books, book chapters, or papers published in refereed journals within the four years preceding a given RAE. If the member of staff has published more than four papers, then the department will select the four papers that show the author in the best light.

A standard scale is used by panels of assessors to rate each institution's submission, from 1 to 5+, depending upon how much of the institution's research is considered to reach national or international levels of excellence. An institution's subsequent research funding is based upon the quality rating it obtains in each unit of assessment. The results of the RAE are made public, and provides an indication of the relative quality of research across higher education institutions.

In a study of the impact of the 1992 RAE on English higher

education institutions, McNay (1997) outlines the process:

> 'For the 1992 exercise, submissions were made by institutions for those units of assessment active in research. These submissions listed all research active staff with details of their publications and research output: patents, inventions, productions in performing and visual arts, etc. The best two in each case were marked with an asterisk. Institutional submissions also included, for each academic area, descriptive sections on performance and plans. Quality was judged by a series of panels covering 72 units of assessment (academic areas, mainly related to traditional disciplines) on a scale 1–5 with 5 as the top grade indicating a body of work all of national excellence with a majority achieving international standards of excellence'.

The calculation of research funding for each unit of assessment is based on the quality rating obtained by the department on the 1–5 scale and the number of research active staff. Hence, a department obtaining a grade 5 will get four times as much income for each research active staff member than one obtaining a grade 2.

Example of RAE assessment criteria

The following example is a summary of the 1996 RAE assessment criteria for the unit of assessment (UOA) number 68, Education (HEFCE, 1995):

- The diversity of research in education includes curriculum, teaching and assessment materials where these have been developed through research and have been published.
- The Education panel's collective judgement is based primarily upon the quality of publications, and the vitality of the department's research culture.
- No general rule is applied to ranking books, book chapters, papers in refereed journals, and papers in refereed conference proceedings, as the relative significance differs between different areas of research.
- Panels recognize that co-authored publications may provide valuable evidence of inter-disciplinary research, and of research teams working collaboratively with or across institutions.

Health-related research and the RAE

A task group was set up by the Department of Health and HEFCE, following the 1996 RAE, to address concerns about the operation of the RAE with regard to health-related research and the impact of funding decisions on institutions doing such research (RAE, 1999b). The task group reviewed the units of assessment, assessment criteria, and panel membership for health-related research, and also the assessment of research directly relevant to the health service, e.g. primary care and health services research. The task group undertook consultation on these issues, and the proposals arising from this are being taken forward.

The RAE mechanism has been criticised for separating teaching and research, particularly in the classification of academic staff into research active and non-research active staff. Nevertheless, the RAE is clearly a significant aspect of continuing professional development in nurse education, with important implications for career development. McNay (1997) found that 43 per cent of higher education staff felt that their career planning had been significantly affected by the RAE.

The website address for the RAE is http://www.rae.ac.uk.

WRITING FOR PUBLICATION

Publications are an important form of continuing professional development, as well as a significant generator of funds and kudos for the educational institution. Publications will enhance an individual's curriculum vitae, and possibly influence shortlisting and employment prospects. The term *publications* encompasses a wide range of activities:

- sole authoring of books;
- editorial authorship of books involving a number of contributors;
- writing chapters in edited books;
- writing journal papers or articles;
- writing open, distance and flexible learning study materials;
- writing material for electronic media, e.g. CD-ROM, Internet.

Writing and editing books

Publishing is a commercial enterprise, and like any other commercial enterprise, profitability is a major consideration. When presented with a book proposal from a prospective author, publishers have to estimate the market and projected sales targets. Hence, a proposal must have something special that makes it capable of attracting sales in a very competitive market, and it is more likely to be accepted for publication if it meets one or more of the following criteria:

- It addresses a need that has developed out of some professional policy decision, e.g. clinical supervision, or clinical governance.
- It addresses an aspect of nurse education not previously addressed in the literature, i.e. a 'first in the field'.
- It adopts a different or novel approach to the subject, making it more attractive to potential readers than existing titles.
- It contains contributions by acknowledged experts in the field, i.e. it includes 'star names'.
- It is written by an author who already has one or more successful publications with the same company.

If a teacher is interested in writing a book, the first consideration is whether she will be the sole author, or the editor for a number of contributors. In both cases, the work can be shared with one or more authors/editors. However, the more authors/editors that are involved, the less any individual's royalty payments. Royalties are paid on the sales of a book, usually ten per cent, and are paid each year at the end of the tax year.

At first glance, becoming the editor of a book seems a fairly easy way of getting into print; the idea is quite seductive that one simply needs to find a few people who will each contribute a chapter on some aspect of the book's theme, add an introductory chapter oneself, and you have a book under your belt! However, the reality is very different; I speak from experience when I say I would rather write a dozen sole-authored books than be the editor of one multi-contributor text!

The editor's job requires a combination of characteristics, including vision, literary skills, administrative skills, and above all interpersonal communication skills. Vision is required if one is to come up with an idea for an edited book that will make a significant contribution to professional knowledge or debate, and at the same time more or less guarantee sufficient sales to meet the publisher's targets. It is also required when deciding the structure of the book and the decisions about who should be invited to contribute a chapter or chapters. Editing a book is a complex business, and good administrative skills are essential to maintain communication with the contributing authors. The more contributors one has in a book, the more difficult the task of editing becomes. The very fact that contributors are chosen for their expertise will inevitably mean that they have other priorities that get in the way of manuscript deadlines, and one of the most frustrating aspects of editing is the chasing-up of chapter drafts from contributors. This is where interpersonal communication skills come in; a mixture of friend-liness, respect and assertiveness will go a long way in encouraging recal-citrant authors to submit their manuscripts, but as a last resort the editor can always enlist the assistance of the publisher to send a more formal reminder to them.

Writer's block

One of the problems encountered by professional writers from time to time is the so-called 'writer's block', a psychological state in which an experienced writer becomes unable to write, sometimes for considerable periods of time. This phenomenon is more likely to occur in the case of sole-authored works, where the workload is considerably greater than that involved in contributing one or two chapters to an edited volume. The everyday workload of teachers in nurse education makes major demands on their time, and commonly spills over into their private time in evenings and weekends. Hence, the added demands of authoring a book can be very stressful, particularly as deadlines approach and slippage occurs. This stress can be compounded by feelings of guilt about neglecting family responsibilities, and the demands of writing may mean that insufficient time is available for recreational pursuits that are so important for 're-charging the batteries'.

There are a number of strategies that may help prevent or eliminate writer's block. It is important to ensure that, wherever possible, writing is done when you are fresh and alert. Writing is a creative activity, and it is very difficult to be creative if you are exhausted in the evening after a heavy day's work. Maintaining regularity of writing is also important, because the more one slips behind in the writing schedule, the more pressure and guilt we feel; this in turn may cause further blocking, so writers should try to do even a small amount of writing each day if possible.

Some publishers prefer to meet with their authors on a regular basis throughout the period of writing, so as to maintain contact and to monitor the author's progress. Whilst this may not be welcomed by every author, I find that meetings with my publisher once per term serve as mini-deadlines that help to keep me focused and on schedule.

Writer's rights

Given the ubiquity of photocopying, authors and editors of books need to know their rights in relation to their intellectual property. Chapter 9 (p. 257) discusses the legal position with regard to photocopying of books and journal articles, and identifies the restrictions on the amount and type of material that can be copied. The Authors Licensing and Collecting Society (ALCS) exists to collect fees for photocopying and to pass 50 per cent of these on to those authors who are members, and the other 50 per cent to the publisher. Membership involves a small annual fee, and fees from photocopying are then passed to members. ALCS has issued a declaration of academic writers' rights (ALCS, 1998) that covers the following areas:

1. It acknowledges the role of the academic author as a communicator.
2. It emphasizes the academic author's aspiration to be a full partner in the communication process with academic employers, publishers, libraries and users.
3. It emphasizes that a fair balance needs to be struck between the needs of academic authors, educational institutions, publishers, learned societies, etc.
4. A contract should be used to specify the uses of an academic author's work, and they should not be made to transfer copyright.
5. Most academic authors wish to get a fair share of revenues for their work.
6. The moral rights of authors are important, e.g. the right of the author to be identified as the author of the work, and the right to prevent the work being altered or amended without permission.

Until recently, fees for photocopying only applied to books, but since 1997 it is now possible for authors of journal articles to receive 25 per cent of the photocopying fee, provided that the publisher does not own less than 90 per cent of the photocopying rights.

Writing for professional journals

Writing an article for a professional journal is usually the first step that teachers take into the world of publication. Unlike book publications, journals are rated according to the degree of prestige they carry, so the most prestigious journals are also the most difficult ones in which to get an article published. Indeed, the RAE takes the title of the journal into account when rating publications in higher education institutions. Most journals offer a guide for contributors that covers such aspects as word length, a requirement for the manuscript to be on both hard copy and disk, referencing format, illustrations and charts, and information about the review process.

Troubleshooter's checklist for prospective authors

Alton-Lee (1998) offers the following checklist for prospective authors, based upon the critical feedback given to authors by reviewers. The checklist identifies 13 weaknesses demonstrated by prospective authors, and these are given in rank order of occurrence, from most common to least common, in the 142 studies researched.

1. lack of methodological transparency, adequacy, or rationale: insufficient information given;
2. unjustified claims: based on insufficient evidence, or in spite of evidence;
3. shortcomings in format: title, abstract, presentation of data, style, etc.;
4. theoretical shortcomings: failure to provide, articulate or develop theoretical perspectives;
5. data analysis problems: inadequate or lacking in substance;
6. inadequacies in literature reviews: insufficient, dated, not linked to subsequent studies;
7. insufficient clarity of focus: focus not clear at outset, focus changed, no statement of research question or purpose of study;
8. conceptual confusion: need to take more care with definitions, and use of metaphor;
9. parochial blinkers: ensure that local contexts, policies and practices are made meaningful to readers in different regions or countries;
10. does not add to the international research literature: need to ensure that the manuscript extends or develops the international literature in the area of study;
11. failure to link findings to the research literature: authors had not linked their findings to the relevant research literature;
12. lack of critical reflections on implicit assumptions: authors are challenged to focus critically on unexamined issues implicit in their manuscripts such as gender, political and economic resource issues, etc.;
13. victory claims: reviewers rejected overly-optimistic outcomes and achievements as lacking in credibility.

An interesting study that surveyed the views of editors of nursing journals about the process for submission and review of articles is described by Wildman (1998). Data was received from 22 journals, 16 of which routinely submitted articles to referees or reviewers. In terms of the quality of papers submitted, the data showed that there were two main aspects that made a manuscript immediately appealing to editors: relevance; and presentation. There were three main grounds that would cause editors to immediately reject a manuscript: irrelevance; poor presentation; and failure to adhere to guidelines.

The most common problems with manuscripts included poor academic work, poor use of English, non-adherence to guidelines, inappropriate references, poor presentation and unaltered coursework. The points most frequently raised with authors about the suitability of their manuscripts for publication included a requirement for better editing to improve understanding, amendments to meet journal requirements, attention to writing style, a need to be more critical, and an alteration of the title. Based upon the study, and the literature, the author offers a checklist for successful publication that includes the following helpful points.

Prospective authors should:

- Consider discussing their work with the journal editor before submitting it for publication.
- Use a 'critical friend' to read the article before submission.
- Be prepared to accept constructive criticism from editors and reviewers.
- Celebrate when the article is accepted, but be prepared for a long wait before it is published.

Presenting papers at conferences

Presenting papers at conferences is considered to be an essential component of continuing professional development in higher education. Conferences are advertised a long time in advance, accompanied by a request for submission of papers. Guidelines on the length of papers are issued by the conference organisers, and if a paper is accepted it is allocated a slot in the conference timetable. Papers are usually read by the presenter, but there is no hard and fast rule about the style of presentation. Conference organisers often make conference papers available to delegates on registration, or alternatively, the papers are published soon after the event.

Writing open, distance and flexible learning study materials

The foregoing discussion about writing books and academic articles will apply to a greater or lesser extent to the writing of open, distance and flexible learning study materials, depending upon whether or not the materials are written for a commercial publisher or an academic institution. In the former case, they can be considered to be like any other commercial publication, but in the latter there are a number of issues that differ significantly from ordinary publishing.

Copyright issues

The employing institution holds the copyright of any open, distance and flexible learning study materials produced by staff in the course of their employment, even though individuals are named as the author of such work. Hence, all such materials must carry the copyright symbol and text in the recommended form of words to ensure full protection of the copyright.

Corporate identity rules

All higher education institutions have corporate identity rules whose purpose is to ensure that business stationery, business cards and promotional and other material produced by the institution conforms consistently to the correct image. The rules include such aspects as the institution's crest, logo and corporate colours; the corporate typeface, front and back covers, and the corporate house style for letters, memoranda and facsimile.

Issues around the writing of open, distance and flexible learning materials are discussed in Chapter 11 (p. 280)

INSTITUTE FOR LEARNING AND TEACHING IN HIGHER EDUCATION

The Institute for Learning and Teaching in Higher Education (ILT, 1999a) has already been described in Chapter 12 (p. 299) in relation to educational quality assurance, so this section will focus on the issue of membership as an aspect of continuing professional development.

Eligibility for membership of the ILT

Membership of the ILT is open to individuals who teach or support learning in higher education, and eligibility is based upon evidence relating to five broad categories of professional activity (ILT, 1999b):

1. teaching and/or support of learning;
2. contribution to the design and planning of learning activities;
3. assessment and giving feedback to students;
4. developing effective learning environments and student support systems;
5. reflective practice and personal development.

Benefits of membership

The benefits of becoming a member are described by the ILT as follows:

1. publications, e.g. a refereed journal, magazine and electronic newsletter, and books;
2. events, e.g. regional and national events, conferences, and workshops;

3. CPD undertaken as part of the individual's commitment to remain in good standing, i.e. to remain eligible for membership;
4. networking, e.g. actual and virtual contacts with a wide range of groups;
5. access to research data, e.g. databases of research on aspects of learning and teaching;
6. members discounts, e.g. conferences and books.

Routes to membership

There are two broad routes to membership, the initial route and long-term routes.

Initial routes to membership

The initial route for experienced individual staff will be based upon a statement of professional experience, supported by two referees. There is also an initial route for the accreditation of existing CPD programmes. Both these routes will be available for not less than two years.

Long-term routes to membership

There will be three main routes to membership once the ILT is fully established:

1. *Institution-based programmes.* Individuals successfully completing an ILT-accredited CPD programme will be eligible for membership.
2. *Individual APL route.* Both individuals and groups may offer evidence that they have met the criteria for membership via an APL portfolio.
3. *Institutional APL route.* Higher education institutions can be accredited by the ILT to assess APL portfolios of evidence on behalf of the ILT.

The assessment of both individual applications and institutional programmes will be carried out by panels of experienced practitioners drawn from the higher education sector.

REFERENCES

Authors Licensing and Collecting Society (1998) Academic writers, academic rights, *ALCS News*, Spring 1998, ALCS.

Alton-Lee, A. (1998) A troubleshooter's checklist for prospective authors derived from reviewers' critical feedback, *Teaching and Teacher Education*, 14(8), 88–90.

Dearing, R. (1997) *Higher Education in the Learning Society*, *The Report of the National Committee of Inquiry into Higher Education*, HMSO, London.

DfEE (1997) *National Advisory Group for Continuing Education and Lifelong Learning for the 21st Century*, DfEE document reference: PP62/31326/1197/43, HMSO, London.

DfEE (1998a) *The Learning Age: a renaissance for a new Britain*, HMSO, London.

DfEE (1998b) *Higher Education for the 21st Century. Response to the Dearing Report*, HMSO, London.

HEFCE (1995) *Research Assessment Exercise: Criteria for Assessment*, HEFCE, London.

Institute for Learning and Teaching (1999a) *Frequently Asked Questions about the Institute for Learning and Teaching.*, www.ilt.ac.uk/faqs.html.

Institute for Learning and Teaching (1999b) *Accreditation and Membership of the ILT,* www.ilt.ac.uk/accredit.html.

McNay, I. (1997) *The Impact of the 1992 Research Assessment Exercise on Individual and Institutional Behaviour in English Higher Education*, Anglia Polytechnic University, Chelmsford.

RAE (1999a) *What is the RAE 2001?*, www.rae.ac.uk/About Us/default.htm.

RAE (1999b) *Interdisciplinary Research and the Research Assessment Exercise. Report from the Joint Department of Health/Higher Education Funding Council for England Task Group on Health-Related Research and the Research Assessment Exercise*, www.rae.ac.uk/Pubs/tg1rep.htm

UKCC (1992a) *Code of Professional Conduct for the Nurse, Midwife and Health Visitor*, 3rd edn, UKCC, London.

UKCC (1992b) *The Scope of Professional Practice*, UKCC, London.

Wildman, S. (1998) Publishing your work in nursing journals, *Professional Nurse*, **13**(7), 419–22.

22 Continuing professional development: the workplace context

In Chapter 21, continuing professional development (CPD) was discussed in the context of the university, but there are also important CPD issues relating to clinical and community practice that have a bearing on the role of the nurse teacher. This chapter addresses: the UKCC PREP standards; *A Higher Level of Practice*; the ENB Higher Award; clinical governance; National Institute for Clinical Excellence (NICE); clinical effectiveness and evidence-based practice; and reflective practice.

UKCC PREP STANDARDS

The most significant development in recent years relating to CPD in nursing is the UKCC Post-Registration Education and Practice (PREP) standards:

> *'PREP is a set of UKCC standards which all registered nurses, midwives and health visitors must meet in order to renew their registration. By meeting the standard, you are demonstrating that you have maintained and developed your professional knowledge and competence'* (UKCC, 1999a).

The PREP requirements consist of two separate elements relating to registration:

1. In order to be able to renew their registration, nurses, midwives and health visitors must have undertaken CPD over the previous three years. This element is called the PREP (CPD) standard.
2. In order to be able to renew their registration, nurses, midwives and health visitors must have worked in some capacity in relation to their nursing, midwifery or health visiting qualification for at least 750 hours during the past five years. Alternatively, they must have completed an approved 'return to practice' course.

The continuing professional development standard

The PREP (CPD) standard consists of three requirements:

1. a requirement to undertake at least five days (35 hours) of learning activity relevant to the nurse, midwife or health visitor's work during the three years prior to renewal of registration. If the practitioner is not working, the learning activities will relate to non-working commitments;
2. maintenance of a personal professional profile (PPP) that records the learning activities;

3. compliance with any request for auditing of the practitioner's profile by the UKCC.

When registration is renewed every three years, the practitioner is required to make a declaration that s/he has met the requirements.

Personal professional profile

There is considerable debate within the literature between the concepts 'profile' and 'portfolio'. Hinchliff (1998) for example, declares that 'the UKCC are using the terms in a confused and confusing way'. She goes along with the distinction that a portfolio is a private collection of material that provides evidence of CPD, whereas a profile is a selection from a portfolio to meet the specific needs of interested parties such as employers or the UKCC; this leads her to conclude that:

> *'The UKCC is, therefore, more correctly asking practitioners to keep a personal and private portfolio, from which they will extract a personal professional profile for the purposes of assuring UKCC that they have met the PREP requirements'.*

Whilst there is no UKCC-approved format, a properly-constructed PREP profile should contain six main elements:

1. factual information about the nurse, e.g. qualifications, employment, etc.;
2. self-appraisal of professional performance, i.e. reflection and evaluation;
3. action plans and outcomes;
4. record of formal learning, e.g. courses, study days, etc.;
5. record of informal or unstructured learning, e.g. reading books and journals; observing other practitioners, etc.;
6. record of hours worked within the three-year period between registrations.

There will clearly be a great deal of material collected over a three-year period, so it is essential to review the contents periodically. Redfern (1998) calls this process 'profile maintenance and gardening', and sums it up as follows: 'From time to time it is important to do some weeding and tidying up and to put on the bonfire things we do not need to keep in our profile any more'.

One of the interesting phenomena that has followed the introduction of PREP has been the plethora of profile formats produced (and often sold) by a variety of agencies including NHS trusts, publishers and statutory bodies. For example, the ENB has produced an electronic professional portfolio that claims the advantage of being more easily kept up to date.

Richardson (1998) undertook a study of 121 nurses, midwives and health visitors in relation to PREP profiles, and the following are some of her findings:

- 23 per cent of respondents did not have a profile;

- 56 per cent made regular entries, and 32 per cent had made no entry or had only placed certificates in their profile;
- 66 per cent agreed that profiling had many benefits;
- 83 per cent agreed that profiling was time-consuming.

Formal monitoring of how nurses, midwives and health visitors meet the PREP requirements begins in 2001, and will not need access to independent information from the workplace. Sanctions for non-compliance will be decided in advance of this date, and the forms and associated guidance will be piloted (UKCC, 1999b).

Teasdale (1998) nicely sums up the purpose of PREP:

'Some nurses continue to see PREP as a complex, form-filling exercise designed by the UKCC to keep them away from patients or even to force them into early retirement. It is nothing like this. PREP is a straightforward requirement that all nurses keep themselves updated for the protection of their patients and the promotion of good quality nursing care'.

The PREP (CPD) audit

In order to audit nurses, midwives, and health visitor's compliance with the PREP (CPD) standards, the UKCC will, each month from April 2001, be taking a sample of evidence of compliance. Individuals in the sample will be asked to complete a PREP (CPD) form describing the nature and outcomes of one of the learning activities they have undertaken over the past three years. The UKCC will be auditing how the individuals in the sample have utilized in their work the learning acquired from the activity.

UKCC: 'A HIGHER LEVEL OF PRACTICE'

In autumn 1998, the UKCC completed a consultation process within the profession on its proposals for recognizing a higher level of practice within post-registration education (UKCC, 1998). The definitive document is scheduled for release towards the end of 1999. The term 'a higher level of practice' applies to those nurses, midwives and health visitors who are working at a higher level of practice than initial registration. The underlying rationale for the proposals is as follows:

1. *The changing nature of health care.* The nature of health care is continually changing as a result of advances in research, technology and practice, and also of more local delivery of care to users. The boundaries between health care professional are becoming less distinct.
2. *Safeguarding the public.* The public interest must be protected in the light of developments in clinical practice, and the introduction of clinical governance, whilst recognizing the need for flexibility of service provision.
3. *The need to regulate a higher level of practice.* There is confusion

amongst the public, employers and professionals about the current system for recognizing post-registration qualifications, and the current arrangements for recording these is voluntary. The UKCC intends to introduce arrangements for recognizing a higher level of practice by the year 2001.

The UKCC core principles

The following core principles have been produced by the UKCC in relation to a higher level of practice.

A higher level of practice based on clinical competence

The UKCC's responsibility to safeguard the public has led to their wish to recognize and regulate practitioners working at a higher level of practice. The criterion for recognition will be a demonstrable attainment of clinical competence supported by appropriate post registration education.

A UK-wide standard

It is intended to set a generic standard for a higher level of practice that applies across all health care settings throughout the UK. This will describe the level of practice rather than the area where the specialism is practised. The standard will cover assessment, planning, implementation and review of clinical practice at a higher level, and will include clear criteria for achievement.

Regulation of a higher level of practice

The UKCC intends to develop a system of regulation for those practitioners working at a higher level of practice. This would require all such practitioners, as part of the three-yearly registration cycle, to notify the UKCC of their intention to:

1. be recognized as practising at a higher level;
2. continue to practise at this level.

When recognition has been achieved, it will be recorded on the register. There will be a series of pilot projects to test the rigour, practical implications and assessment costs.

The English National Board for Nursing, Midwifery and Health Visiting Framework and Higher Award

In 1992 the ENB framework and higher award for continuing professional education for nurses, midwives and health visitors came into operation, and aims to assist practitioners to develop the knowledge and skills necessary to meet the changing needs of the population. The framework is a partnership between the practitioners, managers, and educationalists, and there are four stages to be considered when a practitioner commences the framework:

1. *Review*. The practitioner reviews their expertise and achievements

with their current client group in relation to the key characteristics, and index for the higher award if desired.

2. *Contract.* With the collaboration of the manager, a contract is entered into with the educational institution to identify learning outcomes for the award.

3. *Delivery.* The practitioner then participates in the educational activities to achieve the learning outcomes, including maintaining an individual professional portfolio.

4. *Assessment.* Achievement of learning outcomes is demonstrated by assessment, and recorded in the portfolio.

5. *Quality assurance.* Practitioners, educationalists and managers will review the relevance and effectiveness of the learning experiences undertaken.

Ten key characteristics are identified as representing the knowledge, skills and expertise necessary for the provision of quality care to meet changing health needs, and the integration of all these can be recognized by the higher award. This is at a minimum of first degree level and requires demonstration of mastery of the ten key characteristics into a field of professional practice. The ten key characteristics are given in Table 21.1.

Table 22.1	1. Professional accountability and responsibility
The 10 key characteristics (ENB, 1991)	2. Clinical expertise with a specific client group
	3. Using research to plan, implement and evaluate strategies to improve care
	4. Team working and building, multidisciplinary team leadership
	5. Flexible and innovative approaches to care
	6. Use of health promotion strategies
	7. Facilitating and assessing development in others
	8. Handling information and making informed clinical decisions
	9. Setting standards and evaluation quality of care
	10. Instigating, managing and evaluating clinical change

The outcomes for the higher award can be achieved through a range of activities such as in-service courses, open learning, self-instruction, and taught courses. Practitioners working towards the higher award are required to maintain a personal professional portfolio.

There are similarities between the ENB framework and higher award and the UKCC's PREP standards, and the board sees the former as providing a firm foundation for the latter's implementation (ENB, 1995). The board has also approved large numbers of specialist practitioner programmes, some two thirds of which are in the community area and the remaining one third in the acute area (ENB, 1997).

An initial evaluation of the implementation of the framework and higher award was commissioned by the ENB, involving postal surveys of nurses, nurse managers, practitioners, tutors, and clinical supervisors, and case studies and telephone interviews of institutions delivering the Higher Award (ENB, 1998). The findings fall into two main categories;

those relevant to CPD in general, and those specific to the framework and higher award.

1. *Findings on CPD in general.* The study highlighted the importance ascribed to CPD in the maintenance of a skilled workforce, the maintenance of standards of care, and in the recruitment and retention of staff. It also confirmed the problems staff experience in obtaining study leave and funding for CPD, particularly part-time staff and those on night duty. Self-funding was seen to be the norm, and managers considered it was reasonable for staff to attend in their own time, or to pay their own fees.

2. *Findings specific to framework and higher award.* The principles of the framework and higher award were endorsed, including the importance of a practice-relevant degree, the use of AP(E)L, and the ten key characteristics. However, the findings also indicated that the necessary infrastructure for the higher award was in a rudimentary state of development, and that the post-launch follow-up on how to operationalize the system was inadequate. Limited awarenesss and understanding of the framework and higher award was evident amongst some practitioners and managers, and unclarity about the meaning of degree level practice. There was a perception that the value and credibility of the higher award was less than that of traditional degree programmes, and the portfolio was subject to particular criticism.

McHale (1998) describes a small pilot study on the impact of the higher award on clinical practice, and concludes that successful candidates are more confident, use reflective practice more effectively, and use new ways to plan and evaluate the delivery of care, and to manage resources. She emphasizes the point that, in contrast to other degree programmes, the higher award portfolio provides evidence that the candidate is operating at degree level. The study acknowledges that the actual impact of the higher award on patient care is difficult to measure, but suggests that it is likely to be enhanced by working through the higher award programme. At the time of writing, the ENB is formulating an action plan for a revised continuing education framework, but is awaiting the publication of the UKCC document *A Higher Level of Practice* before making recommendations.

CLINICAL GOVERNANCE

The government white paper *The New NHS: Modern, Dependable* (DoH, 1997) introduced a new quality initiative called clinical governance, which has important implications for professional practice and teaching.

Clinical governance is a framework that unites a range of quality initiatives including clinical effectiveness, evidence-based practice, reflective practice, and quality improvement processes such as clinical audit. The aim of clinical governance is to assure and improve clinical standards at local level throughout the NHS.

The white paper also created a new quality body called the National Institute of Clinical Excellence, whose purpose is to appraise new and existing interventions, and to disseminate evidence-based guidance. It may be helpful at this stage to offer a range of definitions of the term *clinical governance*, in order to identify its key components. The dictionary definition of the term *governance* means 'the act of governing', and hence clinical governance means that clinicians become responsible for the act of governing the service. The following definitions expand on this.

Definitions of clinical governance

DEPARTMENT OF HEALTH, 1997: 'Clinical governance is a new initiative in this white paper to assure and improve clinical standards at local level throughout the NHS. This includes action to ensure that risks are avoided, adverse events are rapidly detected, openly investigated and lessons learned, good practice is rapidly disseminated and systems are in place to ensure continuous improvements in clinical care'.

UKCC, 1999c: 'Clinical governance is a government initiative which is designed to improve standards of care for patients and clients. The government has stated that clinical governance will provide a framework through which NHS organizations will be accountable for continuously improving the quality of their services and safeguarding high standards of care by creating an environment in which excellence in clinical care will flourish. It means that, for the first time, NHS organizations and individuals will have a statutory duty to achieve quality improvement'.

HARVEY, 1998: 'Clinical governance is much more than a set of bureaucratic systems: it's also about a shift in culture and attitude in the health service. It's a new way of working that will affect nurses working on a ward or in the community as much as it affects nurse executives, or your trust board members. Put simply, it means putting doctors and nurses in charge of the way things are done ... and making both clinicians and managers accountable for the quality of patient care'.

Activities relating to clinical governance

Cook (1999) outlines the main activities relating to clinical governance:

- research and development: primary research; implementing research findings; critical appraisal of research evidence;
- risk management: health and safety assessment; clinical risk assessment; staff training; policy/procedure/protocol development;
- quality initiatives: continuous professional development; standard setting; complaints handling; user/patient involvement;

- clinical effectiveness initiatives: standard setting; evidence reviews; identification/production of clinical guidelines.
- audit: criterion-based audit; significant-event audit.

Cook points out that all nurses will need to acquire the skills to carry out these elements of clinical governance, including auditing skills, disseminating good practice, and appraising research findings.

The implementation of clinical governance differs somewhat between NHS trusts and primary care groups (PCGs).

In the former, the chief executive is responsible for ensuring that the trust is meeting its quality responsibilities; in the latter, a senior professional member takes responsibility for planning and implementation throughout the PCG.

As mentioned earlier, the clinical governance framework brings together a number of quality initiatives, some of which are already well-established, and others that are new. The following sections will address a selection of these initiatives.

NATIONAL INSTITUTE FOR CLINICAL EXCELLENCE

This new quality body was created as part of the white paper initiatives, and is designated as a special health authority directly responsible to the Health Secretary and the Secretary of State for Wales. The National Institute for Clinical Excellence (NICE) has representation from the nursing profession, as well as other health care professionals, patients and user groups. Its functions include the following (Shuttleworth, 1999):

- advising on best practice in existing treatment options;
- appraisal of new interventions;
- advising the NHS on implementation of new interventions;
- dissemination of evidence-based guidance on management of diseases and conditions;
- elimination of variations in standards of care and treatment;
- development of clinical audit methodologies.

CLINICAL EFFECTIVENESS AND EVIDENCE-BASED PRACTICE

These two concepts, although often discussed as separate entities in the literature, are effectively the same, and focus on the importance of evidence as the basis for practice.

Clinical effectiveness is very much part of the clinical governance framework, and emphasises the need for practitioners to be clinically effective in their practice. This development reflects the shift in culture consequent upon the white paper, from the quantity-focused provision of care towards a quality-focused, evidence-based approach to health care.

Evidence-based practice is a term derived from evidence-based medicine (EBM), and is also referred to as evidence-based nursing

(EBN). Maggs (1998) nicely sums up this approach:

> *'Evidence-based practice offers, it is claimed, the opportunity of addressing clinical problems through rigorous selection of "best available evidence", from sources such as randomized controlled trials (RCTs), systematic reviews and meta-analyses, and from primary research, and applying those findings in the clinical situation'.*

Clinical effectiveness

Adams (1999) outlines the requirements for clinical effectiveness:

> *'To be clinically effective involves primarily ensuring that your practice is based on the best available evidence of effectiveness and meets your clients' requirements. Furthermore, that you implement any change to practice within a framework of review and evaluation. Once you have achieved clinically effective practice it is important to share your experiences with others so that they may also benefit from it'.*

Stages in achieving clinical effectiveness

Adams (1999) describes a practitioner's achievement of clinical effectiveness as involving six stages:

1. *Question your routine practice*. This involves selecting an aspect of clinical practice, and then asking specific questions such as: 'what evidence is there for the way I currently practice this aspect'? 'Could it be performed more effectively?'
2. *Find the best evidence*. This stage involves searching for the best evidence for the chosen aspect of practice. Such evidence can be acquired from colleagues, journals and books, electronic databases such as the Cochrane database of systematic reviews, and the internet.
3. *Interpret your evidence*. This stage involves a critical appraisal of the sources of evidence acquired in Stage 2. This requires a thorough understanding of research principles and methodology, and skills in interpreting the evidence.
4. *Put your evidence into practice*. The evidence is applied in the practitioner's day-to-day practice.
5. *Evaluate clinical change*. This involves determining the impact of the change on patient/client care, e.g. audit.
6. *Disseminate successful outcomes*. It is important to make known to other professionals any successful outcomes, so that good practice is disseminated.

An alternative model for nurses to evaluate their clinical effectiveness is offered by McClarey (1997), consisting of six steps:

1. *Is there any research available which could be used? Is this the highest level of evidence available?*. This involves the identification

of an area of practice, and investigating whether or not it is based on evidence or tradition. Step 1 involves searching databases and other sources of evidence.

2. *Is this a practice which should be research-based?* This requires a consideration of whether or not the chosen area of practice is, or should be, research-based. If no evidence is available, the practitioner should bring this to the attention of those in the service with responsibility for prioritizing research.

3. *Has the research been incorporated into a systematic review?* If the identified evidence is in the form of a systematic review it has greater credibility. A systematic review brings together a range of research focusing on a given topic.

4. *Are there guidelines, standards or concensus statements for implementing this evidence?* Although evidence may be available, there may be no guidelines or standards. If this is the case, the latter will need to be developed at local level.

5. *How can I implement a proposed change in practice?* Successful implementation requires collaboration, consultation and multi-professional agreement, using publicity, conference presentations, and forums.

6. *Is anything else needed to ensure care is clinically effective?* Auditing should be carried out to ascertain the impact of the change on patient/client care, and continuation audit to ensure that the improvement is maintained.

REFLECTIVE PRACTICE IN NURSING

Reflective practice has been the dominant model for professional practice in both the nursing and teaching professions, but pinning down the concept is not straightforward (Quinn, 1998). Definitions in the literature range from simple to complex, and two examples will illustrate this:

'The concept of reflective practice is mainly associated with the idea of reflection on experience' (Johns, 1996).

'Reflective practice then is more than just thoughtful practice, it is the process of turning thoughtful practice into a potential learning situation and, significantly enough, it is the utilization of good theory in practice in what must always be a situation of probability – but the professional reflective practitioner is always trying to ensure that the outcome of any action is close to what is anticipated by the theory and the previous experience combined' (Jarvis, 1992).

Although reflection is not specifically mentioned in the UKCC Code of Conduct (UKCC, 1992), Palmer (1994) draws the inference that:

'it could be suggested that it will be the responsibility of each practising nurse, midwife and health visitor to introduce reflection

> *into their professional practice if reflection is considered a necessary requisite for the evaluation and development of professional practice'.*

The nature of reflection

Reflection is essentially a psychological construct that is closely related to a range of other internal mental (cognitive) processes such as thinking, reasoning, considering and deliberating (Gregory, 1997). The term is used in two ways:

1. In a general sense, as synonymous with thinking and deliberating;
2. In a specific sense, as the recollection of past experiences and mental states by *retrospection*, i.e. 'looking back'. (The word reflection is derived from the Latin *reflectere* meaning to bend back.)

The nature of reflective practice: Schon's approach

Perhaps the single most influential interpretation of reflective practice is that of Donald Schon, whose approach has influenced thinking about professional practice in a number of professions, not least those of teaching and nursing.

The publication of Donald Schon's books *The Reflective Practitioner: How Professionals Think in Action* (Schon, 1983) and *Educating the Reflective Practitioner: Towards a New Design for Teaching and Learning in the Professions* (Schon, 1987) had a considerable impact on both the teaching and the nursing professions, providing as it does an alternative rationale for professional practice.

Schon's focus is the relationship between academic knowledge as defined in universities, and the competence involved in professional practice. He argues that professional practice is based upon a technical rationality model which makes erroneous assumptions about the nature of practice, and in so doing reduces its important in relation to theory. Technical rationality views professional practice as the application of general, standardized, theoretical principles to the solving of practice problems; in other words, professional practice is problem-solving. This top-down view puts general theoretical principles at the top of the hierarchy of professional knowledge and practical problem-solving at the bottom, leading to what Schon termed the pre-eminence of theory and the denigration of practice.

Problem-setting

Within the technical rationality model, professional practice is viewed as a process of instrumental problem-solving, with the assumption that problems are self-evident. Schon, however, argues that in reality practitioners are not presented with problems *per se*, but with problem-situations. These must be converted into actual problems by a process of problem-setting, i.e. selecting the elements of the situation, deciding the ends and means, and framing the context. Technical rationality also fails to take account of the fact that problems encountered in professional practice are rarely standard or predictable.

Knowing-in-action

Schon uses this term to describe the intuitive or tacit 'knowing' that is embedded in professional actions. Intuition is a mental process commonly termed the 'sixth sense', and refers to a process by which an individual comes to a conclusion about something in the absence of sensory inputs, and without consciously thinking about it. For example, skilled practitioners constantly make intuitive judgements about situations without being able to specify exactly the criteria they base those judgements on; this is often termed 'thinking on your feet'. Schon maintains that, although this intuitive 'knowing' is implicit within our actions, it is possible for practitioners to access this by reflecting on what they are doing while they are doing it.

Reflection-in-action

Reflection-in-action occurs when the practitioner is confronted by a novel puzzle or problem-situation which s/he attempts to resolve. This resolution occurs when the problem is *re-framed*, i.e. seen differently during the actions. The process of reflecting upon the intuitive 'knowing' that is implicit in a practitioner's actions, whilst at the same time carrying out those actions, together constitutes reflection-in-action.

It is important to emphasize that the reflection is inherent in the action itself, and not in any thinking going on at the same time. Reflection-in-action is non-rational and non-linear, and is embedded in the action. Richardson (1990) succinctly captures this phenomenon: 'Schon found intelligence in the act itself rather than in attempting to make the act seem intelligent'. Schon suggests that reflection-in-action is triggered more commonly by surprising results, whereas anticipated results are less likely to be thought about. Reflection-in-action occurs within what Schon terms the action-present, i.e. the timescale in which any action by the practitioner can still influence a situation.

Reflection-on-action

This is the type of reflection that is referred to in the models of reflection discussed in the previous section of this chapter and involves retrospection on past experiences, the aim of which is to generate knowledge for future practice. Reflection-on-action contrasts markedly with reflection-in-action, the latter occurring whilst the practitioner is engaged in actions rather than thinking about it later.

Knowledge-in-action

This is practical professional knowledge, and develops by the process of reflection-in-action. It docs not rely on a series of conscious steps in a decision-making process; instead it is inherent in the action itself. It is not possible to ascertain this knowledge-in-action by talking to a practitioner, as it is not a conscious process, but expert knowledge can be elicited by observing the practitioner reflecting-in-action.

Characteristics of reflective practitioners

This notion of the reflective practitioner, according to Schon, contrasts markedly with the prevailing model of professional practice, the technical rationality model.

According to Schon, the reflective practitioner is characterized by a range of personal qualities and abilities, such as the ability to engage in self-assessment to criticize the existing state of affairs, to promote change and to adapt to change, and the ability to practise as an autonomous professional. He also distinguishes between the effective and the ineffective practitioner; the former is able to recognize and explore confusing or unique events that occur during practice, whereas the latter is 'burned-out', i.e. confined to repetitive and routine practice, neglecting opportunities to think about what s/he is doing

Although Schon's ideas on reflective practice have been widely accepted within the nursing profession, his approach has been criticized for a lack of empirical support. Muncie and Russell (1989) point out the there is 'virtually no elaboration of the psychological realities of reflection-in-action', e.g. What makes it begin? What happens when it begins? How do we know when it is occurring?

Jones (1999) suggests that approaches based on reflection may be more appropriate for current health-care provision. She argues that nursing models are not integral to patient care, and points out that qualified nurses often disregard the contribution of nursing models to their delivery of care.

> *'Models may be viewed as unnecessary academic exercises that increase nurses' workload. In reality, they are inadequately used, incompletely implemented and poorly understood by other practitioners'.*

The use of reflection-on-action, the author argues, constitutes an alternative professional framework for the provision of nursing care.

Strategies for teaching reflective practice

Boud, Keogh and Walker's Model of Reflection

The Boud, Keogh and Walker (1985) model is a three-stage model to assist learners to reflect upon experiences:

1. *Returning to the experience*. In this stage the learner mentally 'replays' the experience, describing what happened in a descriptive, non-judgmental way.
2. *Attending to feelings*. This stage is about getting in touch with the learner's own feelings about the experience, utilizing any positive feelings about the experience and removing any feelings that may obstruct the reflection.

3. *Re-evaluating the experience.* This stage is broken down into four sub-stages, each of which is designed to enhance outcomes of reflection. In re-evaluating the experience, it is important that any new information arising from experience and reflection makes an *association* with the learner's existing knowledge and attitudes. These associations are then put together by *integration* into new ideas or attitudes, which are then tested by *validation* to determine whether there are any inconsistencies or contradictions. The fourth sub-stage, *appropriation*, occurs when the new knowledge and attitudes become an intrinsic part of the learner's identity, and this will depend upon the significance placed upon any given experience and associated reflections.

The Boud, Keogh and Walker model demonstrates a relatively rational approach to the process of reflecting upon experience, and as such as been adopted widely in nursing as a tool for teaching practitioners how to reflect. It is worth noting, however, that in a more recent paper (Boud *et al.*, 1993) the authors emphasise that systematic reflection is not the only way in which individuals' learn from experiences:

> 'What we can say is that learning from experience is far more indirect than we often pretend it to be. It can be prompted by systematic reflection, but it can also be powerfully prompted by discrepancies or dilemmas which we are "forced" to confront'.

They go on to conclude:

> 'Much as we may enjoy the intellectual chase, we cannot neglect our full experience in the process. To do so is to fool ourselves into treating learning from experience as a simple, rational process'.

Gibbs reflective cycle

Figure 22.1 illustrates Gibbs' (1988) reflective cycle. It is interesting to note that, although at first sight it looks similar to the Kolb cycle, it is

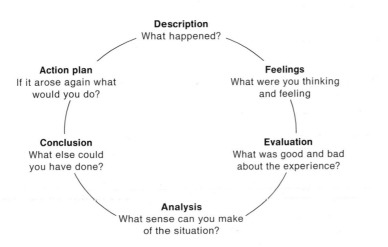

Figure 22.1

Gibb's reflective cycle

actually much closer to the Boud, Keogh and Walker model. Gibbs uses the term 'description' rather than 'returning to the experience'; the emphasis on dealing with good and bad feelings is similar in both cycles; Gibbs' term *analysis* is less specific than 're-evaluating the experience' in the Boud *et al.* (1993) model, but in his reflective cycle Gibbs makes more overt the action planning component of reflection.

Johns' model of structured reflection

Johns (1992) uses the concept of guided reflection to describe a structured, supported approach that helps practitioners learn from their reflections upon experiences. The approach involves the use of the model of structured reflection, one-to-one or group supervision, and the keeping of a structured reflective diary. The model of structured reflection involves a series of questions which help structure the practitioner's reflections. There is one core question and five cue questions, as shown in Table 22.2.

Table 22.2

Johns' model of structured reflection

Core question – What information do I need access to in order to learn through this experience?
Cue questions
1.0 *Description of experience*
1.1 *Phenomenon* – describe the 'here and now' experience
1.2 *Causal* – What essential factors contributed to this experience?
1.3 *Context* – What are the significant background actors to this experience?
1.4 *Clarifying* – What are the key processes (for reflection) in this experience?
2.0 *Reflection*
2.1 What was I trying to achieve?
2.2 Why did I intervene as I did?
2.3 What were the consequences of my actions for:
– Myself?
– The patient/family?
– For the people I work with?
2.4 How did I feel about this experience when it was happening?
2.5 How did the patient feel about it?
2.6 How do I know how the patient felt about it?
3.0 *Influencing factors*
3.1 What internal factors influenced my decision making?
3.2 What external factors influenced my decision making?
3.3 What sources of knowledge did/should have influenced my decision making?
4.0 *Could I have dealt better with the situation?*
4.1 What other choices did I have?
4.2 What would be the consequences of those choices?
5.0 *Learning*
5.1 How do I *now* feel about this experience?
5.2 How have I made sense of this experience in light of past experiences and future practice?
5.3 How has this experience changed my ways of knowing:
– empirics?
– aesthetics?
– ethics?
– personal?

Johns' model is more detailed than any of the models outlined above, and there are both advantages and disadvantages to this. The nursing literature indicates that nurses need to be taught how to reflect, and the detailed questions that practitioners are required to ask of themselves in the Johns' model certainly provides a comprehensive checklist for reflection. The disadvantage of such a detailed structure is that it imposes a framework that is external to the practitioner, leaving little scope for inclusion of her/his own approach. It is also open to criticism on the grounds of complexity, although other models can be criticized on precisely the opposite grounds, i.e. they may appear simplistic and self-evident.

Reflective writing

Reflective writing is the term given to a range of written reflections including profiling, portfolios, reflective journals, reflective diaries, personal letters and narratives. Reflective writing, in this sense, refers to the retrospective analysis of past experiences, and comprises an important learning strategy in nurse education at both pre-registration and post-registration levels. One of the values of reflective writing is that the record is permanently available for further reflection on future occasions. The UKCC post-registration education and practice requirements endorse the importance of reflection in the requirement that every practitioner maintains a personal professional profile. The profile 'is based on a regular process of reflection and recording what you learn from every day experiences, as well as planned learning activity' (UKCC, 1997).

Reflective writing, in the form of a personal professional portfolio, is one of the UKCC's PREP requirements for continuing registration (UKCC, 1997). Professional portfolios have been discussed earlier in this chapter (p. 559).

Critical incident analysis

Critical incident technique (Flanagan, 1954) provides a useful strategy for helping practitioners to reflect. Benner (1984) identified critical incidents in nursing as comprising any of the following:

- those in which the nurse's intervention really made a difference in patient outcome;
- those that went unusually well;
- those in which there was a breakdown;
- those that were ordinary and typical;
- those that captured the essence of nursing;
- those that were particularly demanding.

Benner's study provides a useful framework for reflecting upon and analysing critical incidents, leading to new insights into practice; descriptions of critical incidents should cover the following:

- the context of the incident;
- a detailed description of it;
- why the incident was critical to the practitioner;
- what the practitioner's concerns were at the time;

- what they were thinking about during the incident;
- what they felt about it afterwards;
- what they found most demanding about it.

Wood (1998) offers a four-stage model for analysing critical incidents:

1. description of what took place during the incident;
2. analysis of communication skills used and clarification of the underpinning moral values;
3. exploration of potentially effective alternative strategies to those skills actually employed, including moral justification for proposed alternatives;
4. identification of implications for practice.

Critical incident technique is not without its problems; Rich and Parker (1995) explore the morality of using critical incident technique as a teaching and learning tool. They point out that if students' critical incidents contain reference to dangerous behaviour or unprofessional conduct, the tutor or lecturer may be deemed to be in breach of the UKCC code of conduct if s/he does not report the behaviour to the appropriate authorities.

REFERENCES

Adams, C. (1999) Clinical effectiveness: a practical guide, *Community Practitioner*, **72**(5), 125–7.

Benner, P. (1984) *From Novice to Expert: Excellence and Power in Clinical Nursing Practice*, Addison-Wesley, London.

Boud, D., Keogh, R. and Walker, D. (1985) *Reflection: Turning Experience into Learning*, Kogan Page, London.

Boud, D., Cohen, R. and Walker, D. (eds) (1993) *Using Experience for Learning*, Open University Press, Milton Keynes.

Cook, R. (1999) Clinical governance: the role of community practitioners, *Community Practitioner*, **72**(4), 83–5.

Department of Health (1997) *The New NHS – Modern, Dependable*, HMSO, London.

English National Board for Nursing, Midwifery and Health Visiting (1991) *Framework for Continuing Professional Education for Nurses, Midwives and Health Visitors: A Guide to Implementation*, ENB, London

English National Board for Nursing, Midwifery and Health Visiting (1995) *The Future of Professional Practice: the Board's Response to PREP*, ENB, London.

English National Board for Nursing, Midwifery and Health Visiting (1997) *Annual Report 1996-1997*, ENB, London.

English National Board for Nursing, Midwifery and Health Visiting (1998) Evaluation of the implementation of the framework for continuing professional education and the higher award (initial evaluation), *Research Highlights 33*, ENB, London.

Flanagan, J. (1954) The critical incident technique, *Psychological Bulletin*, **51**, 327–58.

Gibbs, G. (1988) *Learning by Doing: A Guide to Teaching and Learning Methods*, Further Education Unit, Oxford Polytechnic, Oxford.

Gregory, R.L. (1997) (ed.) *The Oxford Companion to the Mind*, Oxford University Press, Oxford.

Harvey, G. (1998) Improving patient care: getting to grips with clinical governance, *RCN Magazine*, Autumn 1998.

Hinchcliff, S. (1998) Lifelong learning, in *Continuing Professional Development in Nursing: A Guide for Practitioners and Educators*, F. M. Quinn (ed.) Stanley Thornes, Cheltenham.

Jarvis, P. (1992) Reflective practice and Nursing, *Nurse Education Today*, **12**(3), 174–81.

Johns, C. (1992) The Burford nursing development unit holistic model of nursing practice, *Journal of Advanced Nursing*, **16**, 1090–8.

Johns, C. (1996) Using a reflective model of nursing and guided reflection, *Nursing Standard*, **11**(2), 34–8.

Jones, K.N. (1999) Reflection: an alternative to nursing models, *Professional Nurse*, **14**(12), 853–5.

Maggs, C. (1998) A philosophy of continuing professional education in nursing, in *Continuing Professional Development in Nursing: A Handbook for Practitioners and Educators*, F.M. Quinn (ed.), Stanley Thornes, Cheltenham.

McClarey, M. (1997) Clinical effectiveness and evidence-based practice, *Nursing Standard*, **11**(52), 33–7.

McHale, C. (1998) ENB higher award: evaluation of its impact on practice, *Nursing Standard*,**12**(34), 44–6.

Muncie, H. and Russell, T. (1989) Educating the reflective teacher: an essay review of two books by Donald Schon, *Journal of Curriculum Studies*, **21**(1), 71–80.

Palmer, A. (1994) Introduction, in *Reflective Practice in Nursing: The Growth of the Professional Practitioner*, A. Palmer, S. Burns and C. Bulman (eds), Blackwell. Oxford.

Quinn, F.M. (1998) Reflection and reflective practice, in *Continuing Professional Development in Nursing: A Handbook for Practitioners and Educators*, F.M. Quinn (ed.), Stanley Thornes, Cheltenham.

Redfern, E. (1998) The power of the professional profile, in *Continuing Professional Development in Nursing: A Guide for Practitioners and Educators*, F.M. Quinn (ed.), Stanley Thornes, Cheltenham.

Rich, A. and Parker, D. (1995) Reflection and critical incident analysis: ethical and moral implications of their use within nursing and midwifery education, *Journal of Advanced Nursing*, **22**, 1050–7.

Richardson, A. (1998) Personal professional profiles, *Nursing Standard*, **12**(10), 35–40.

Richardson, V. (1990) The evolution of reflective teaching and teacher education, in *Encouraging Reflective Practice in Education*, T. Clift, W. Houston and M. Pugach (eds), Teachers College Press, New York.

Schon, D. (1983) *The Reflective Practitioner: How Professionals Think in Action*, Basic Books, New York.

Schon, D. (1987) *Educating the Reflective Practitioner: Towards a New Design for Teaching and Learning in the Professions*, Jossey Bass, San Francisco.

Shuttleworth, A. (1999) NICE puts clinical governance on the agenda, *Professional Nurse*, **14**(9), 605.

Teasdale, K. (1998) Getting to grips with PREP, *Professional Nurse*, **13**(10), Profile Pack.

UKCC (1992) *Code of Professional Conduct for the Nurse, Midwife and Health Visitor* 3rd edn, UKCC, London.

UKCC (1997) *PREP and You*, UKCC, London.

UKCC (1998) *A Higher Level of Practice: Consultation Document*, UKCC, London.

UKCC (1999a) *The Continuing Professional Development Standard*, UKCC, London.

UKCC (1999b) *Register*, No 27, Spring 1999.

UKCC (1999c) Making the connection: professional self-regulation and clinical governance, *Register*, No. 27, Spring 1999.

Wood, S. (1998) Ethics and communication: developing reflective practice, *Nursing Standard*,**12**(18), 44–7.

INDEX